Clinical
Retinoscopy

Clinical
Retinoscopy

AK Jain DNB, MNAMS
Assistant Professor
Department of Ophthalmology
Rajshree Medical Research Institute
Bareilly, UP

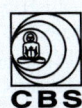

CBS Publishers & Distributors Pvt Ltd

New Delhi • Bengaluru • Chennai • Kochi • Kolkata • Mumbai
Bhopal • Bhubaneswar • Hyderabad • Jharkhand • Nagpur • Patna • Pune • Uttarakhand • Dhaka (Bangladesh)

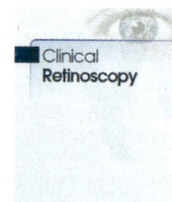

Clinical
Retinoscopy

ISBN: 978-93-88178-78-5

Copyright © Author and Publisher

First Edition: 2019

Published by Satish Kumar Jain and produced by Varun Jain for

CBS Publishers & Distributors Pvt Ltd

4819/XI Prahlad Street, 24 Ansari Road, Daryaganj, New Delhi 110 002, India.
Ph: 23289259, 23266861, 23266867   Fax: 011-23243014   Website: www.cbspd.com
e-mail: delhi@cbspd.com; cbspubs@airtelmail.in.

Corporate Office: 204 FIE, Industrial Area, Patparganj, Delhi 110 092
Ph: 4934 4934   Fax: 4934 4935   e-mail: publishing@cbspd.com; publicity@cbspd.com

Branches

- **Bengaluru:** Seema House 2975, 17th Cross, K.R. Road,
  Banasankari 2nd Stage, Bengaluru 560 070, Karnataka
  Ph: +91-80-26771678/79   Fax: +91-80-26771680   e-mail: bangalore@cbspd.com
- **Chennai:** 7, Subbaraya Street, Shenoy Nagar, Chennai 600 030, Tamil Nadu
  Ph: +91-44-26680620, 26681266   Fax: +91-44-42032115   e-mail: chennai@cbspd.com
- **Kochi:** 42/1325, 1326, Power House Road, Opposite KSEB Power House,
  Ernakulam 682 018, Kochi, Kerala
  Ph: +91-484-4059061-65   Fax: +91-484-4059065   e-mail: kochi@cbspd.com
- **Kolkata:** 6/B, Ground Floor, Rameswar Shaw Road, Kolkata-700 014, West Bengal
  Ph: +91-33-22891126, 22891127, 22891128   e-mail: kolkata@cbspd.com
- **Mumbai:** 83-C, Dr E Moses Road, Worli, Mumbai-400018, Maharashtra
  Ph: +91-22-24902340/41   Fax: +91-22-24902342   e-mail: mumbai@cbspd.com

Representatives

• Bhopal 0-8319310552	• Bhubaneswar 0-9911037372	• Hyderabad 0-9885175004	• Jharkhand 0-9811541605
• Nagpur 0-9021734563	• Patna 0-9334159340	• Pune 0-9623451994	• Uttarakhand 0-9716462459
• Dhaka (Bangladesh) 01912-003485			

Printed at Goyal Offset Printers, GT Karnal Road, Industrial Area, Delhi, India

to
_____

my beloved family members
for their support, encouragement and love

Preface

Refractive anomalies are one of the most common clinical problems encountered in the field of ophthalmology throughout the world and remain one of the difficult challenges to understand hence, a deep knowledge for correction of refractive anomalies is a prerequisite for the successful ophthalmic practice. This book *Clinical Retinoscopy* has been written to provide the complete information about correction of refractive errors. The present text is written in simple, concise and lucid manner with supportive illustrations in the form of ray diagrams, figures and tables so that reader can acquire the profound knowledge about the subject with the help of diagrammatic representation of the respective topic.

This book comprises four sections including total 15 chapters where each section contains the diagrammatic illustrations related to text for easy understanding of the readers. Section I deals with the basic concepts of retinoscopy and also depicts the evolution of retinoscopes down the era. For mastering the art of refraction, optics of various kinds of retinoscopes and refraction tools is explained in details. Detailed retinoscopy methods and various reflexes encountered during retinoscopy are also explained in simpler and illustrated manner. Chapters on retinoscopy contain the diagrams representing the actual reflexes seen in patient's eye, hence reader can master the technique of retinoscopy by reading this book.

Sections II and III deal with the visual rehabilitation related to the management of different kinds of refractive anomalies. In Section II spectacles are explained in relation to the manufacturing of lenses and fitting of lenses in frames. Various designs of spectacle lenses are also explained in an illustrated manner for easy understanding of readers. Section III is all about contact lenses. In this section starting from manufacturing till fitting and complications related to contact lenses is covered in six chapters. After reading these chapters the readers will be proficient in evaluation, fitting and maintenance of contact lenses in all age groups.

In the end, Section IV contains problem-based learning, where various problems related to refraction encountered during practice and their possible solutions has also been discussed in detail. This section will help the students to master the art of retinoscopy and prescribe glasses in difficult clinical situations.

I hope this book will help teachers, residents, ophthalmologists and optometrists to widen their knowledge about refraction and management of refractive errors. The knowledge and information gained from this book will assist the readers to comprehend the basic concepts of retinoscopy in relation to various refraction anomalies of the human eye.

Author believes that careful review and evaluation can create a better one and there is always scope of improvement. If there are any mistakes, printing errors, suggestions and feedback from readers about the book, please mail your feedback to dramitjain75@gmail.com.

AK Jain

Acknowledgments

It is my great pleasure to express my gratitude to all those, whose blessings and contribution has made this endeavor possible. First and foremost, I would like to thank God, the 'Almighty', who has provided me the strength to undertake this work and complete it successfully.

I take pride in acknowledging the guidance of Prof AK Gupta (former Dean, Maulana Azad Medical College, New Delhi), ICARE Eye Hospital and Postgraduate Institute, Noida, who has been so helpful and cooperative in giving his support at all times to achieve my goal.

I also thank all my teachers, colleagues and students from Saraswathi Institute of Medical Sciences, Hapur; Santosh Medical College, Ghaziabad; ICARE Eye Hospital and Postgraduate Institute, Noida; Sharp Sight Centre, Delhi; Narinder Mohan Hospital, Ghaziabad, SHRC, Jaipur colleagues for their kind cooperation and valuable suggestions to complete this project. I am also thankful to Dr Sparsh Gupta, Dr Ashish Mehta, Dr Swati Gupta, Dr Roopak Tandon and Dr Vikrant Sharma for their help and cooperation.

My acknowledgement would be incomplete without thanking all my family members for their indubitable support, love and encouragement in all my endeavours. I owe my special thanks to my wife Dr Seema and lovely sweet daughter Harshita Jain for their great patience, understanding and for giving me unlimited happiness and pleasure.

I would like to thank Mr Satish Kumar Jain (CMD), Mr Varun Jain (Director), CBS Publishers & Distributors, and their management team for the enthusiastic cooperation, professional skills, and suggestions and to finish this task in an impressive manner. I would like to take this opportunity to thank Mr YN Arjuna (Senior Vice-President—Publishing, Editorial and Publicity), Mrs Ritu Chawla (AGM Production), Mr Vikrant Sharma and Mr Ram Murti, for preparing the book material in a press-ready form. My thanks go to artist Mr Sumit Sharma whose artistic representations created the magical illustrations.

Last but not the least I thank all my patients who make me knowledgeable enough to write such a impressive book on clinical refraction.

AK Jain

Contents

Retinoscope and Retinoscopy

Retinoscopy: An Overview

INTRODUCTION

History of retinoscopy goes back to 1859, when initial observations about the images were made by Sir William Bowman which finally led to the basis of present day clinical retinoscopy. Sir William Bowman observed a linear shadow (linear fundus reflex) while he was doing examination of the fundus of a patient who had an astigmatic refractive error. He used a plane mirror ophthalmoscope for examination of astigmatic eye and illuminated this plane mirror ophthalmoscope with the help of a burning candle and this light was then focused on the patient's eye. Thus, it was Bowman who first described this method to detect astigmatic error in a patient of keratoconus and he established the basis for assessment of refractive status by objective means. Because prior to this observation made by Bowman, refractive status of patients was corrected by subjective methods only. Finally, H. Parent in 1880 established the quantitative refraction test by measuring refractive error using lenses and coined the term retinoscopie.

Retinoscope used in earlier times had simple mirrors either plane or concave to reflect the light coming from of a candle. The candle light created a "spot of light" which in turn produced shadows instead of linear reflection from eye of the patient.

Gradually it was tried and understood by various scientists working on this, that a linear streak of reflected light can be produced by utilizing slit-shaped mirrors as shown in Fig. 1.1.

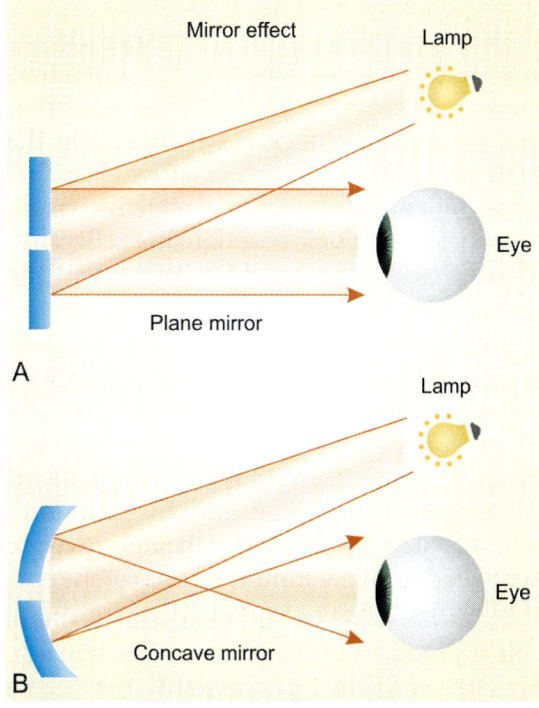

Fig. 1.1: Mirror effects on light. A. Plane mirror emits parallel, uncrossed rays; B. Concave mirror converge rays at a point, from which light rays cross and diverge hence produces an opposite reflex or reversed motion

Pioneers of Retinoscopy

In the year 1873, French ophthalmologist Ferdinand Cuignet compared various reflexes in the eyes by using a simple mirror ophthalmoscope. When he observed through the peephole of his plane mirror he noticed that the reflexes varied in different patients. He thought that this phenomenon might be happening because every person has different refractive status. This became the basis for a *qualitative* test.

Cuignet observed that when the light from the plane mirror is moved across the pupil then the reflexes from the fundus also move with light movement. Occasionally, the movements of fundus reflex was in the same direction as that of mirror light, but most of the time it was in the opposite direction. He thought that the cornea was responsible for the production of these reflexes in the eyes and hence coined the term for his method as keratoscopie ('kerato' means cornea).

He further observed these reflexes in details in terms of the reflex sizes, brightness of reflex, speed and direction of the reflexes in relation to the movement of projected light. On the basis of his observations Cuignet classified these patients with various refractive errors as myopia, hyperopia or astigmatism. Because of this contribution in field of retinoscopy, he is known as Father of retinoscopy.

Subsequently, in the year 1878, M. Mengin explained that the source of the reflex produced during retinoscopy was not the cornea (as per Cuignet) but reflexes were produced from the fundus of the eye. Based on his postulation Mengin introduced the term retinoscopie considering that the reflexes were generated from the fundus (retina) of the eye.

H. Parent (1849–1924) in the year 1880 was able to produce the quantitative refraction test. He utilized the lenses to quantify the degree of various types of refractive errors suggested by Cuignet. Parent coined the term retinoscopie which later changed to skiascopie (which means shadow) for his quantitative technique. Apart from abovementioned terms various other names were suggested for the techniques done to study the reflexes from the eye were

- Shadow test (proposed by Priestley Smith, an Ophthalmologist from Birmingham)
- Skiaskopie (Egger translated the word shadow in Greek and coined this term)
- Pupilloskopie (korescopy)
- Umbrascopy
- Scotoscopy
- Dioptroscopy

The electric retinoscopes commonly used in the beginning of 20th century had spiral filament bulb with a rotating sleeve. These spiral filaments used to give the spot of light which was not in line or very sharp. Later on, Jacob Copeland introduced a bulb in retinoscope which had linear filament. The light produced by this bulb was sharp, bright and linear. This change in bulb became the basis for the discovery of Copeland's streak retinoscope which passed many phases of development to reach the present day retinoscopes.

Over the last 100 years many improvement and modifications in the design and functioning of retinoscope in terms of viewing system of retinoscope, meridians of bulb filament and control of light vergence, etc. had been done. During this period of development the Retinoscope handles and sleeve design were made handy, compact, more comfortable and user friendly, with better battery power.

Various Theories of Retinoscopy

Though the technique of retinoscopy was put to an effective clinical use during the 19th and 20th centuries, however, the principle of retinoscopy was still a debatable issue among scientists. The most popular theories regarding the principle of retinoscopy emerged during this period were:

- The far point theory (proposed by Landolt)

- The observer pupil theory (proposed by Wolff)
- The photokinetic theory (proposed by Haass)

Out of these theories the far point theory proposed by Landolt is most widely accepted theory and forms the basis for understanding the principle of retinoscopy till date. Eminent scientists like Priestly-Smith, Donder, Gullstrand, Wolff, Haass and others also put theories for optics and mechanism of retinoscopy.

In the year 1903, scientist Duane started use of cylindrical lenses in cases of astigmatism. He developed method to use cylindrical lenses while performing retinoscopy to neutralize the reflexes. Most widely accepted far point theory of Landolt which still forms the basis for understanding the principle of retinoscopy was challenged by theories proposed by Wolff (observer pupil theory) and Haass (photo kinetic theory).

In initial phases, for illumination of retina gaslight was used as a light source. This light source was later on replaced with an incandescent lamp. Examiner used a mirror retinoscope to reflect the rays from the gaslight into the patient's eye, while studying the fundus reflex through the peephole of mirror retinoscope.

Gradually, a miniature bulb was developed which could be placed inside the instrument. This was the model of an early luminous retinoscope. These small electric bulbs projected a spot of light to illuminate the retina much similar to present day's Ophthalmoscope. Later on, various designs of retinoscope came with variable vergence. These vergences were produced by the use of either plane or concave mirror. These mirrors were also fitted in the same instrument.

Over a period of nearly 100 years the initially designed spot retinoscopes have not changed much in their design. There were several limitations in function and handling of these instruments but still they remain in use till recently. However, streak retinoscopy in reality is more accurate, much simpler and faster than other techniques of retinoscopy. With time the importance of a linear fundus reflex as compared to spot reflex especially, in the patients having astigmatism was recognized. Many researchers stressed on the importance of linear reflex and by using various types of slit-shaped mirrors they tried to create a linear beam (or streak) of light, which lead to development of streak retinoscope. This streak retinoscope simplified the procedure of refraction in astigmatism. With further advancement an electric retinoscope which consisted of a rotating slit was produced which allowed the examiner to compare various ocular meridians simultaneously.

RETINOSCOPE: AN OVERVIEW

Retinoscope as a Tool

Retinoscopy is also known as skiascopie. This terminology is more accurate because it indicates that the shadows (reflexes) from the fundus are being observed by use of an instrument.

Retina by itself is a thin and transparent structures, hence it cannot casts a shadow. So the structures get illuminated by the light are retinal pigment epithelium and choroid. These structures reflect the light and shadows or reflexes of this reflected light are seen by the instrument called retinoscope. Previously, spot retinoscopes were used which are now replaced by streak retinoscope in modern era and designed by many manufactures commercially. All these brands of retinoscopes have slight difference in their appearance and design of instrument but the basic principles remains more or less similar in all commercially available instruments.

Parts of Retinoscope

Though from external appearance the retinoscope looks like a simple instrument with head and handle. It has several smaller units which are compiled to perform various functions.

To know the retinoscope in better way we can broadly divide this instrument into two parts as shown in Fig. 1.2.

- Head piece
- Handle piece

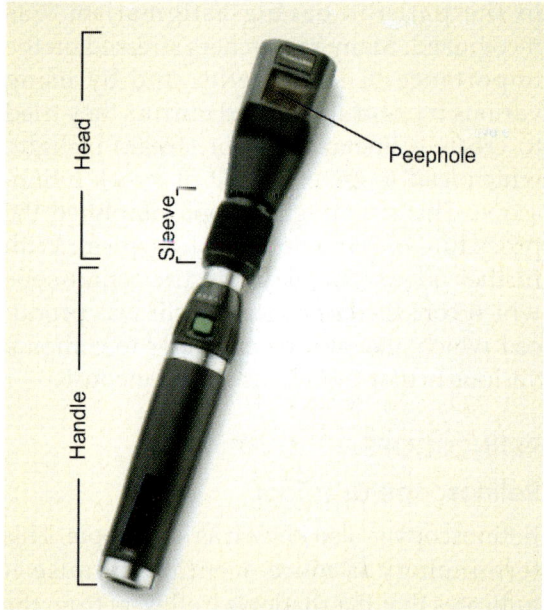

Head
Sleeve
Handle
Peephole

Fig. 1.2: Retinoscope

Head piece: It is the upper portion of retinoscope which consists of
- A peephole, through which examiner looks the retinal reflex.
- A sleeve which rotates the projected streak of light, hence increases or decreases the width of projected beam.
- A socket for source of illumination, i.e. bulb at its terminal end.
     This head piece is fixed by the socket system into the handle.

Handle piece: It is the lower portion of retinoscope and has an elongated hollow tube where battery is inserted inside. This battery may be rechargeable or non-rechargeable. This handle is fixed with head piece by socket locking system.

Internal Components of Streak Retinoscopes

Various commercially designed streak retinoscopes basically have two main components:
- Light projection system
- Examiner observation system

Light projection system: The projection system is the one which provides illumination to the retina and involve the following major components.

Light source: In majority of designs a small bulb having a linear filament is used as light source. This filament produces a line or streak of light because the design of this filament is linear or straight. This bulb is fixed with sleeve in such a manner that by turning sleeve up or down the bulb also moves up and down and as it comes near to the lens the light is divergent and as it goes away from the condensing lens the projected beam is convergent. In simpler words, the width of projected beam is narrowed or widened by moving the bulb up or down using the sleeve.

Condensing lens: Plus power convex lens placed between the light source and reflecting mirror is called condensing lens. This plus lens condenses the light ray, hence named condensing lens. Streak of the light which is produced from the bulb (having linear filament) is a highly diverging ray, hence a plus lens is used to control the vergence of streak. This condensing lens produces a positive effect on vergence of the projected light rays. The rotating sleeve present between the head and the handle of retinoscope helps to change the relative position of the condensing lens and the bulb and thus vergence of emitted light streak can be altered by either raising or lowering the sleeve according to the convenience of the examiner. As this condensing lens lies in the path of light streak, hence it focuses the rays from the bulb onto the mirror.

Mirror: The mirror (mostly plane mirror) causes bending of the light rays which emerges from the bulb, so that it is projected inside the patient's eye. The light from bulb filament emerges in upward direction towards the ceiling and has an axis parallel to the floor, which is then bended and reflected by the mirror. Although 100% of the emerged light from the bulb filament is not reflected by the mirror but to a certain extent some of light rays pass via the mirror. These bypassed light rays give an opportunity to the examiner to view inside the patient's pupil. These light rays are coaxial to the path of the reflex streak. As this reflecting mirror is placed at prefixed angle inside the head of retinoscope, the path of emerging light is at right angle to the axis of the retinoscope handle.

Focusing sleeve: Sleeve is a hollow cylinder, can be mounted in the head or over the handle of retinoscope. Function of sleeve is to narrow or widen the width of light streak and it also changes the direction of the light streak by rotation movement. This is used to control the amount of light projected inside the eye and also controls the direction of eye examination. The sleeve when moved up or down, the distance between the bulb and lens varies, hence it allows the retinoscope to project the rays which are either divergent (plane mirror effect) or convergent (concave mirror effect). Because of this function it is also called the vergence control of retinoscope.

In most of the commercially available retinoscopes, the sleeve changes the focus (vergence) by moving the bulb up or down keeping the lens at a fixed place. But in some commercially available retinoscopes, the condensing lens (rather than the bulb) is moved up or down to change the vergence. The movement of lens can also be done by raising or lowering the sleeve.

As discussed later in this chapter, that instruments which use a fixed bulb system and movable condensing lens, they work just the opposite way as compared to those retinoscopes which use a fixed lens and movable bulb in up or downward direction.

In present day retinoscopes, the sleeve controls both the factors, i.e. rotation of the light streak in different axes and vergence of light focused by the streak. In all types of retinoscopes, we progressively increase the vergence of the light beam from diverging rays (plane mirror effect) through parallel rays to converging rays (concave mirror effect), as we move the sleeve from top to bottom or vice versa.

Electric current source: This is provided by a battery in the handle (e.g. rechargeable single battery or replaceable small batteries). There are a few models of retinoscope, which use electric connections for providing the current source to the bulb.

> **Note**
>
> In a nutshell, the projection system is simple to understand. The retinoscope emits rays of light to illuminate the retina. By rotating the sleeve the projected streak is rotated and by moving the sleeve up or down the projected ray can be made divergent or convergent.

Examiner observation system: The observation system enables examiner to see the reflex from the retina. The illuminated retina reflect back some of the light rays and these few rays then go into retinoscope and pass through a small hole in the mirror and later on they reach at the back end of the head of retinoscope. This small hole in the mirror is called the peephole. Thus, examiner can see the retinal reflex through this peephole. When examiner move the retinoscope up or down, while still looking through the peephole, he/she can observe the up and down movement of the light streak.

Generally, these rays when emerge from the patient's retina, they pass through various optical components of the eye and thus get affected by the various eye components of the patient. The manner in which these reflected rays get affected tells the examiner about the optics of the patient's eye.

Optics of Peephole

Usually people think the peephole of retinoscope as the hole which is present on the examiner's side of the retinoscope (we see the emerging reflected light through it). But in reality, peephole is the "hole" present in the center of the reflecting mirror inside the retinoscope. As examiner peep (see) through this hole it is called peephole. This peephole can be manufactured in the following ways

- One way is that a small circular portion of the mirror can be left unsilvered and the remaining area is silvered so that the light is not reflected from this small unsilvered area.

- Other way is that the mirror is partially silvered, so that this mirror will act as a beam splitter.

Size of peephole is a major contributing factor in designing of retinoscope because a very large size peephole will reduce the amount of valuable light reflecting into the patient's eye. To decrease the chances of these internal reflections producing glare and polarization, some manufactures of retinoscope have introduce various types of filters which are fixed in between the peephole of the retinoscope and the true peephole.

This true peephole is the one which allows the observer to see inside the patient's eye by maintaining a coaxial relationship between his eye and the light emerging from the peephole of retinoscope. This coaxial (having same axis) relationship among the observer's eye and emitted light streak from patient's eye is very important and prerequisite to view a red reflex inside the eye of patient as shown in Fig. 1.3.

Tilting of the retinoscope in sideways will allow the examiner to see some area of the red reflex of retina present in alignment with retinoscope peephole, whereas a few area of red reflex which are not in line, get cut off.

> **Note** _____
>
> If this coaxial relationship of light is not maintained, then examiner will see only a black pupillary area inside the patient eye, instead of a red reflex.

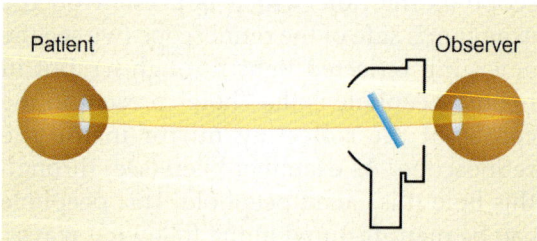

Fig. 1.3: Observation system illustrating the path of light through mirror from patient's retina to observer's retina

> **Note** _____
>
> In a nutshell, the observation system of retinoscope is simply to observe the reflected light ray from illuminated retina through a peephole in mirror.

These cut-off areas will be seen as a dark shadows inside the patient's pupil, whereas remaining area which are coaxial will be seen as red glow.

Optics of Retinoscope

Figure 1.4 is a diagrammatic cross-sectional representation of streak retinoscope. Bulb emits light from its filament, which passes through a convex lens (condensing lens) and then this light hits the plane mirror. From the mirror light rays get reflected outside the retinoscope toward the patient's eye. The examiner observes a portion of these reflected light rays via an aperture in mirror called peephole.

The arrows shown in Fig. 1.4 on sides of retinoscope are representing two types of movements done by the sleeve of retinoscope, i.e. up or down and rotation. The straight arrow represents the vertical movement of

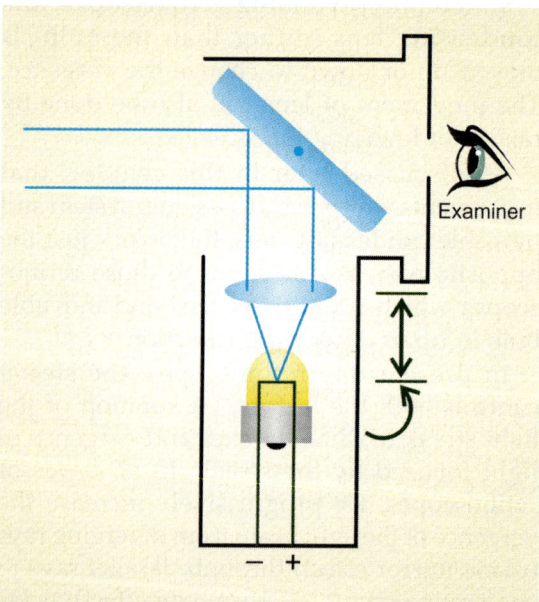

Fig. 1.4: Optics of retinoscope showing positions of bulb, condensing lens and mirror

sleeve where upward or downward movement will change the vergence of the emitting light rays by altering the distance between filament of bulb and convex lens. The curved arrow represents the bulb, which can be rotated both clockwise and anticlockwise; to move the orientation of reflex either vertical or horizontal, as per requirement.

In our diagrammatic illustration the filament of bulb is considered to be present at the focal point of convex lens, hence the light rays emerging after reflecting from the mirror are parallel in nature.

Two types of retinoscope are available
- Type I: In this type of retinoscope, the bulb is moved up or down with the movement of sleeve, whereas convex lens remain fixed.
- Type II: In this type of retinoscope, the convex lens is moved up or down with the movement of sleeve, whereas bulb remains fixed.

Type I retinoscope

Optics and cross section view of the first type of retinoscope in which the bulb moves up or down and convex lens remains fixed is as follows:

As shown in Fig. 1.5A, when sleeve of retinoscope is moved in downward direction, the bulb moves downward (away from lens) and the effect produced is similar to a concave mirror which means emerging light rays will be convergent in nature.

As shown in Fig. 1.5B, opposite will happen when sleeve is moved up, i.e. the bulb will move up (nearer to lens) and produces plane mirror effect, hence emerging light rays will be divergent in nature.

Type II retinoscope

Optics and cross section view of the second type of retinoscope in which the lens moves upward or downward and bulb remains fixed.

As shown in Fig. 1.6A, when lens is moved up (away from bulb), an effect similar to a concave mirror is produced and hence emerging light rays are convergent when sleeve of retinoscope is moved in upward direction.

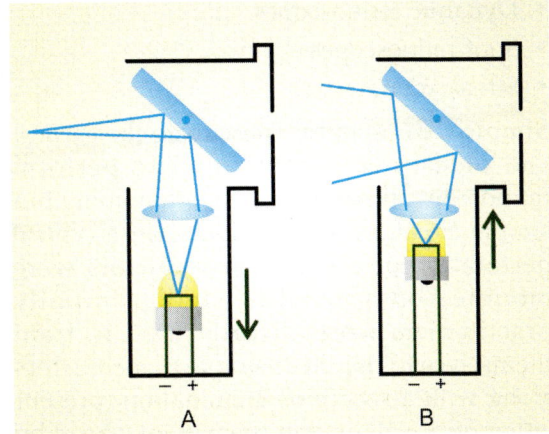

Fig. 1.5A and B: Optical effects by the movement of retinoscope bulb. A. Bulb moving downwards; B. Bulb moving upwards

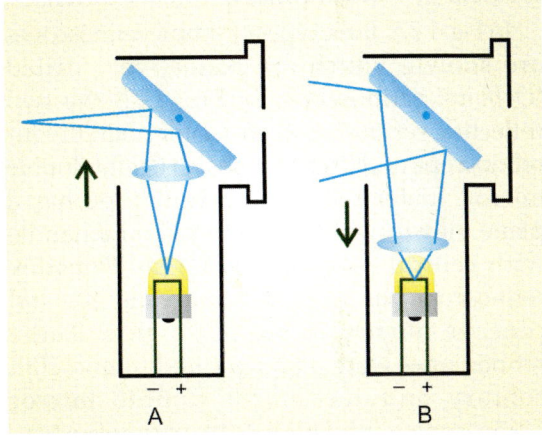

Fig. 1.6A and B: Optical effects by the movement of retinoscope lens. A. Lens moving upwards; B. Lens moving downwards

Opposite effect happens as shown in Fig. 1.6B, when sleeve is moved down, the lens moves downward (nearer to bulb) and produces plane mirror effect and hence emerging light rays are divergent in nature.

Various Types of Retinoscopes

Retinoscopes took a long revolutionary path to reach present day's sleek retinoscope models. Various types of retinoscopes are
- Simple retinoscopes
- MacNab retinoscope

- Dynamic retinoscopes
- Spot retinoscopes
- Streak retinoscopes

Simple retinoscopes: These were the earliest and oldest instruments used to perform retinoscopy. Initially, these were nothing but simple circular mirrors which had a central perforation or a hole. These mirrors were mounted on a metallic handle. Initially practitioners worked really hard to train themselves to use these simple plane mirrors along with a source of illumination (present either on a wall or over the patient's head by a light mounted on patient's chair). The practitioners observed the red reflex from patient's eye and tried to neutralize these reflexes with the help of various concave or convex lenses.

In Fig. 1.7A, three types of simple retinoscopes are shown, which are collectively called 'Orthops' retinoscope. In Fig. 1.7B the two reflecting retinoscopes are Lister plain mirror retinoscope and Priestley- Smith Bright double mirror. Lister reflecting retinoscope has a plane mirror, which is mounted on a handle with central peephole, whereas Priestley retinoscope has plane mirror on one side and concave mirror on the other side. These retinoscopes were manufactured in mid 20th century and the bright double mirror retinoscope is used till date by various institutions for teaching and learning purposes.

MacNab retinoscope: In year 1909, an Ophthalmologist Angus MacNab (1876–1914) had designed a retinoscope for study purposes. MacNab's retinoscope was a unique kind of retinoscope. It has an ivory handle with a gilt screw to fix. This retinoscope had an axis indicator wheel (marked from 0 till 180 degrees) with gear underneath the peephole of retinoscope. This axis wheel was operated by use of gears and had a central peephole as shown in Fig. 1.8.

Once the red reflex is neutralized in one meridian and if there is a movement in other meridian, then this meridian was neutralized by use of the axis wheel. This was a sophisticated retinoscope and needed continuous practice to master this instrument. Actually, this retinoscope was an improvement over the existing simple retinoscope because an astigmatism error can also be neutralized by use of this retinoscope.

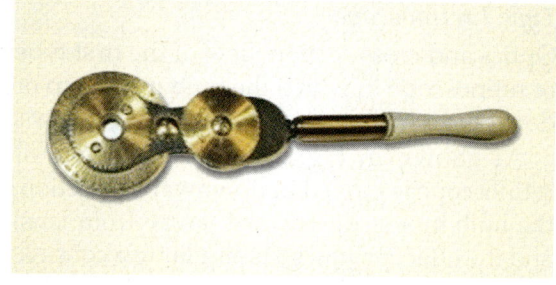

Fig. 1.8: MacNab retinoscope

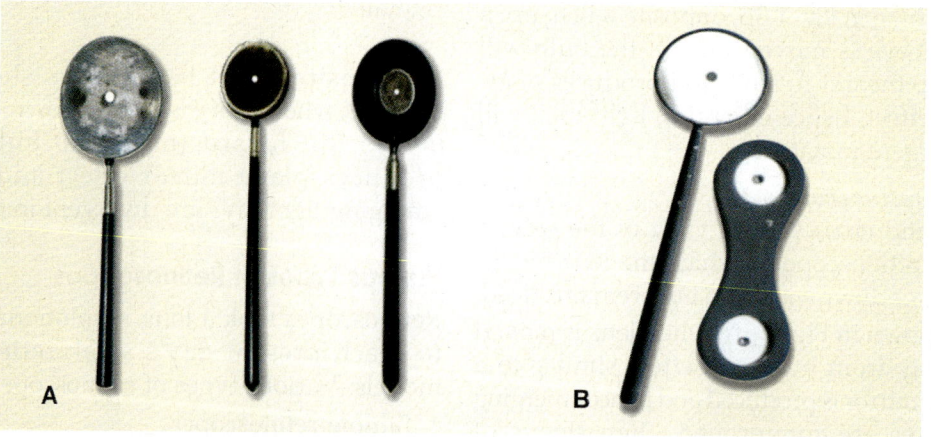

Fig. 1.7A and B: A. Orthops retinoscope; B. Reflecting retinoscopes

Dynamic retinoscopes: In earlier days, when performing retinoscopy with simple retinoscopes patients were instructed to fixate on a target situated at far distance and their accommodation was kept relaxed. This method of retinoscopy was called static retinoscopy because accommodation is at rest and no change of refractive status can occur due to accommodation during retinoscopy. Usually, to relax the accommodation of patient various mydriatics or cycloplegics drugs were used sometimes, even high convex lenses in the fellow eye were used to relax the accommodation.

Dynamic retinoscopy was a revolutionary thought in the field of retinoscopy. In the year 1902 scientist AJ Cross first identified the basic principle of this technique. Dynamic retinoscopy is defined as "retinoscopy done when the patient is instructed to fixate on a near object with both the eyes (binocularly)". Initially, any simple object like a reading book was used as the near object to fixate binocularly which can be easily held by the patients at desired distance. Over a period of time gradually retinoscopes were designed in such ways that near fixation targets were incorporated into the retinoscope itself.

The two popular types of dynamic retinoscopes were present in the era of 1930s. These were Margaret Dobson retinoscope and Turville-Pascal Dynascope.

Margaret Dobson retinoscope: As shown in Fig. 1.9A, the Margaret Dobson dynamic retinoscope had a spiral filament fitted inside the retinoscope bulb to produce a spot of light and emerging rays were made slightly divergent by using a plane mirror before they were reflected into the eye of the patient. This instrument was specially designed so that when patient try to compensate for achieving the binocular fixation, the working distance of retinoscope is compensated automatically.

A revolving disc present on the retinoscope had eight targets; out of these seven targets were near fixation charts which were designed to be examined from a reading distance of 30–35 cm. The eighth target designed for patient was a simple blank chart. This blank slot of target was designed to decrease the illumination from all other near targets and hence will convert this dynamic retinoscope into an old traditional static type of retinoscope. The fixation target shown in above retinoscope picture is that of a horse. These kinds of pictures were used to perform retinoscopy in children so that while doing the retinoscopy the examiner can ask simple questions to child such as whether this horse has a tail or can you see the beautiful eyes of the horse. These simple questions will help child as well as examiner in fixating the object and relax their accommodation.

Turville-Pascal dynascope: The Turville-Pascal retinoscope or 'Dynascope' (Dynamic retinoscope) (Fig. 1.9B) was introduced in the year 1931. It was designed by the collective efforts of both scientists, who worked together with an aim to remove different errors supposedly introduced by the retinoscope itself in the process of dynamic retinoscopy.

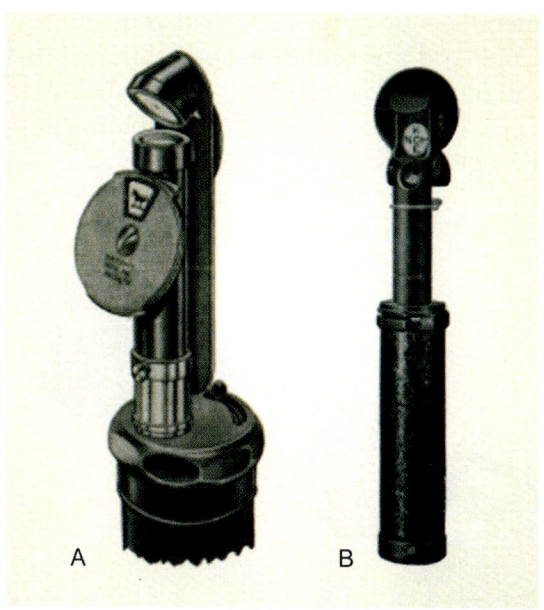

Fig. 1.9A and B: Dynamic retinoscopes. A. Margaret Dobson retinoscope; B. Turville-Pascal dynascope

Spot retinoscopes: In the year 1901, first electric retinoscope was introduced by Wolff (Fig. 1.10). This newly designed self-illuminated retinoscope was fitted with a small bulb which emitted a spot of light inside the patient's eye. In the subsequent years various other vergence models of retinoscopes were introduced which were capable of producing the vergence to spot light, either getting reflected from a plane mirror (more common) or a concave mirror (less common).

Streak retinoscopes: The fundus reflexes produced in an astigmatic eye are linear, thus for accurate detection of astigmatism it was better to use a rectangular streak of light than a spot light. To produce this type of streak early researchers tried to produce their own reflecting mirrors having a slit in the middle and this helped in conversion of a spot light into a linear beam. Jack C Copeland (Father of streak retinoscopy) introduced the first streak retinoscope having variable vergence around 1920. His streak retinoscope was designed to produce its own linear light beam which could have been rotated in all the ocular meridians by a sleeve. In mid 20th century, Copeland's retinoscope popularly called Pulzone streak retinoscope as shown in Fig. 1.11 was commercially available in entire European countries.

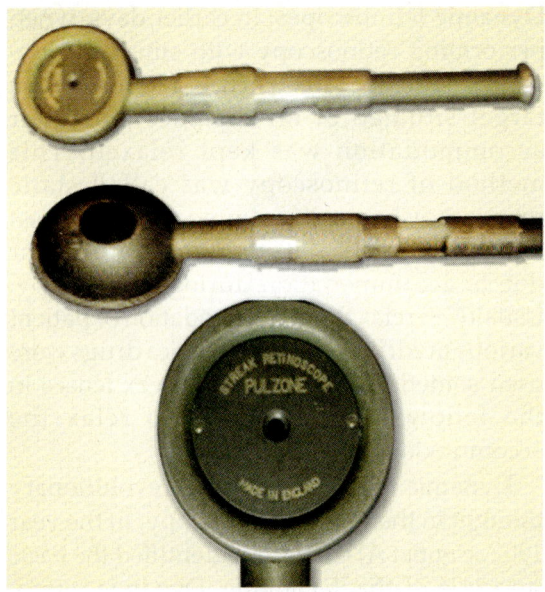

Fig. 1.11: Pulzone streak retinoscope

Commercially two types of retinoscope are manufactured such as

- Bausch and Lomb, Copeland and Copeland-Optec 360: In these retinoscope designs convex lens (condensing lens) is kept fixed, whereas with the movement of sleeve the source of light, i.e. bulb can be moved upwards (towards the lens) or downwards (away from the lens). When sleeve present on the retinoscope handle is raised, the light beam is emitted as a divergent beam and opposite occurs when sleeve is lowered, i.e. a convergent beam is produced.
- Retinoscopes made by companies such as Welch Allen, Heine (Fig. 1.12), Neitz, and Keeler: In these retinoscope designs the source of light, i.e. bulb is kept fixed, whereas the convex lens (condensing lens) can be moved upwards (towards mirror) or downwards (towards bulb) by raising or lowering the sleeve. When sleeve present on the retinoscope handle is raised, the light beam is emitted as a convergent beam and a divergent beam is produced by lowering of sleeve.

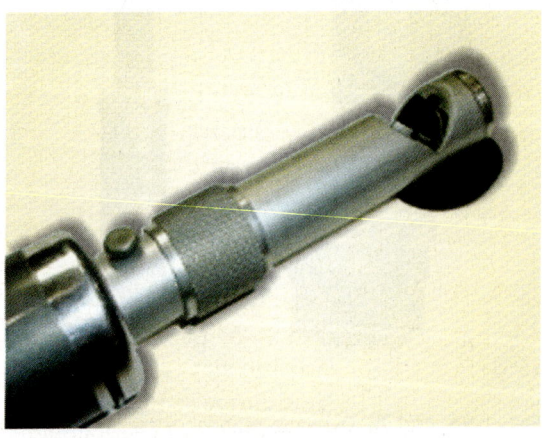

Fig. 1.10: Spot retinoscope

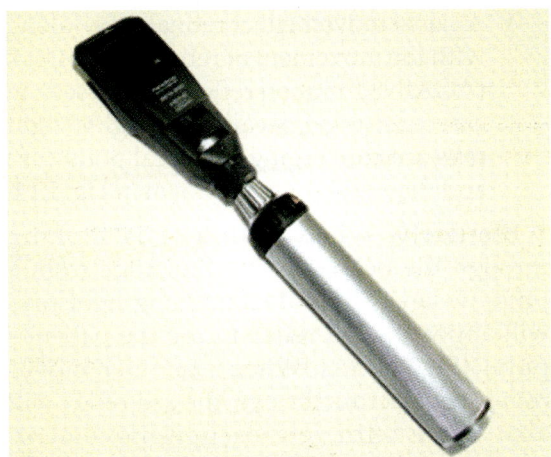

Fig. 1.12: Heine streak retinoscope

RETINOSCOPY

Principles and Techniques of Retinoscopy

The principle is to observe the different kind of retinal reflections (reflex) obtained from patient's eye when light beam produced from retinoscope illuminates the internal portion of patient's eye. The examiner observes the relative movement of the retinal reflexes when he/she moves the streak or spot of light beam either in vertical or horizontal meridians from corner to corner of patient's pupil. Then examiner tries to neutralize these retinal reflexes manually by placing trial lenses of different power in front of the eye in a trial frame.

Retinoscopy is a technique used to calculate the amount of refractive error by an objective means. Objective refraction test is done by performing retinoscopy under the effect of mydriasis. Retinoscopes' light source is utilized to illuminate the fundus of patient's eye while examiner will observe and measure the reflected rays of light from the retina. Retinoscopy may be followed by various subjective tests to calculate an accurate amount of refractive correction required for the patient.

Over many decades retinoscopy has proved to be an excellent method to evaluate the refractive status of an eye and is considered as a clinically effective method to assess an accurate refractive correction needed by patient in very less time without compromising the quality of result.

Retinoscopy Reflex

Various images obtained while performing retinoscopy need evaluation for the calculation and estimation of refractive status of the eye. As discussed above, when fundus is illuminated with the retinoscope light source and examiner observes the emerging rays coming from the retina (as if retina is luminous), the optical system of eye exerts various types of vergence to these emitting rays. For example, when retina is illuminated with parallel rays (by plane mirror), the rays reflected from the retina will emerge from the eye according to the refractive status of eye as follows

- Reflected light rays will emerge from the eye as parallel rays in case of emmetropia.
- Reflected light rays will emerge from the eye as divergent rays in case of hypermetropia.
- Reflected light rays will emerge from the eye as convergent rays in case of myopia.

The emitting rays will behave differently if we illuminate the retina with rays which are not parallel.

The optics of retina in different ocular status, i.e. emmetropia, hypermetropia and myopia, assuming that the entering light rays were parallel in all three ocular states, can be understood by graphic representation as shown in Fig. 1.13. In an emmetrope (Fig. 1.13A), the focal point is at infinity, in hypermetrope

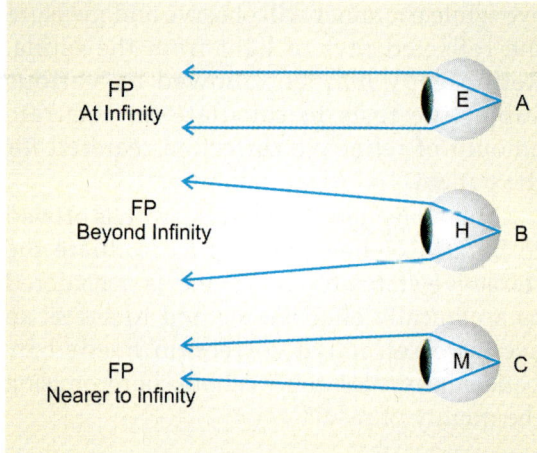

Fig. 1.13A to C: Emerging rays pattern and focal point (FP) for emmetropic (E), hypermetropic (H) and myopic (M) eyes

(Fig. 1.13B) it is beyond infinity, whereas in myope (Fig. 1.13C) the focal point is at lesser distance than infinity.

Consider that examiner is sitting at infinity distance and looking through the peephole of retinoscope. Various observations in three basic conditions as mentioned above will be as follows

- Retinal reflex moves along with the movement of retinoscope streak (WITH motion reflex) in case of emmetrope and hypermetrope because emerging light rays are not converging to a focal point as shown in Fig. 1.14.

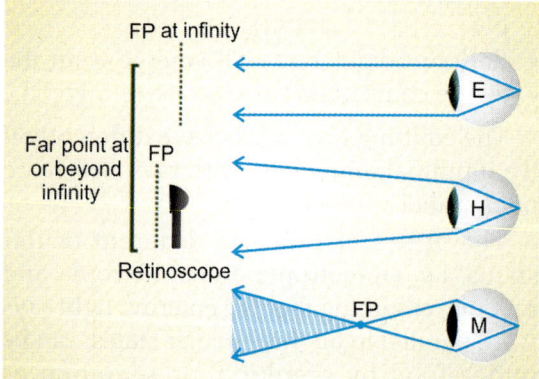

Fig. 1.14: Different types of retinal reflex considering that retinoscope is situated at infinity

- Against movement of retinal reflex along with the movement of retinoscope streak (AGAINST motion reflex) will be seen in case of myope because emerging light rays are converging to a focal point (FP) and then diverging as shown in Fig. 1.14.

Similarly, when examiner is looking through the peephole of retinoscope from a finite distance, then the emerging light rays will appear as red reflex inside the patient's pupil (Fig. 1.15A). When examiner moves retinoscope across the eye, the red reflex will also move with retinoscope movement. Suppose the emerging light rays are parallel or diverging, then the red retinal reflex will move in the same direction as of the retinoscope streak (intercept), this is called with movement (Fig. 1.15B). In contrast, if emerging light rays meet at focal point and are diverging, then the retinal reflex will move in opposite direction, as that of retinoscope streak; this is called against movement (Fig. 1.15C).

📖 *Note* _____

An interesting way to interpret this condition is that, if we observe against movement we are beyond the focal point and if we see with movement, then focal point is beyond us.

Practically, optical infinity is considered beyond 20 feet or 6 meters distance but it is impossible for an examiner to sit at this far distance and then observe the retinal reflex or add the correcting lenses in trial frame. For practical convenience either one meter or 66 cm distance is advocated to observe the retinal reflex, from where reflex appears brighter and examiner can easily add or remove lenses in/from the trial frame.

When examiner observes from 1 meter distance, then in case of emmetrope and hyperopes still the examiner will observe with movement reflex (Fig. 1.16) because focal point in both these cases is beyond the examiner. However, in case of myope (for example,

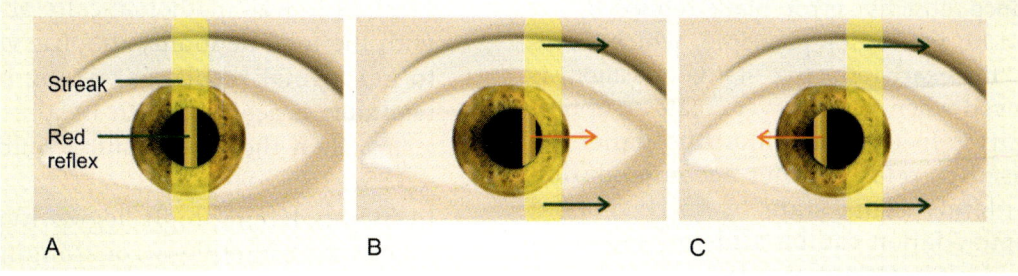

Fig. 1.15A to C: Red reflex motion with retinoscope streak (intercept). A. In center with streak; B. With movement; C. Against movement

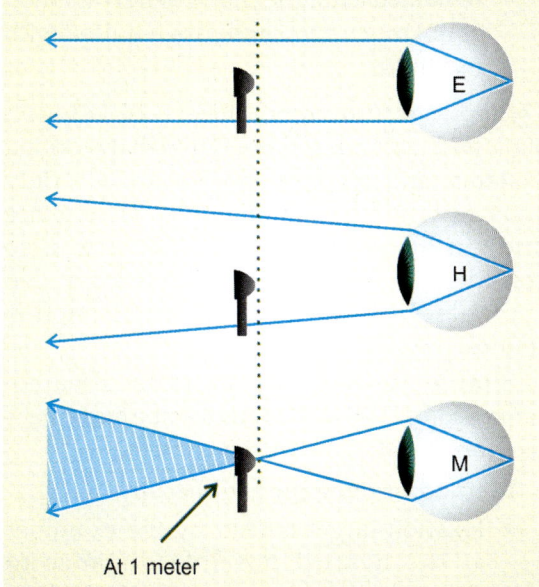

Fig. 1.16: Different types of retinal reflex considering that retinoscope is situated at one meter distance.

having one dioptre refractive error) following typical reflexes are observed with various positions such as

- Suppose examiner leans forward with retinoscope: With movement of reflex is seen
- When examiner goes backward: Against movement reflex will be seen
- However, with retinoscope exactly at one meter distance no movement of reflex or a neutrality reflex will be seen because focal point in our example is at one meter distance.

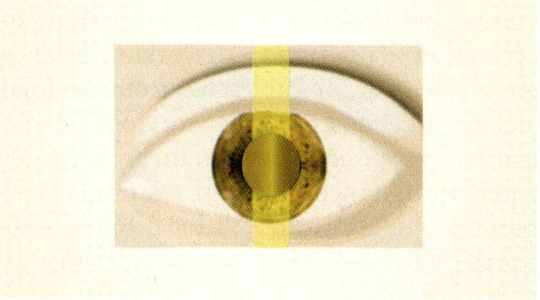

Fig. 1.17: Neutrality of red reflex

A neutrality of red (retinal) reflex is seen when peephole of retinoscope coincides with focal point. This reflex is the one which fills the entire pupil with light (Fig. 1.17). At this point there is no streak of light and also there is no movement of retinal reflex either with or against. At this point the retina of eye is in conjugate with the peephole of retinoscope. As retinal reflex reverses its direction from with movement to against movement, this focal point is also called reversal point in retinoscopy.

Methods of Retinoscopy

Retinoscopy methods can be grouped mainly as

- Static retinoscopy
- Mohindra near retinoscopy
- Dynamic retinoscopy

Static retinoscopy: This is the most widely and routinely performed retinoscopy technique to estimate the accurate amount of distance refractive error. Static retinoscopy is based on Foucault's principle, which states that "the exact refractive status of patient is achieved when the observer create an optical infinity". In this technique the patient is advised to relax his/her accommodation completely. This state of fully relaxed accommodation can be achieved either by providing a distant fixation target to the patient or by using cycloplegics in cases of hypermetropes and children.

To obtain the patient's exact refractive status, the dioptric power equivalent to cycloplegic (if used) and also working distance are mathematically subtracted from the total amount of retinoscopy. The working distance lens has power equivalent to the focal length equal to distance between examiner and patient. For example, +1.00 dioptre lens equates for one meter of working distance.

Mohindra near retinoscopy: This technique is also used to measure distance refractive error in a non-accommodative state, however, this technique differs from dynamic retinoscopy. This is a very useful technique to assess refractive state of eye in infants.

Steps of retinoscopy technique are

- The examination room must be dark as much as possible. Underlying principle is simple that the dim light emitting from retinoscope will act as a fixation target for the child so that accommodation will not get stimulate.

- Sometimes this technique can be performed over the shoulder of parents while parent is holding the infant or feeding the infant. The examiner performs retinoscopy from 50 cm distance and two principal meridians of retinal reflexes, i.e. horizontal and vertical are neutralized separately by using spherical or a combination of spherical and cylindrical trial lenses.

- Originally, Mohindra used a −1.25 D lenses for adjustment; this dioptric value

of −1.25 D was mathematically added with the total neutrality dioptric value to get a final result. For example, if neutrality is achieved with +4.50 /−1.75 × 90°, then the final result would be + 3.25/−1.75 × 90°.

- In infants having high degree hypermetropic refractive error, Mohindra retinoscopy showed less accurate results when compared with cycloplegic retinoscopy. Although Mohindra technique remained a unique child-friendly method as not much cooperation is required with the child.

Dynamic retinoscopy: Difference between static and dynamic retinoscopy is that working distance and accommodation are not only equated with lens power rather convergence and information processing are also considered in the dynamic retinoscopy. No cycloplegia is required to perform this retinoscopy.

Simple method to perform a dynamic retinoscopy is by using retinoscope and a near fixation target, say reading chart.

Method of dynamic retinoscopy

- Fixation target is held by the examiner at the nearest possible distance to peephole of retinoscope, without blocking the aperture of peephole.

- Darken the examination room and a light is directed towards the reading chart so that patient is able to read this chart. Examiner holds the reading chart and retinoscope at the normal reading distance.

- If distant vision correction is present, then patient is instructed to wear the distance vision glasses. Then patient is instructed to fixate on a distant target wearing distance correction (if present) and fundus reflexes are observed in both the eyes, usually with motion is seen.

- Now the patient is instructed to suddenly fixate on the reading chart from the distance target, while examiner continues the retinoscopy. Usually the previously observed with motion will either swiftly converts into the state of neutralization or may appear as against motion.

- Suppose neutralization of reflex is incomplete, then patient is instructed again to fixate on the previous distant target, so that the retinoscopy reflex will quickly change back into with motion.

- Examiner gradually moves nearer to the patient and simultaneously instructs him/her to sustain their fixation for longer duration on near target. This increases the efforts of accommodative system and helps the examiner to estimate about the sustainability of accommodative efforts.

- Plus lenses are now added to neutralize the reflex.

The results of dynamic retinoscopy can be interpreted as:

- Normal when reflex seen is rapid, complete, and steady.
- Abnormal when reflex seen is incomplete, sluggish and shows momentary accommodation and/or accommodative lag.

Various techniques to execute dynamic retinoscopy are:

- Bell retinoscopy
- Nott retinoscopy (NR)
- Book retinoscopy
- Stress point retinoscopy
- Monocular estimate method (MEM)

Bell Retinoscopy

In previous days originally a cat bell was used as the target to perform the technique of dynamic retinoscopy, hence was named as Bell retinoscopy. Although nowadays Wolff wand is used as target to perform this technique. As shown in Fig. 1.18, Wolff wand target has a gold or silver metal ball of ½ inch diameter mounted on one or both ends of a rod.

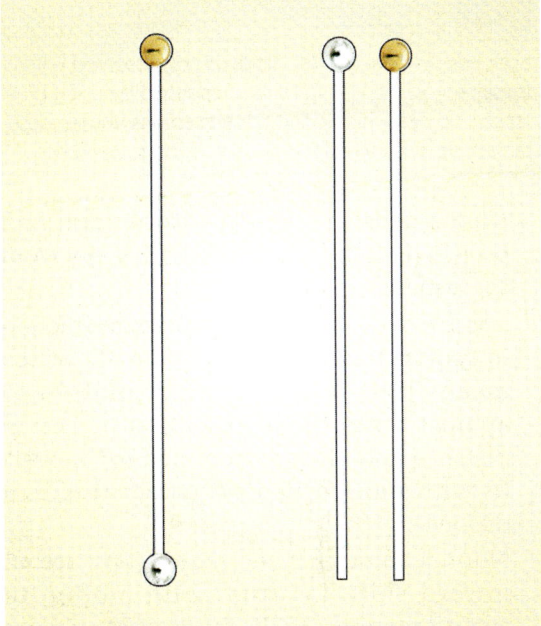

Fig. 1.18: Wolff wand target for bell retinoscopy (*courtesy*: Bernell Corporation)

Procedure of retinoscopy

- Examiner holds the retinoscope at 50 cm distance from the patient and observes the fundus reflex. Now examiner gradually moves the ball towards the patient, while patient is instructed to look at the ball continuously. Simultaneously, examiner continues to perform the retinoscopy and observe the movements of reflex in relation with the movement of ball target.

- As the ball moves closer, usually a fast with motion is observed, gradually reflex changes to neutral and then against.

- Now when examiner gradually moves the ball away from the patient a reverse order of changes in reflex, i.e. from against to neutral and then with motion will be observed by the examiner.

- Firstly record the distance between ball and the patient's nose at which a change from with motion to against motion had occurred while ball was moved towards the patient.

- Secondly, record the distance between ball and the patient's nose at which a change

📖 *Note*

Suppose lag of accommodation is not observed within these ranges, then procedure is repeated by using plus lenses. Lenses which bring the recordings within these ranges are acknowledged as near vision prescription.

from against motion to with motion had occurred while ball was moved away from the patient.

- These two distances are recorded as fraction in centimeters. For example, 36/42 which means first recording with motion to against motion had occurred at 36 cm distance and change from against motion to with motion had occurred at 42 cm distance.
- Normal values for bell retinoscopy are an inward shift, i.e. from with motion to against motion is in the range of 35–42.5 cm and an outward shift, i.e. from against motion to with motion is in the range of 37.5–45 cm.

Nott Retinoscopy

Nott retinoscopy (NR) is a unique method of retinoscopy. Here an internally-illuminated cube is used as a target which contains high contrast cartoon images (usually in black and white color). This cube is attached on a retractable tape measure and is viewed from a 40 cm distance in a dim illumination as shown in Fig. 1.19.

The target is kept stationary (D1) and examiner moves in backward direction holding retinoscope, while observing the reflex till it becomes neutralized. This distance between the examiner and the child (D2) is recorded and accommodative response is equal to the inverse of this final distance.

Book Retinoscopy

In book retinoscopy various changes in retinoscopic reflex are observed depending upon the involvement level or interaction of child, who continuously read a book as target. These changes in retinoscopic reflexes could be

- A bright, sharp edged pinkish colored reflex with motion is seen, while child is reading freely and easily.
- A bright, sharp and dark pink colored reflex having fast against motion is seen, while

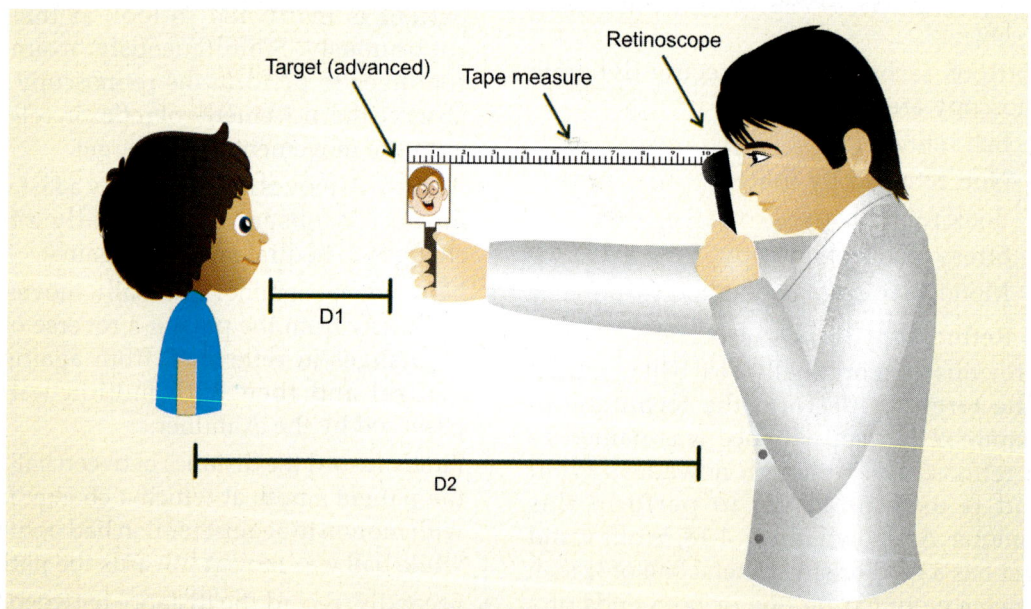

Fig. 1.19: Method of Nott retinoscopy. D1—fixed distance; D2—final distance

child is reading on instructions of examiner, means maintain the reading task in spite of being stressed.

- A dull brick red colored reflex having slow against motion is observed, while child is reading with frustration.

Stress point retinoscopy

Harmon and Kraskin described stress point retinoscopy. As discussed above, in Bell retinoscopy a change in motion of reflex was observed, whereas in stress-point retinoscopy a change in reflex quality is observed. Following three types of observations can be seen when near point stress is observed

- A change in radial pulse of subject
- An inner canthal twitch
- A color change in retinal reflex

Harmon distance: It is measured from the elbow to the knuckle of middle finger as shown in Fig. 1.20.

Test procedure

- Examiner initially observes the fundus reflex, then patient is instructed to focus on a Wolff ball as near target.
- Now examiner slowly moves Wolff's ball closer to the patient and simultaneously

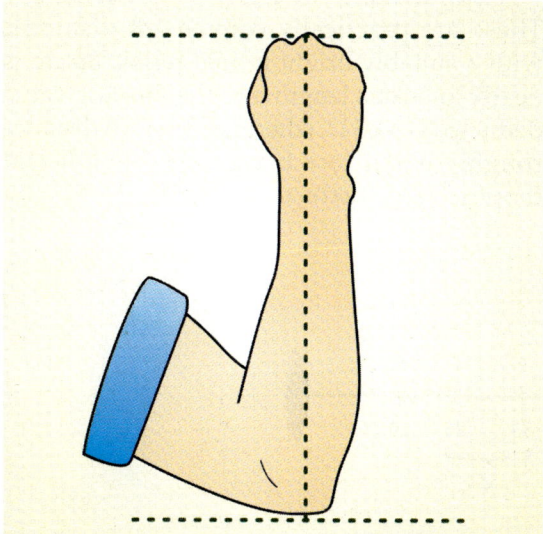

Fig. 1.20: Harmon distance

Note

A retinoscopy reflex is called popping reflex when reflex initially brightens, then becomes dull and again becomes bright.

observes that at what distance the patient's fundus reflex pops.

Interpretation: Normally, in children the stress point should be 10 cm nearer than Harmon distance of that subject, whereas normally in adults the stress point is 20–22.5 cm away from the face. For example, suppose in a 10 years old child, Harmon distance is 22 cm and a stress point is 18 cm. When stress point is measured again with add of + 1.0 DS lens, the stress point becomes 14 cm, whereas with add of +1.5 DS lens, it becomes 24 cm. In this case + 1.0 DS lens is serving as counter-stress lens, whereas +1.5 DS lens is inducing a new stress pattern. Hence, we will prescribe + 1.0 DS lens for near work to this child.

Monocular estimate method

Monocular estimate method (MEM) is performed in an entirely different way than that from other methods of dynamic retinoscopy. Most of the near dynamic retinoscopy methods are performed by inserting a lens and its effect on the performance is observed.

MEM is a distinctive method where lenses are principally used to confirm the observations done by the examiner. A fixation card is attached to the retinoscope and under normal illumination conditions examiner views retinal reflexes through a central aperture from a distance of 40 cm.

Techniques of Retinoscopy

- Dry retinoscopy
- Wet retinoscopy

Dry retinoscopy: Most widely used technique to perform the retinoscopy is dry retinoscopy. Dry simply means that no mydriatic is used while performing the retinoscopy. Hence, a correction from total refraction is done only for distance, for example, if we are doing retinoscopy

Clinical Inference

- In low degree hypermetropes dynamic retinoscopy may show a rapid, complete but unsteady or discontinuous accommodation which confirms a diagnosis of an accommodative insufficiency and should be treated by prescribing glasses.
- In non ocular causes a brisk normal dynamic retinoscopy response is present but if symptoms persist then an addition of reading glasses (small power) can be used in cases of a fallaciously normal dynamic retinoscopy.

from 66 cm distance, then simply +1.5 D is deducted from the total refractive amount obtained at neutralization and if doing from 50 cm, then +2 D is deducted from total refractive error.

Wet retinoscopy: When mydriatic is used to perform retinoscopy, it is called wet retinoscopy or cycloplegic refraction. Normally in clinical practice tropicamide with phenylepherine drops are used to perform retinoscopy. These drugs produce pupillary dilatation but are weak cycloplegics, hence when strong cycloplegic effect is needed as in cases of very young child or high degree hypermetropes, then atropine, homatropine or cyclopentolate is used. Here a correction is done for both distance and mydriasis, for example, if retinoscopy is done from 66 cm distance by using atropine, then +1.5 D for distance and +1 D for atropine is deducted from total refractive value obtained by neutralization. For homatropine +0.75 D and for cyclopentolate +0.5 D is deducted.

> **Note**
>
> No correction for cycloplegic is needed when tropicamide is used for retinoscopy.

Retinoscopy Working Distance

If retinoscopy is performed at 25 cm distance; the retinal reflex will be bright and it is easy to reach the patient, but at the same time chances of the distance error is very high. If it is performed at 100 cm distance, the retinal reflex will be dim and it is difficult to reach the patient for changing trial lenses, however, the distance error is very low.

As shown in Fig. 1.21 space (X) of 8 cm width at 25 cm retinoscopy distance is representing 1 D difference, whereas same 8 cm space (Y) is representing only 0.09 D difference near 100 cm distance. So when retinoscopy is done at 25 cm distance then an error of few centimeters in distance estimation can bring a large change in results (by 0.50–1.0 D), whereas a distance error of equal magnitude gives negligible change in results (by 0.05–0.1 D) at 100 cm distance.

Considering these advantages and disadvantages of near and far working distances, most of the examiners compromise for a working distance of either 66 cm or 50 cm. These are practically convenient distances with a suitably bright retinal reflex. 66 cm is nearly an arm's length and the dioptric value deducted is +1.5 D, whereas 50 cm is a distance roughly equal to a bend arm's length and dioptric value deducted is +2 D.

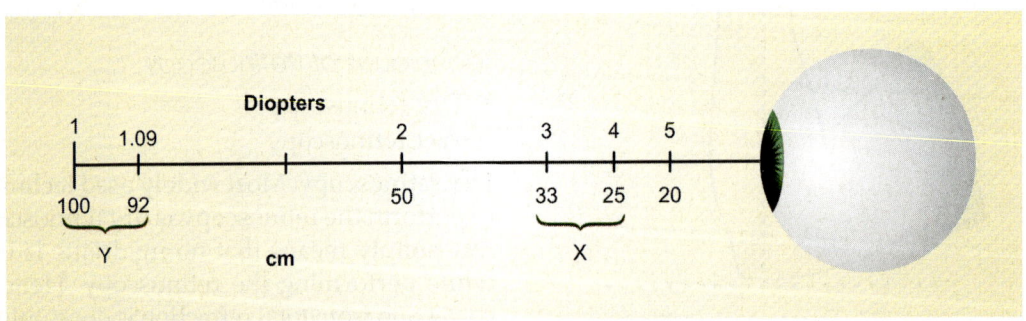

Fig. 1.21: Retinoscopy distance (cm) with corresponding dioptric power (D)

Retinoscopy Reflexes and Neutralization

INTRODUCTION

Reflexes in Emmetropes

Normally when retinoscopy is performed from 66 cm distance, an emmetrope will produce "with movement" in both vertical and horizontal meridians. These reflexes can be neutralized by small power plus lenses as shown in Fig. 2.1. For example, with +1.5 DS lens because retinoscopy was done from 66 cm.

Reflexes in Hypermetropes

Various reflexes seen in hypermetrope depend upon the degree of hypermetropia (Fig. 2.2). In low degree hypermetrope the retinal reflex is of small width and fast moving "with

motion", however, as the degree of hyperopia increases the width of reflex increases and speed of reflex decreases.

This 'with motion' can easily be neutralized by using a plus lens whose power depends upon the degree of hypermetropia. For example, as shown in Fig. 2.3, a hypermetrope of +1 DS will get neutralize by adding a +2.5 DS lens when retinoscopy is done from 66 cm distance (without cycloplegic drug).

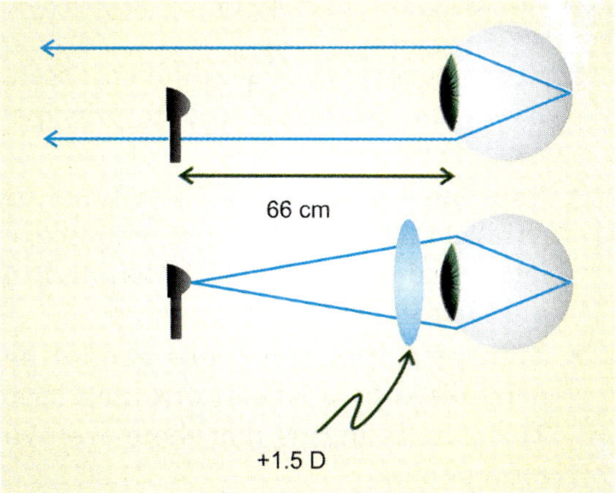

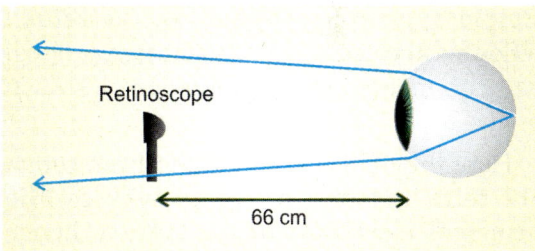

Fig. 2.2: With motion

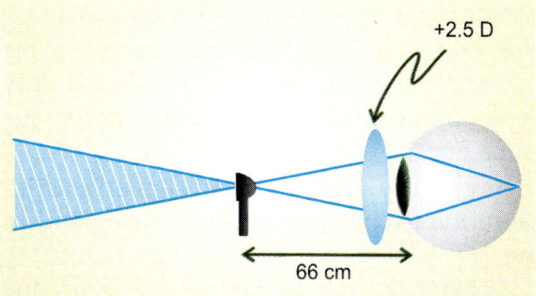

Fig. 2.3: Neutralization with +2.5 DS lens, in case of +1 DS hypermetropia

Fig. 2.1: With motion getting neutralize with small power plus lens in emmetropia

Reflexes in Myopia

Similar to hypermetropia various reflexes are seen in myopes depending upon the degree of myopia. In low degree myopia the retinal reflex is small width and fast moving 'against motion', however, as the degree of myopia increases the width of reflex increases and speed of reflex decreases, although it still remains an against motion as shown in Fig. 2.4.

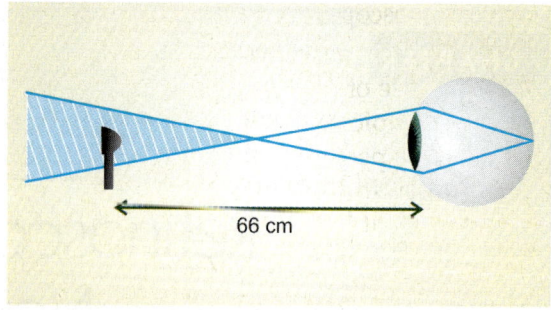

Fig. 2.4: An against motion in myopia

This against motion can be neutralized by using a minus power lens whose power depends upon the degree of myopia. For example, as shown in Fig. 2.5, a myope of –3 DS will get neutralize by adding a –1.5 DS lens when retinoscopy is done from 66 cm distance (without cycloplegic drug).

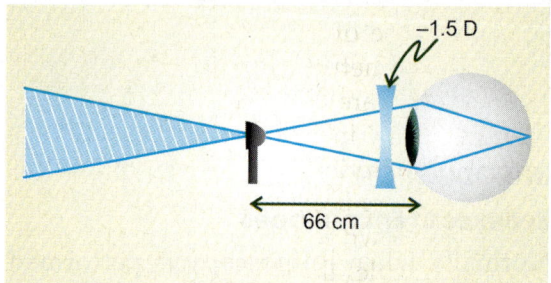

Fig. 2.5: Neutralization with –1.5 DS lens, in case of –3 DS myopia

Reflexes in Astigmatism

Astigmatism is a state of refractive error where a few rays of incident light focus on the retina and a few behind or in front of the retina. Hence, when retinoscopy is done we get different kind of movement of retinal reflexes in different meridians. For example, in case of simple hyperopic astigmatism the retinal reflex may be neutral in 90° meridian and will be 'with motion' in 180° meridian as shown in Fig. 2.6.

Here the light rays emerging from retina are refracted in a different way by the principal meridians of the cornea, hence reflexes behave as if there are two eyes instead of one eye and each of these principal meridians is acting like a separate eye. Once the retinoscopy has been performed on the eye with one principal meridian, then simply repeat the retinoscopy second time on the same eye.

Several phenomena observed while performing retinoscopy in case of astigmatism are

- Eye will show two types of reflexes one in each principal meridian as shown in Fig. 2.6.

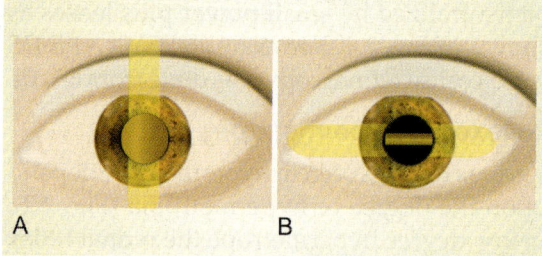

Fig. 2.6: Astigmatic reflex. A. Neutral reflex at 90° meridian; B. With motion reflex at 180° meridian

- Retinal reflexes will have different speed, width and brightness in both principal meridians.
- Movement of retinal reflex will not be parallel to the movement of retinoscope intercept; unless scoping along the principal meridian.
- Both principal meridians cannot be neutralized by a single correcting lens. This simply means that there are two focal points.

Various types of astigmatic error will show following reflexes when retinoscopy is done using working lens of +1.5 DS (compensating for a retinoscopy distance of 66 cm) in the trial frame.

- In case of an uncorrected simple hypermetropic astigmatism, one focal point lies at peephole of retinoscope and other is behind it. For example, a neutral reflex at 90° meridian and with motion in 180° meridian will be seen when retinoscopy is done from 66 cm distance using a working lens of +1.5 D as shown in Fig. 2.7.

- In case of an uncorrected compound hypermetropic astigmatism both focal points are behind retinoscope, so 'with motion' in both meridians will be seen when retinoscopy is done from 66 cm distance using a working lens of +1.5 D as shown in Fig. 2.8. However, in our example, the reflex will be more with motion at 180° meridian.

- Uncorrected simple myopic astigmatism cases are similar to simple hyperopic astigmatism, except that in these cases one focal point is in the front and another

point is at peephole. Hence, for example, in these cases 'against motion' at 90° meridian and neutral reflex at 180° meridian will be seen when retinoscopy is done from 66 cm distance using a working lens of +1.5 D as shown in Fig. 2.9.

- Uncorrected compound myopic astigmatism is a state of eye where both focal points are in front of the retinoscope peephole. Hence, in these cases 'against motion' in both 90° and 180° meridians will be seen when retinoscopy is done from 66 cm distance using a working lens of +1.5 D as shown in Fig. 2.10, although there is more against in 90° meridian in our example.

- In case of an uncorrected mixed astigmatic one focal point is in front and

Note _____

Practically during retinoscopy it is very difficult to judge the degree of against motion.

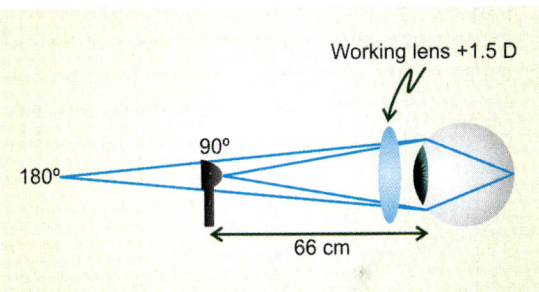

Fig. 2.7: Uncorrected simple hyperopic astigmatism

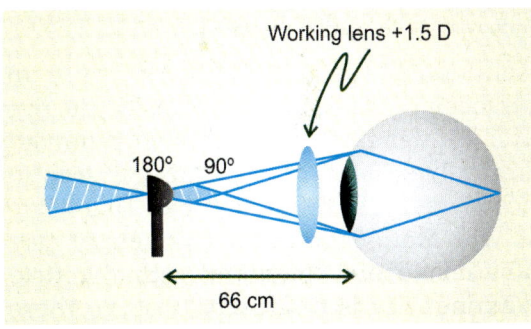

Fig. 2.9: Uncorrected simple myopic astigmatism

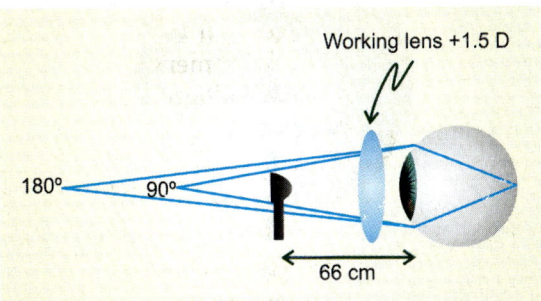

Fig. 2.8: Uncorrected compound hyperopic astigmatism

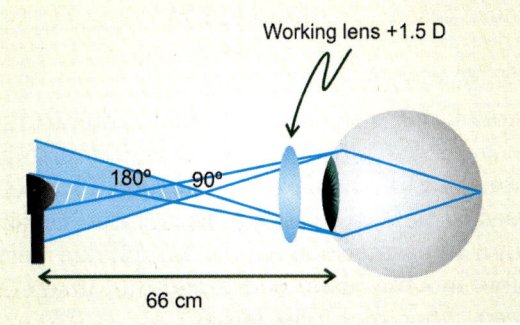

Fig. 2.10: Uncorrected compound myopic astigmatism

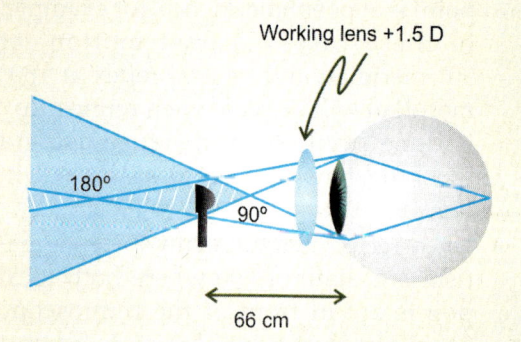

Working lens +1.5 D

180°

90°

66 cm

Fig. 2.11: Uncorrected mixed astigmatism

other point is behind the peephole of retinoscope. On retinoscopy 'against motion' in one meridian and 'with motion' in other meridian, i.e. 90 degree and 180 degree meridians, respectively (in our example) will be seen when retinoscopy is done from 66 cm distance using a working lens of +1.5 D as shown in Fig. 2.11.

Rare Retinoscopy Reflexes

Reflexes in Pseudophakia

Pseudophakia is a state of eye where an intraocular lens is implanted inside the eye after cataractous lens has been removed surgically. The retinoscopy images seen in these cases are of different types. There may be 'with motion' or 'against motion' or may have mixed movements of retinal reflex. Examiner needs to closely observe these reflexes to neutralize them, a wet retinoscopy is preferred over dry retinoscopy in these cases.

Reflexes in Aphakia

Aphakia is a state of eye where cataractous lens is removed surgically without implantation of an intraocular lens. The retinal reflexes seen in these cases are similar to those seen in high hypermetropic cases. In aphakia very slow moving, wide width and dull image is seen, when high plus lenses, say +6–7 D are added then the speed, brightness of reflex

increases and width decreases (similar to a hypermetropic case).

Reflexes of Rare Types

- Scissor movement on retinoscopy means when one arm of retinal image is moving in opposite direction to that of other arm of retinal reflex, like the blades of scissor. Most of the time these images are difficult to assess, but on careful examination one can see that there are two arms of retinal reflex as shown in Fig. 2.12. Usually one arm is thicker and show 'with movement', whereas other arm will be thin and have 'against motion'.

- Oblique movement on retinoscopy means movement of reflex is not in coordination with our retinoscope intercept. In these cases when intercept of retinoscope is moved either horizontally or vertically the retinal reflex moves oblique to the movement of intercept either in 'with' or 'against' motion. Retinal reflex in these cases will appear as shown in Fig. 2.13.

- No movement on retinoscopy examination is considered when practically almost entire pupillary area is filled with reflex and examiner cannot see the boundary of retinal reflex easily. When observer try to move the streak of retinoscope in any meridian, say horizontal or vertical, no appreciable

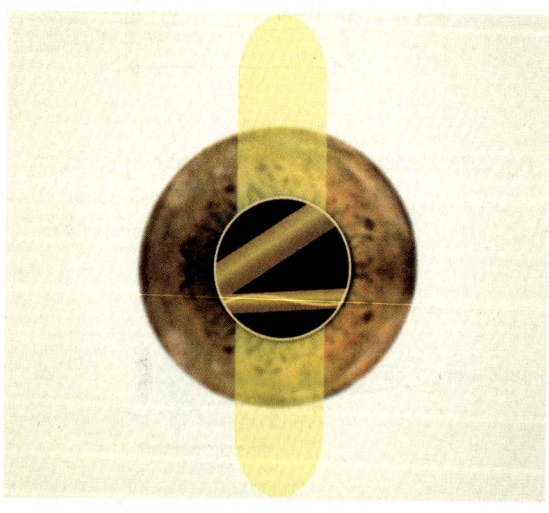

Fig. 2.12: Scissor reflex

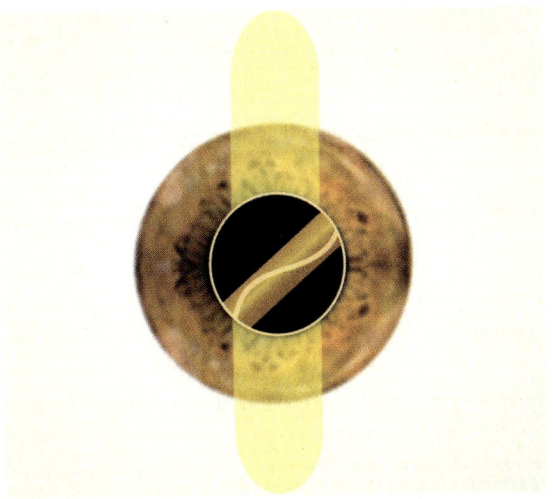

Fig. 2.13: Oblique retinal reflex

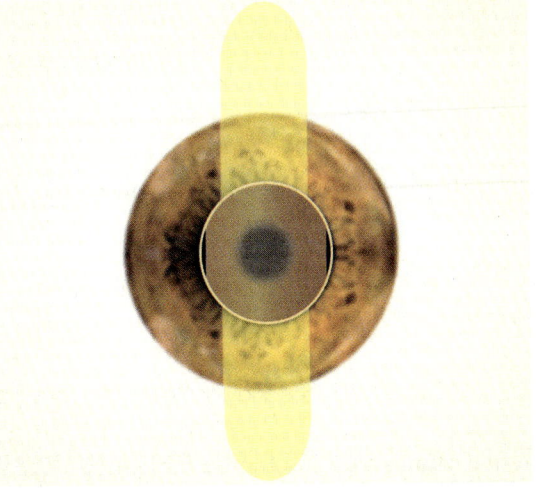

Fig. 2.15: Centrally dark retinal reflex

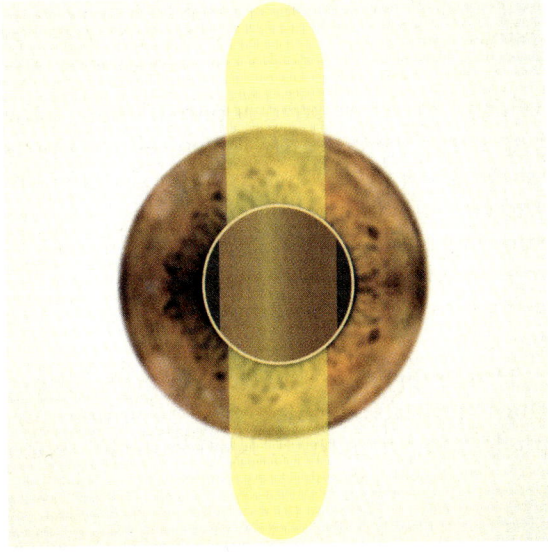

Fig. 2.14: Dim retinal reflex

Interpretation of Retinal Reflexes

Routine Images

To study the reflex in routine refractive error cases these steps must be followed by an observer

- First decide whether retinal reflex is 'with' or 'against' movement which is decided by the location of focal point relative to the observer's eyes, i.e. it is in front or behind the observer.
- Then it is important to judge the amount of 'with' or 'against' movement to decide how far the observer is from neutrality point. Certain identifiable characteristics of moving reflex will help in the estimation of distance from neutrality.
- Indirectly this will help to decide how much correcting lens power will be needed to move the focal point in conjugate to our retina.

Note

This experience in rough estimation of lens power will save much trial and error, and will shorten the time to reach at neutrality.

The moving retinal reflex can be characterized by three main features

Speed: Depending on the distance from focal point, the retinal reflex moves very slowly

movement of retinal reflex will be seen. Clinically, these reflexes are very confusing and appear as shown in Fig. 2.14.

- Centrally dark reflex on retinoscopy means that a dim retinal reflex is seen only on sides of pupil margins and the central area of pupil is dark, which shows no reflex. In these cases bend the retinoscope streak to study the characteristics of these kinds of reflexes, also examiner can lean forward to enhance the brightness of reflex (Fig. 2.15).

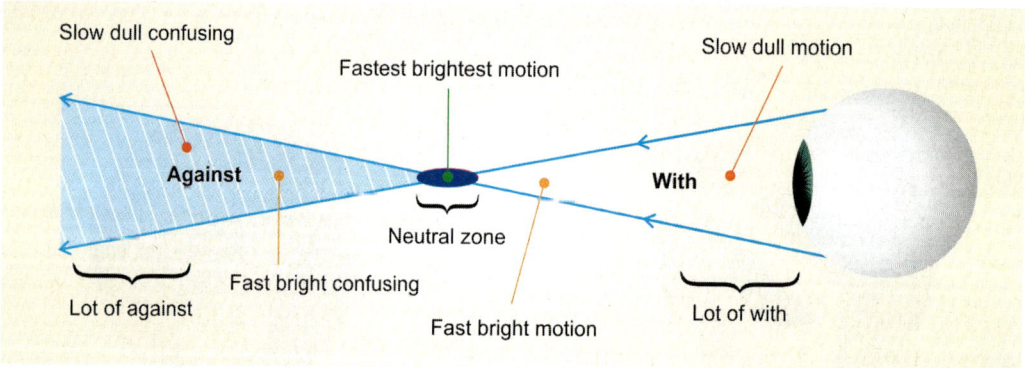

Fig. 2.16: Speed and brightness of reflex at various intervals in relation to position of retinoscope

when retinoscope is situated far from the focal point and it becomes more rapid as retinoscope gets closer to focal point. When neutrality point is reached, the pupil fills with light reflex and no movement of retinoscope streak is seen. In simpler words, large degree refractive errors will have a slow moving retinal reflex and small degree refractive errors will have a fast moving retinal reflex (Fig. 2.16).

Brightness: The retinal reflex will appear dull when retinoscope is situated far from the focal point and it will become brighter as examiner approaches at the neutrality point. Hence, refractive errors of large degree will have a dull reflex and small degree refractive errors will have a brighter reflex (Fig. 2.17).

Note

In Fig. 2.16, against portion is shown as cross-matched because against retinal reflex is dimmer as compared to with reflex at any comparable distance from the focal point.

Width: The width band of retinal reflex in the pupillary area is narrow when retinoscope is situated at a far distance from the focal point, width of the band broadens as the observer approaches near the focal point and ultimately reflex width will fill the entire pupil when the refractive error gets neutralized as shown in Fig. 2.17.

However, in clinical practice these characteristic of reflex may be sometimes misleading in nature. For example, when

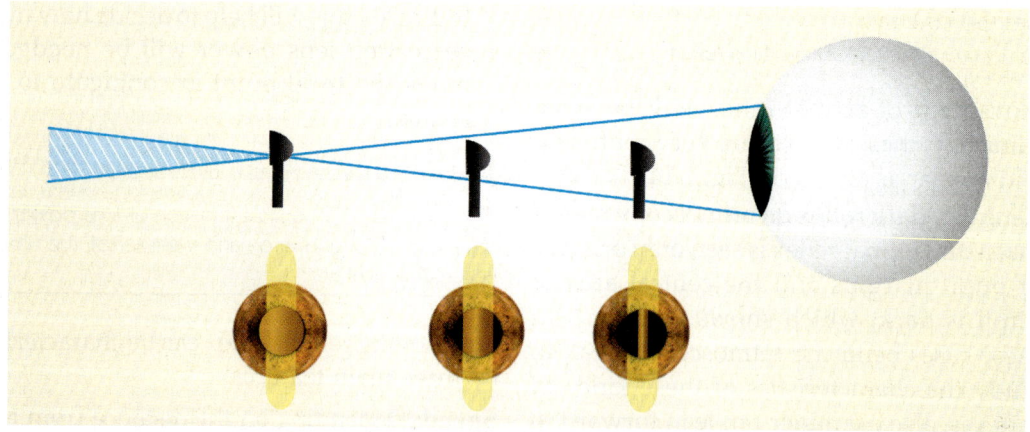

Fig. 2.17: Change in width of retinal reflex with distance of retinoscope

retinoscope is situated very far away from neutrality point then the retinal reflex appears to become widen as if approaching the neutrality as discussed above. This state is termed pseudoneutrality and is commonly seen in very high degree of refractive errors, means when position of the retinoscope is a long way from the focal point.

However, with continuous practice of retinoscopy it becomes easy for examiner to find out the distance of focal point as observer becomes able to judge speed, brilliance and width of retinal reflex simultaneously. For example, when examiner notices enough 'with movement' having vast width and moving slowly, automatically he/she will add a lot of plus lenses to drag the focal point towards retinoscope. On the other hand, if a little 'against' small width and fast moving reflex is seen then he/she will add a little minus lenses to push out the focal point.

Rare Images

Sometimes detection of high refractive errors appears difficult by retinoscopy, however, it is not so difficult. Once the examiner is able to identify the type of error and does retinoscopy after partially correcting them, then these error starts appearing as routine small refractive errors and examiner can easily neutralize these errors as routine reflexes. For example, suppose if an aphakic patient is presented to clinic for retinoscopy. Patient is already wearing a +11 DS power spectacles and still is not able to see clearly. On retinoscopic examination, the retinal reflex seen in this patient is peculiar and it is little difficult to assess the movement or margins of reflex. Simply, add + 8 or +9 D spherical lens in the trial frame (as the patient is aphakic) and again observe the retinal reflex. Now it will be a nice smooth with reflex which can easily be neutralize by adding more plus power lenses gradually.

It is very important to recognize presence of high spheric error because sometimes they may remain unrecognizable due to presence of

- Hazy media disguise: In presence of hazy media, the high degree errors may present either as no reflex or a very dull reflex showing no appreciable movements. When examiner place either a weak plus or weak minus lens and notices that there is no change in the reflex, then probably it is a case of an opaque media. However, when these types of situation are encountered during retinoscopy, then simply add strong plus lenses or minus lenses up to the power of 5.0 to 7.0 D directly. Reassess the retinal reflex whether there is any change in the reflex movement or not. If it is a case of very high error, then definitely a recognizable reflex will be seen after adding of strong lenses.

- Neutrality disguise. These are also called as motionless reflex (pseudoneutrality) which covers the full pupillary area, means mimicking as if observer is approaching the neutrality point (Fig. 2.18). To confirm this type of disguise simply move forward about 15–20 cm and now again assess the movement. If the characteristics of reflex do not

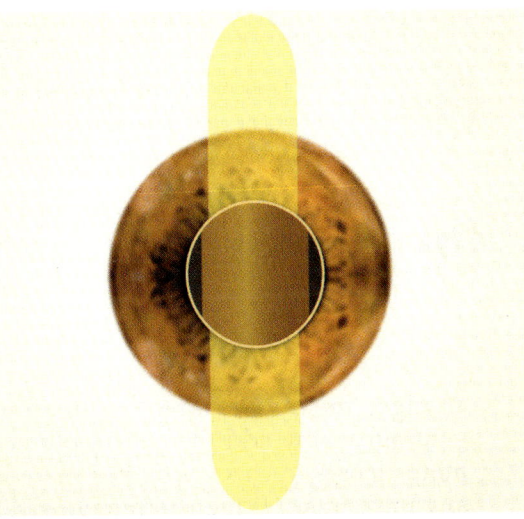

Fig. 2.18: Retinal reflex showing neutrality disguise

Table 2.1: Routine retinal reflexes and their interpretations

Retinal reflex	Characteristics	Interpretation
	Small width fast moving bright with reflex	Emmetropia or Hypermetropia/Myopia (less than 1D)
	Small width fast moving very bright against reflex	Myopia
	Medium width medium speed bright with reflex	Hypermetropia
	Medium width medium speed bright against reflex	Moderate degree myopia
	Large width slow moving dim with reflex	High degree hypermetropia
	Large width slow moving dim against reflex	High degree myopia
	Medium width medium speed dim reflex oblique to retinoscope streak	High degree astigmatism usually regular type
	Very large width no appreciable movement very dim reflex	High degree hypermetropia or myopia/ Aphakia
	Two reflexes moving against each other like blades of scissor one bright with and one dim against reflex	High degree irregular astigmatism, e.g. keratoconus

change, means we are not near to neutrality, now add the strong plus or minus lenses to check whether there is any movement. If high refractive error is present, then there will be a definite reflex movement after adding the strong power lenses.

Various retinal reflexes encountered during regular retinoscopy examination and their interpretation is shown in Table 2.1.

Neutralization of Various Reflexes

Neutralization State

Neutralization state is defined as the state achieved when the focal point of the emerging light lies at the peephole of retinoscope. At this point the movement of reflex is not seen and is called neutral reflex. Trial correcting lens which is applied by the examiner to achieve this state of neutralization is the measurement of error of refraction. Hence, to achieve the state of neutrality the aim of the examiner is to bring the focal point to the peephole of retinoscope while simultaneously remains at the working distance.

Figure 2.19 tells about the approach which should be followed by the examiner to achieve this point of neutralization, while maintaining the working distance. If the examiner with retinoscope is situated in the cone of emerging light (Fig. 2.19) and the focal point is behind the examiner (Fig. 2.19A). Now as the examiner adds the convex lens, the focal point starts moving towards retinoscope and the retinal reflex gradually gets widened (Fig. 2.19B). After adding another plus power lens as the focal point reaches to the peephole of retinoscope, then the retinal reflex will fill the entire pupillary area and no movement can be appreciated. This is called the neutralization state of reflex (Fig. 2.19C).

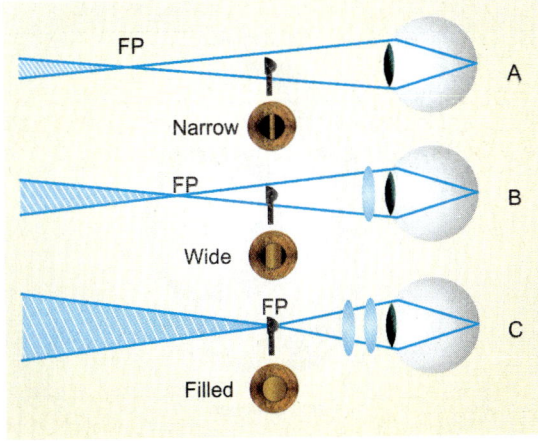

Fig. 2.19: Achieving neutralization state

Note

In case of 'with motion' plus lenses are added; because the focal point lies behind the retinoscope and we need to pull it towards the peephole of retinoscope. On the other hand, in case of 'against motion' minus lenses are added, because the focal point lies in front of the retinoscope and we need to push it towards the peephole of retinoscope.

Although in routine practice of retinoscopy especially for beginners it is difficult to approach the neutralization state from 'against motion'. To simplify this, one can overcorrect 'against motion' by adding extra minus lenses so that the retinal reflex gets converted into 'with motion'. Now this 'with motion' can be neutralized by adding plus (means reducing minus) lenses, in smaller steps, say 0.25 D power. This approach to achieve neutralization is superior and easier as compared to neutrality achieved by gradually increasing the power of minus lenses.

Avoid against movement: Practically while neutralizing any retinal reflex, 'against motion' creates more difficulty than 'with motion' so always try to avoid these against motions.

Study these following reflexes carefully:

As shown in Fig. 2.20B that 'against motion' appears first at the side of pupil opposite to the streak of retinoscope. When streak is moved across the pupil, this reflex moves in a reverse direction across the entire pupil and finally get disappear on the opposite side of the retinoscope streak. Because of this opposite, fast and disappearing property of 'against motion', it is difficult to quantify the three basic characteristics (speed, brilliance and width) of reflex with 'against motion'. For example, speed of the reflex cannot be assessed easily when it moves in a reverse direction. Similarly, as the 'against motion' moves always away from the illuminated retina, its brightness is reduced and hence reflex margins become hazy. Because of these blurry reflex margins, the width of the reflex is also difficult to appreciate clearly.

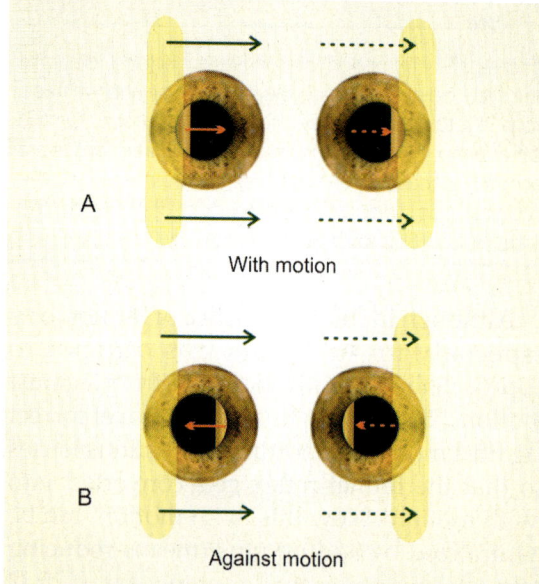

A

With motion

B

Against motion

Fig. 2.20: Reflex movement. Compare retinoscope streak with retinal reflex and notice both types of movements: A. With motion; B. Against motion

Another problem with 'against reflex motion' is that it also poses difficulties during neutralization. The movement of 'against motion' opposite to streak of the retinoscope appears highly irregular especially, near neutrality state. 'Against motion' is usually dull, confusing, difficult to evaluate and measure, hence a general concept is that "when observer is unable to identify the type of reflex, then it is taken for granted that it is against reflex".

On the other hand, as shown in Fig. 2.20A 'with motion' reflex can be identified easily and is more feasible. The 'with reflex' is bright, crispy, rarely confusing and can be assessed without difficulty. A 'with motion' is highly dependable, easily agreeable and never contrary, hence one can quickly learn to recognize its degree, width and speed which helps to neutralize it faster and accurately. Therefore, whenever performing retinoscopy always first recognize 'with movement' if by chance 'against motion' is seen, then immediately convert it into 'with motion' by adding minus lenses.

"Always work with a WITH and against an AGAINST"

Rules to be followed to Achieve Neutralization

Rule 1: Suppose if 'with motion' is observed, then add plus lenses or reduce minus lenses until neutralization is attained.

Rule 2: Suppose if 'against motion' is observed, then add minus lenses or reduce plus lenses until 'with motion' is seen and then follow the rule 1 for neutralization.

Rule 3: For neutralization, always use plane mirror or keep sleeve up at working distance.

In the abovementioned rules the terms add plus (or minus) lenses or reduce minus (plus) lenses have been used. Remember the fact that "adding plus power is the same as that of reducing minus power or vice versa". By doing this basically we are changing the vergence of the emerging light rays which depend on the starting point. This concept can be understood by phenomenon of dioptric continuity which can be elucidated with the help of a lens power wheel (Fig. 2.21) used in a lensometer. Rotation of this wheel in clockwise direction from any point will result in increase of minus power or decrease of plus power, while opposite occurs when rotated in counterclockwise direction, i.e. increase of plus or decrease of minus power. The signs and numbers mentioned on this wheel are irrelevant, only the direction of rotation of wheel has value.

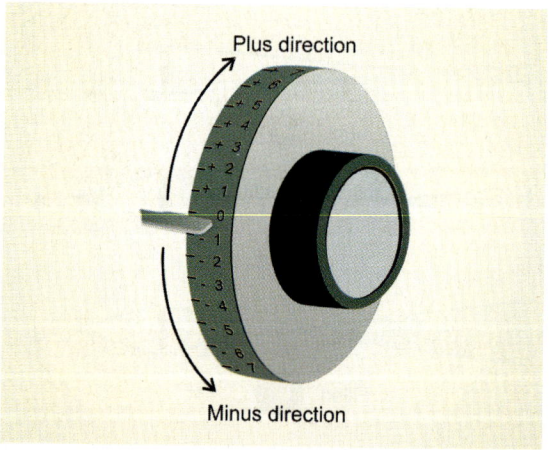

Plus direction

Minus direction

Fig. 2.21: Lens power wheel showing dioptric continuity

Thus, either neutralizing case of myopia or a hypermetropia, the basic principle of neutralization remains the same. In case of 'with motion' the plus power lenses are added to increase the convergence of emitting light rays until there is no movement of reflex. Similarly, in 'against motion' minus power lenses are added to increase the divergence of emitting rays until 'with movement' is seen (then reduce the divergence of rays until neutralization state is reached).

"With motion is key to the neutrality or endpoint of retinoscopy and the power of lens with which it is achieved is the measure of refractive error".

Interpretation of Neutrality

In reality, neutrality is not a point rather it is area or zone created as a result of spherical aberrations and many other factors. Size of this zone varies with the size of pupil and working distance.

Size of pupil: The width of neutral zone is directly proportional to the size of pupil. As the size of pupil increases, the width of this neutral zone also increases. In Fig. 2.22, we can see that there is no pupil in the eye thus the zone of neutrality is magnified due to spherical aberration. Axial rays are focused in nearest focal point (FP1) and peripheral rays on distant focal point (FP2). While doing retinoscopy on a dilated pupil, always concentrate only on the central pupillary reflex and avoid the peripheral aberrations.

Working distance: Width of neutral zone is narrowest when the working distance is closer, however, if the neutral zone is very narrow, then an accurate estimation of retinal reflex and working distance becomes so significant that even a minor inaccuracy may produce a major error in evaluation.

As shown in Fig. 2.23, that there is a significant amount of doubt within the neutral zone. Examiner remains indecisive about the presence or absence of reflex, similarly examiner is unable to assess the movement and position of the reflex within this neutral zone. Easiest way to avoid this confusion and stay in a safe (with) zone is to make a judgment of neutrality just before the doubt of movement begins as shown in Fig. 2.24.

In a nutshell accurate judgment of a neutrality state is a skill and basically it is to judge a point just before the zone of doubt appears, means there is still a weak 'with movement'. At this point when observer leans forward with retinoscope a definite and clear 'with motion' will be seen and if bend backwards then in the beginning an uncertain type of reflex movement and on further leaning backwards a confusing reflex suggestive of an early 'against motion' will be seen.

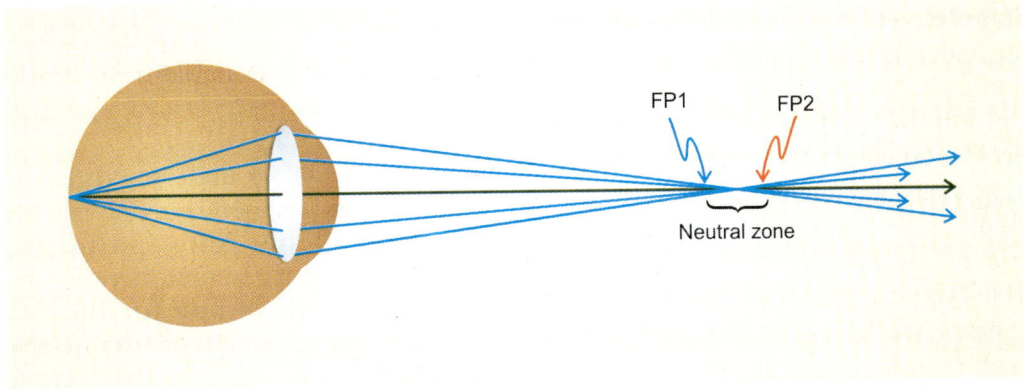

Fig. 2.22: Neutral zone; spherical aberration causes nearer focal point FP1 for axial rays, and a distant focal point FP2 for peripheral rays

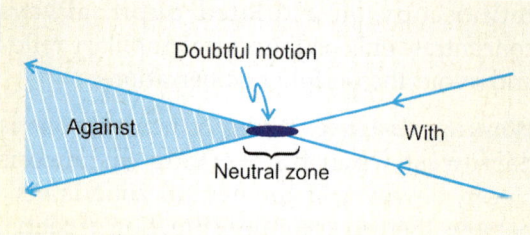

Fig. 2.23: Doubtful motion within neutral zone

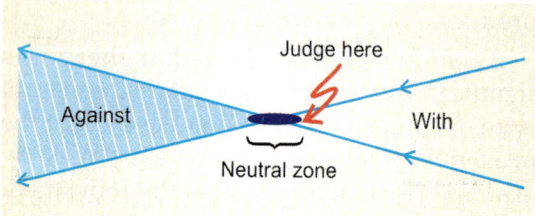

Fig. 2.24: Point of judgment for neutrality

Various Neutralization Methods

Retinal reflex can be neutralized by either only spherical lenses (in cases of spherical and/or astigmatic errors) or by a combination of spherical and cylindrical lenses (in case of astigmatic error).

Neutralizing with Only Spherical Lenses

To understand the neutralization with use of only spherical lenses, consider an example where on retinoscopy at 66 cm 'with motion' at 90° and a larger width slower moving 'with motion' at 180° is seen as shown in Fig. 2.25.

Now place a plus spherical lens (say +4 DS) at the 90° meridian (having lesser 'with motion') to neutralize this meridian. Now, on doing retinoscopy having +4 DS lenses in vertical meridian (90°) no reflex movement is seen, whereas horizontal meridian (180°) will still show 'with motion'. Continue to add plus spheres till this horizontal meridian becomes neutral. Suppose after adding an additional +2 D sphere (above +4 DS) 180° meridian also gets neutralized. These retinoscopy values will be recorded in the form of a retinoscopy cross as shown in Fig. 2.26.

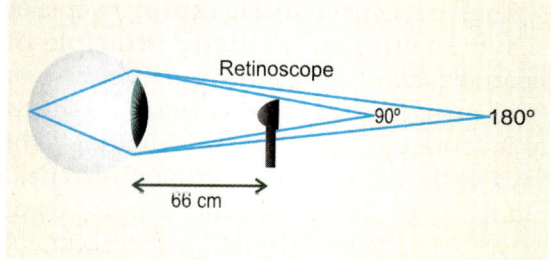

Fig. 2.25: Retinoscopy showing with motion at 90° and more with motion at 180°

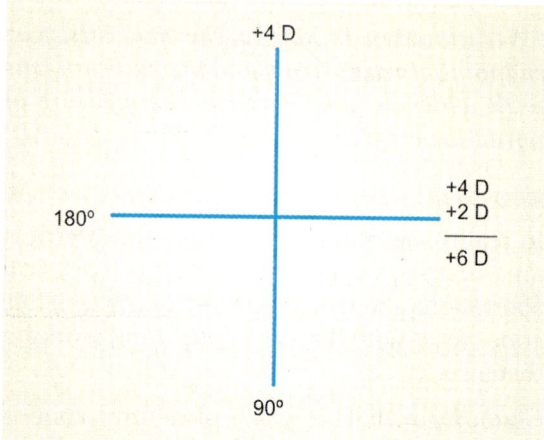

Fig. 2.26: Diagrammatic representation of neutralization with spheres

---

> **Note** _____
>
> Always reduce the working distance from gross sphere in both the meridian spheres.

This can also be represented as gross sphere + 4 Dsph × 90° + 6 Dsph × 180°

Deduction for the working distance (66 cm or +1.5 DS in our example) from this gross refraction will give +2.5 D × 90° +4.5 D × 180° net refraction value.

It is important to understand that when neutralization is done using only spheres, it is necessary to measure and record the spherical value of the first meridian before performing retinoscopy for the second meridian. Hence, in the above example, when 90° meridian is reexamined after completing the neutralization in 180° meridian, this 90° meridian will show 'against motion' because now it is overcorrected by +2 DS. In cases of compound refractive errors when neutralization is done with only spheres both the meridians will not be seen as neutral at the same time.

Neutralization with only spheres is a good technique for children, as they resist wearing trial frame and it is practically very difficult to hold the cylindrical lens on its axis or hold two lenses for a longer duration. A lens rack as shown in Fig. 2.27 is particularly useful while performing this retinoscopy method in clinic or when doing refraction under anesthesia.

Neutralization with Spheres and Cylinders

Consider the same example as discussed above, where 90° meridian gets neutralized with +4D sphere, which is considered as spherical meridian. As per our previous discussion, spherical lenses produce power in all meridians, hence this +4 DS power (in our example) is also working in 180° meridian (which is still having 'with movement'). Add a +2 D cylinder at 180° axis to neutralize this 'with movement'. By adding + 2 D cylinder at 180° axis (horizontal meridian) there is no change in the reflex movement at 90° meridian because cylindrical lenses exert power only in one particular axis. This 180° meridian is considered as cylindrical meridian.

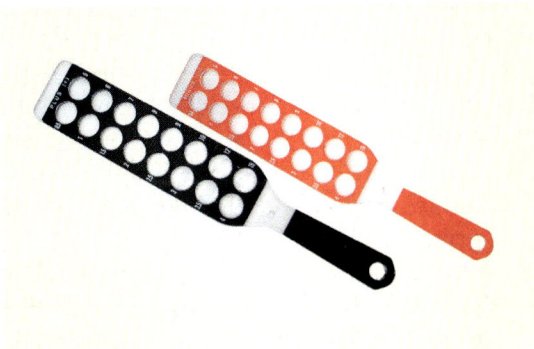

Fig. 2.27: Lens racks. Red color racks have minus lenses and black color has plus lenses. (*courtesy:* Bernell Corporation)

After neutralizing the principal meridians independently when the streak of retinoscope is rotated, both the meridians now appear neutral and show no movement of retinal reflex. This is more accurate method to neutralize compound refractive errors because both the meridians can be seen neutral at the same time.

In our example the gross refraction or lenses in front of eye are +4 DS/+2 DC × 180°.

Always write the spherical power first and then the cylindrical power with axis. As this is the gross refraction deduct the working distance of 66 cm, i.e. +1.5 D from spheres only to get the net refraction +2.5 DS/+2 DC × 180°.

Universally the spherical and cylindrical powers are written in this order hence this net refraction can also be conveniently written as +2.5/+2 × 180° (without any power abbreviations).

> **Note** _____
>
> No correction for working distance or cycloplegic is done from the cylindrical power.

Many readers may get confuse that as cylindrical power works on an axis perpendicular to its position, then why a plus cylinder is added at 180° to neutralize the 'with motion' at the same axis rather it has to be applied at 90° so that cylindrical power will be applicable at 180°. To understand this study the streak meridians and corneal meridians are discussed below.

Streak Meridian versus Corneal Meridian

In reality, the orientation of retinoscopic reflexes does not correspond to corneal meridians. For example, the reflexes seen at 180° or horizontally on retinoscopy in reality are produced by the 90° corneal meridians and vice versa. In other words, retinoscope streak actually tests the power of corresponding corneal meridian. If retinoscope is scooped vertically, i.e. retinoscope streak is at 90° and examiner is moving the retinoscope sideways to judge the movement of reflex, then actually examiner is evaluating the refractive power of the eye at horizontal or 180° corneal meridian. Hence, when a cylinder is placed vertically or at 90°, it is going to neutralize the power of eye at 180°, i.e. perpendicular to the cylinder axis which in reality is the corneal meridian needed to be corrected in this example.

If 90° corneal meridian (say +47 D) has focal point at the peephole of retinoscope, then a neutral reflex will be seen, when the streak is horizontal (testing for 90 meridian). If 180° corneal meridian has only +44 D, so it will show a 3 D with motion when streak is vertical (testing for 180 meridian). Adding +3 DC at 90°, will in reality add power at 180° thus it will neutralize the reflex seen at 90° (Fig. 2.28).

Although it all looks a little confusing, a simple rule to remember is that "simply place a plus cylinder in the same axis where there is with movement". Hence it is very comfortable to neutralize compound refractive errors with a plus cylinder system. Once spherical meridian is neutralized, place the cylindrical axis of trial cylindrical lens on the same axis as that of remaining with reflex axis, this will correct the corneal cylindrical axis properly.

Ocular Meridians

Ocular meridians universally are defined from 1 to 180 degrees in both the eyes as shown in

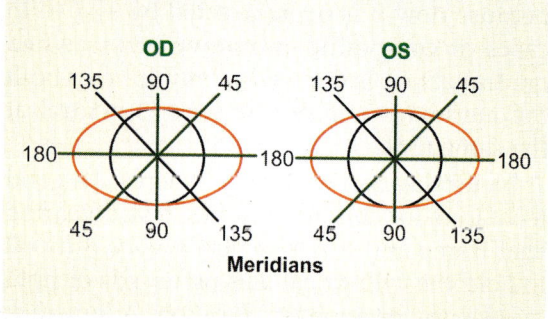

Fig. 2.29: Ocular meridians

Fig. 2.29, there is no meridian labeled as 'zero' and there is nor any angle larger than 180°. Traditionally, right eye is abbreviated as OD (oculus dexter) and left eye as OS (oculus sinister).

Neutralization in Astigmatic Errors

As discussed before astigmatism is a phenomenon when the entire light rays do not refract to a single focal point. In aspheric eye all the ocular meridians refract the light differently because corneal surface is toric in nature. Ocular meridians which refract the light maximum and minimum are called 'Principal meridians'. Each of these principal meridians focuses the arriving light rays to a different point of focus at the back of the eye, which are called principal foci. These principal foci may be in front of the retina, on the retina or behind the retina; but for retinoscopy it is immaterial.

Neutralization of various types of astigmatic errors is done as

- In regular astigmatism the principal meridians are perpendicular or 90° to each other, i.e. 90° and 180° and so on. These can be corrected by cylindrical lenses because they also have their principal meridian perpendicular to each other. For example, if a plus cylinder is placed with its axis in alignment with that of most refracting or stronger meridian, then it will add power to the weaker meridian. Hence, when the correcting cylindrical lens placed in

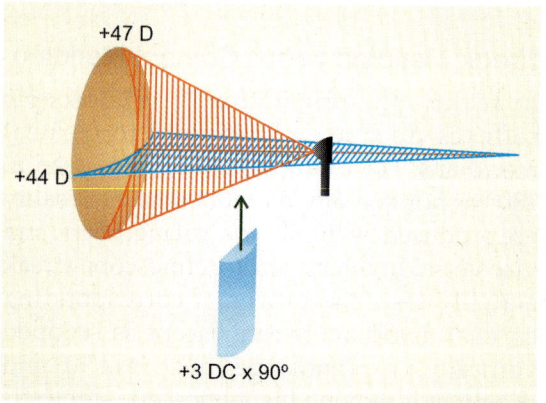

Fig. 2.28: Effect of corneal meridians on emerging rays

proper axis, which equals the corneal cylinder, then the meridians gets balance and astigmatism gets neutralized, as a spherical condition of eye had been created by balancing the corneal cylinder with cylindrical lens power.

- In an irregular astigmatism principal meridians are not perpendicular to each other; hence they cannot be neutralized with cylinders alone. These conditions are usually caused due to corneal irregularities.

- An oblique astigmatism is simply a regular astigmatism, where principal meridians are perpendicular to each other, but are not usual (90°/180°) and it should not be confused with irregular astigmatism. The principal meridians are tilted, for example, at 45°/135°. These can be neutralized with cylinders similar to a regular astigmatism.

- 'With the rule' astigmatism is referred to a condition where correcting plus cylindrical axis is more or less vertical, i.e. between 75° and 105°. 'Against the rule' astigmatism refers to a condition where the correcting plus cylindrical axis is more or less horizontal, i.e. 15° to 165°. These conditions generally describe the location of most refracting corneal meridians and hence the axis of its accompanying plus cylindrical lenses.

- Symmetrical astigmatism is a condition where the total axis of correcting cylinders of both the eyes equals to 180°; means, for example, OD 70° and OS 110°. These can be corrected by cylindrical lenses easily as in regular astigmatism.

- Asymmetrical astigmatism is a condition where the axis of cylinders of both the eyes has no rule, means, for example, OD 75° and OS 25°. These conditions are not abnormal but are rare, hence whenever such conditions are encountered try to reevaluate the retinoscopy.

Simple astigmatism whether it is simple hypermetropic or simple myopic are in fact simple to neutralize because one of the principal meridians is already neutral at working distance and second meridian can easily be neutralized by either plus or minus cylinder.

Figure 2.30 represents example of simple hypermetropic astigmatism where one principal meridian, say 90°, is neutral and other principal meridian, i.e. 180°, is showing 'with motion' at working distance of 66 cm (keeping working lens in the position). We simply need to add a plus cylinder at 180° with gradual increasing in power until with motion gets neutralize.

Figure 2.31 represents an example of simple myopic astigmatism where 180° meridian is

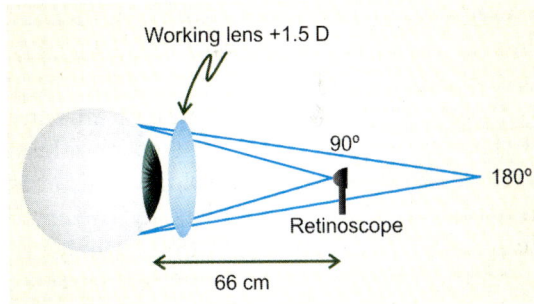

Fig. 2.30: Simple hypermetropic astigmatism

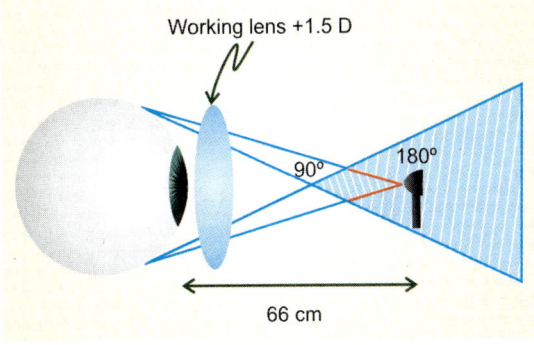

Fig. 2.31: Simple myopic astigmatism

'neutral' and 90° meridian is showing 'against motion' at working distance of 66 cm (keeping working lens in the position). Neutralization in this case is a little complicated, first add minus spheres to push out the focal point of myopic meridian (90°) and neutralize it. This minus sphere has also pushed out the focal point at 180° meridian and converted it into 'with motion' which was initially neutral. Now add plus cylinders at 180° meridian to neutralize this with movement.

Compound astigmatism is a condition where neither meridian is neutral at working distance of 66 cm (keeping working lens in position). This could be of following types

- Compound hypermetropic astigmatism
- Compound myopic astigmatism
- Compound mixed astigmatism

These conditions seem difficult to neutralize, but simply the rules of neutralization are followed to convert these three conditions first into simple hypermetropic astigmatism and then neutralize them accordingly.

Compound hypermetropic astigmatism (Fig. 2.32) can easily be neutralized because both the principal meridians are having a 'with motion' although of different amount. First add plus spheres until the weaker or least with meridian (spherical meridian) becomes neutralized. Now add plus cylinder to neutralize the stronger with meridian (cylindrical meridian). Now rotate the streak of retinoscope in both the directions to confirm that both the meridians are neutral.

In compound myopic astigmatism (Fig. 2.33) both the principal meridians show 'against motion', and it is difficult to assess which meridian is more against or stronger. First add strong minus spheres to push out the focal points beyond retinoscope, this gives a friendly 'with motion' in both the meridians. Now simply proceed as in the case of a compound hypermetropic astigmatism. Slowly reduce the minus spherical powers or add plus spherical powers, until first meridian (more myopic) gets neutralize, add plus cylinders in the opposite meridian (least myopic) to neutralize the remaining 'with motion'.

Mixed astigmatism (Fig. 2.34) is a condition where both 'with and against movement' are seen in different meridians. First add minus spheres until 'against movement' becomes 'with movement', then slowly reduce the minus spherical power or add plus spherical power to neutralize this meridian. Once this is done, then the opposite meridian having

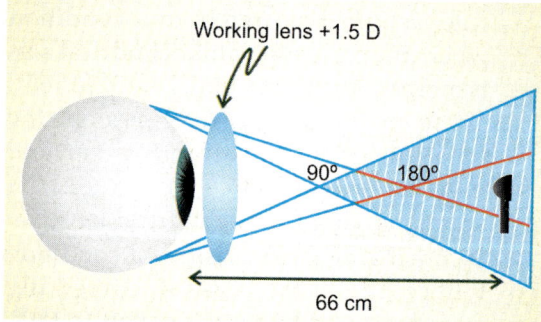

Fig. 2.33: Compound myopic astigmatism

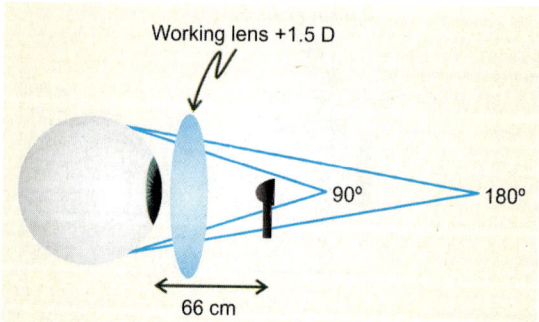

Fig. 2.32: Compound hypermetropic astigmatism

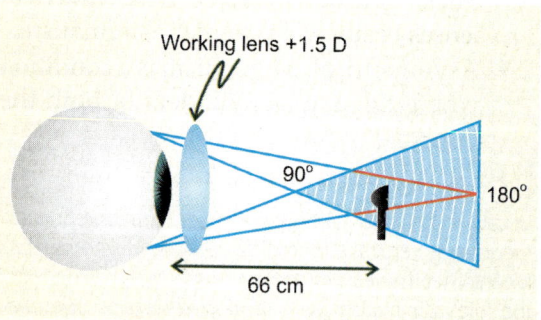

Fig. 2.34: Mixed astigmatism

'with movement' can easily be neutralize by using plus cylinders.

To summarise the principles of neutralization

- First neutralize the least hypermetropic or most myopic meridian with appropriate spheres, means first neutralize the meridian having focal point closer to patient's eye.
- Now neutralize remaining most hypermetropic or least myopic meridian by using plus cylinders, because this meridian will always show 'with movement' means fill the remaining astigmatic interval by using plus cylinders in the opposite meridian which has a focal point farthest from patient's eye.

 Note

However, in these illustrations the actual amount of refractive error is not mentioned, because while performing the retinoscopy amount of refractive error is immaterial. Simply neutralize the reflexes in all the meridians and get the gross refraction, then deduct the values of working distance and cycloplegic (if used) from gross refraction and one can get the actual amount of refractive error.

Estimation of Cylindrical Axis and Power

Estimation of Cylindrical Axis

To understand the direction of cylindrical axis four properties of retinal reflexes are needed to be studied such as

- Break
- Width
- Intensity
- Skew

To follow these properties understanding of the enhancement phenomenon of retinal reflex is important. The position or height of the retinoscope sleeve at which the fundus reflex seen is brightest, sharpest and narrowest is called enhancement position. Usually small cylindrical powers are seen well when retinoscope sleeve is up, i.e. plane mirror

effect. On the other hand, large cylindrical powers are best enhanced when sleeve is down, i.e. concave mirror effect.

Image of retinoscope streak on the surface of eye is called intercept. In low cylindrical powers the retinal reflex is narrowest when intercept is wide, while in high cylindrical powers the reflex is narrowest when intercept is narrow as shown in Fig. 2.35.

Break: When retinoscopy streak is off axis, i.e. not on the correct astigmatic axis (XX' in our example), then a break is seen. Here, intercept and streak are not parallel, hence a broken line is formed which can easily be observed by rotating the retinoscopy streak on either sides of astigmatic fundus reflex as shown in Fig. 2.36A.

This break will disappear when intercept and retinal reflex become parallel, means retinoscope streak is on the correct astigmatic axis, i.e. on XX' axis (at 90° in our example) in Fig. 2.36B. We will place the correcting cylindrical lens on this axis for neutralization in trial fame. To practice, adjust the retinoscopy sleeve at enhancement position and rotate the sleeve about 15° on either side of XX' axis, i.e. at 75° and 105°. A break which will be more clear at the extremes of this arc

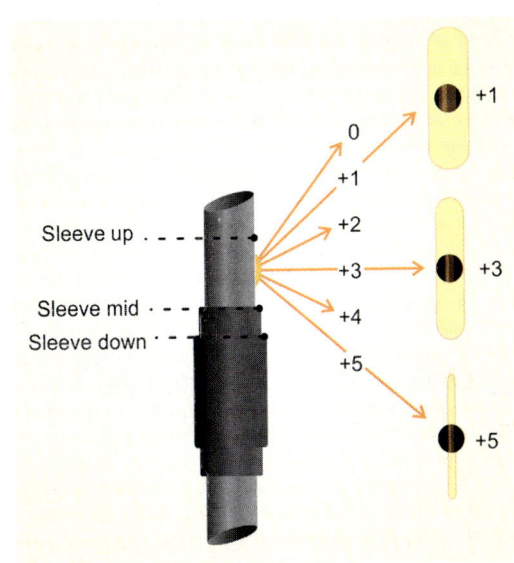

Fig. 2.35: Enhancement and midpoint position

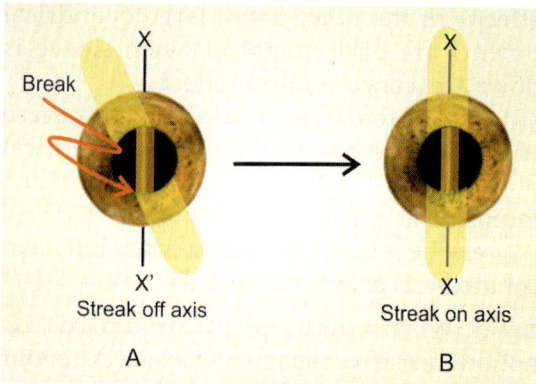

Fig. 2.36: Phenomenon of break

(i.e. 75° and 105°) will be seen and it will be less appreciable when examiner approaches near XX′ axis, i.e. 90°; and no break in intercept will be seen exactly at 90°.

Thickness: Thickness of retinal reflex modifies when examiner rotates the streak on either sides of the correct astigmatic axis. The reflex is narrowest when the streak of retinoscope is on the correct axis and becomes wide as it moves away from the correct axis. For example, if astigmatic axis is 115° (XX in Fig. 2.37), then the width of retinal reflex will change as retinoscope move on either sides of correct axis or will be narrowest at correct axis.

> **Note**
>
> To practice retinoscopy, enhance the retinal reflex and rotate the streak on either side of 115° (in our example for correct astigmatic axis) observe the change in width of retinal reflex.

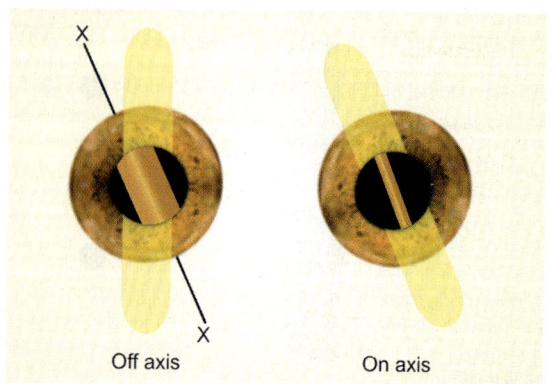

Fig. 2.37: Change in thickness of reflex

Intensity: Retinal reflex intensity varies to some extent when examiner rotates the streak off-axis and it will become very bright when on the correct astigmatic axis. Although, this observation is indistinct and is useful in patients having low degree astigmatism, because small cylinders cannot be enhanced, whereas larger cylinders can be enhanced to high brightness.

Skew: Skew is also called oblique motion and is used to refine the cylindrical axis in small power cylinders. In this case examiner does not rotate the retinoscope streak rather moves his/her head or wiggle the retinoscope streak in a 30° zone. Notice the movement of retinal reflex in comparison of intercept. Retinal reflex will move parallel to intercept if streak is on the correct axis and when the streak is off axis, the retinal reflex and intercept will move in different directions.

As shown in Fig. 2.38, consider that the correct axis of astigmatism is XX (90°), but retinoscope streak is at somewhere X′X′ (say 110°). Now when examiner moves his/her head 'against motion' of retinal reflex in comparison to retinoscope intercept will be seen. This movement of retinal reflex in comparison to movement of intercept is called as skewed motion.

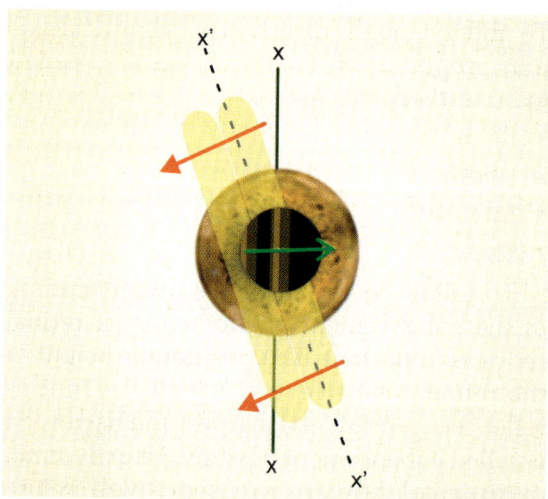

Fig. 2.38: Skewed motion

> **Note** _____
>
> All these four characteristics help in determination of correct cylindrical axis. Break and thickness of retinal reflex help in high degree astigmatic errors, whereas intensity and skew motion help in low degree astigmatic errors.

> **Note** _____
>
> Once a rough estimate of amount of cylindrical power is obtained, then astigmatic errors can be neutralized with routine technique with keeping sleeve up. "An accurate location of cylindrical axis cannot be achieved with an incorrect cylindrical power; an accurate cylindrical power cannot be achieved with an incorrect cylindrical axis".

Estimation of Cylindrical Power

As discussed before, gradually widening of pupillary reflex indicates that the point of neutralization is approaching. To estimate the cylindrical power, first neutralization of spherical power is done and then the width of retinal reflex in the astigmatic axis will give a rough estimate of the amount of astigmatism and hence the power of cylinder requires for neutralizing. As a general rule width of astigmatic reflex is inversely proportional to degree of astigmatism; i.e. thinner the astigmatic reflex, larger will be the degree of astigmatism.

Low degree astigmatism cannot be enhanced, hence width of retinal reflex in astigmatic axis gives an estimate of amount of cylindrical power require to neutralize it. Whereas high degree astigmatic errors can be enhanced, hence width of retinal reflex shows a gradual narrowing along with decrease width of intercept (Fig. 2.39). In these cases the width of intercept required to enhance the retinal reflex gives an estimate of amount of cylinder which is required to neutralize the reflex.

Refining Cylindrical Axis and Power

Refining Cylindrical Axis

The method used to refine the cylindrical axis is called straddling. In this technique the correcting cylinder is placed in the axis obtained by neutralization methods as discussed above. Straddling meridians are situated at 45° away on either sides of the astigmatic axis at which the examiner had placed the correcting cylinders and needs to be compared at sleeve up position. For example, if correct axis of astigmatism is at 90° and examiner had placed the correcting cylindrical lens axis at 100°, then the straddling meridians will be 55° and 145° as shown in Fig. 2.40.

Refining Method

- Place the entire correction of cylindrical power in the position and perform retinoscopy while comparing the width of retinal reflexes in each straddling meridian.

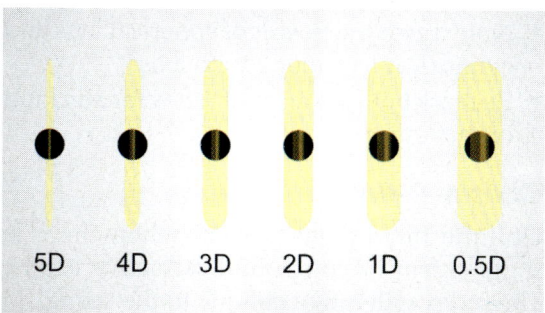

Fig. 2.39: Narrowing of retinal reflex width with decreasing intercept width in cases of high cylindrical power

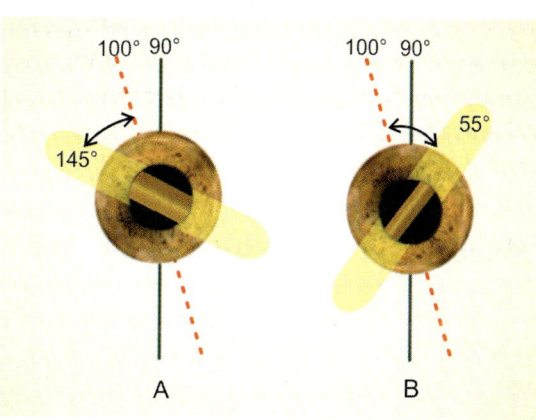

Fig. 2.40: Straddling meridians and respective retinal reflex width

- Slowly move back to about 10 cm distance keeping retinoscope in the position and again compare the width of retinal reflexes in straddling meridians by rotating the sleeve.
- Repeat this procedure by moving back at 10 cm steps till there is widening or neutralization in one of either straddling meridians is seen.
- Note that whether widening is in 55° or 145° axis. Because there is difference in width of reflex at the same distance, it means there is an axis error.
- In our example as shown in Fig. 2.40 widening of reflex is occurring at 145° axis and retinal reflex remains narrow at 55° meridian, then this 55° axis is called guide. Now to correct the axis error, turn the correcting plus cylinder axis towards 55° (initially in 5° steps) means make 100° as 95°.
- Again check the straddling meridians and see if there is any axis error or not.
- If still there is an axis error, then slowly turn the correcting plus cylinder axis towards the narrow reflex axis (guide) in 2° steps (means from 95° to 93°) and so on till there is no difference in width of reflexes.

Refining Cylindrical Power

As a rule an incorrect cylindrical axis will not give a correct cylindrical power and vice versa, hence by rule first refine the cylindrical axis by straddling method and then before refine the cylindrical power. Once axis is refined the power of cylinders can easily be refined by comparing the neutralization state in principal meridians. First neutralize the spherical meridian and then refine the correcting cylinder at the refined cylindrical axis.

Neutralization of Rare Refractive Errors

Scissor Reflex

Scissor movement will be considered when retinal reflex has two arms joined one side (usually nasally) and open on other side (usually temporally). These two arms move in opposite directions to each other when

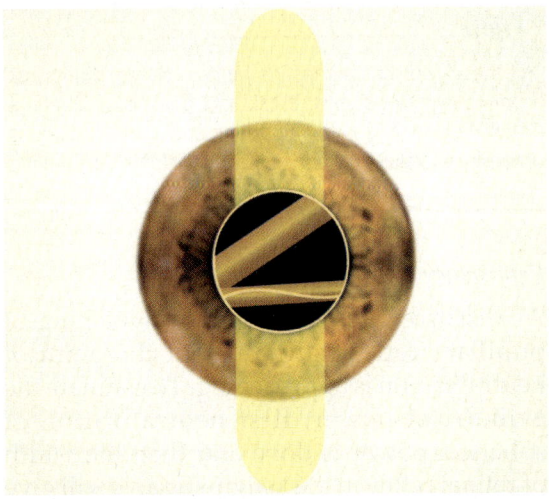

Fig. 2.41: Scissor reflex

examiner moves retinoscope streak in either vertical or horizontal meridians.

- To neutralize this scissor reflex as shown in Fig. 2.41, first see which arm is moving in 'with direction'.
- Then neutralize the movement of the arm which is moving in 'with motion' of scope by using plus spherical power lenses.
- Now focus on the remaining arm and observe its movement, whether it moves 'with or against' the scope and what is the meridian.
- If 'with movement' is seen then add plus cylinder in the meridian where motion is seen till there is no movement of reflex is observed.
- If 'against movement' is seen, then add minus cylinder in that particular meridian of motion till there is no movement of reflex is noticed.
- Note down the power of spherical lens and cylindrical lens along with axis.
- Recheck both the arms of reflex for any kind of movement.

Oblique Reflex

Oblique movement is seen when there is astigmatism or compound refractive errors. The reflex will move oblique to the scope.

- To neutralize this oblique retinal reflex (Fig. 2.42) change the direction of retinoscope

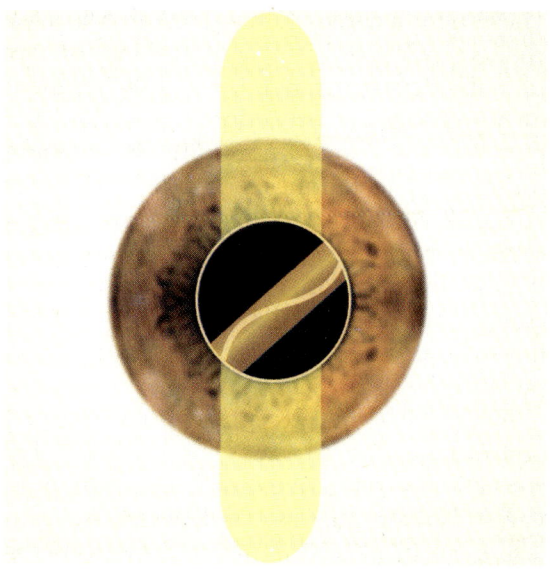

Fig. 2.42: Oblique retinal reflex

intercept parallel to the oblique meridian in which the retinal reflex is moving.

- Notice the movement of retinal reflex with retinoscope movement.
- If movement of reflex is 'with' streak, then add plus cylinder in that particular meridian, till no movement of reflex is seen.
- If movement of retinal reflex is 'against' the retinoscope streak, then add minus cylinder in the same meridian till no further movement of reflex is noticed.
- Sometimes when we scope horizontally the reflex movement is 'with' and in vertical meridian the movement becomes oblique. In these cases first neutralize the horizontal meridian by plus spheres and change the scope parallel to other meridian and see whether 'with or against' movement. If see 'with motion' in oblique meridian, then add plus cylinders and if 'against motion', then add minus cylinders to neutralize this remaining oblique retinal reflex.
- Note the spherical and cylindrical power of lenses with axis.
- Recheck all meridians whether there is any residual movement present or not.

No Reflex

No reflex or very slow or dim reflex (Fig. 2.43) is seen when very high refractive powers are present. Always try to see the margins of this kind of reflexes, and if seen try to notice the movement of reflex with streak whether 'with' or 'against'.

- Suppose slow 'with motion' is seen, then add high plus spherical power lenses (say + 6 D) and again see the movement of reflex. Usually the retinal reflex becomes clearer, thinner and its movement can be appreciated, if it is a case of high hypermetropia or aphakia.
- Suppose very dim retinal reflex is present and no margins are seen, then try high minus spherical power lens (say–6D) and again see the movement.
  - If slow movement seen but not a clear 'with motion', then add more minus spherical power lenses, till movement becomes clearer and crisper with motion.
  - Now add small power plus spherical lenses to neutralize this clearer 'with movement'.
  - Check other meridian and suppose 'with motion' is seen, then add plus cylinder in that particular meridian or if 'against motion' is seen, then add minus cylinder lenses till this movement is neutralized.

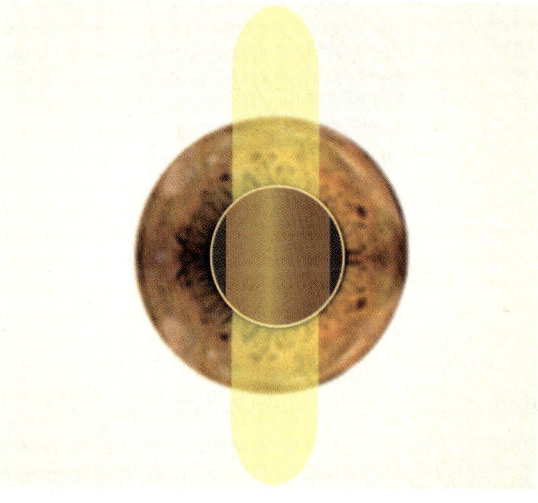

Fig. 2.43: No reflex or very slow or dim retinal reflex

Centrally Dark Reflex

Centrally dark reflex (Fig. 2.44) is seen in media opacity cases like cataract or corneal opacities. Always dilate these patients for retinoscopy, because it is very difficult to appreciate any kind of reflex centrally, however, after dilatation one can see some peripheral retinal reflexes.

- Try to see the sides of reflex motion, which is seen on the periphery of reflex and notice the movement.
- Suppose if 'with motion' is seen in periphery, add plus spherical power lenses and if 'against motion' (rarely appreciable) is seen, add minus spherical power lenses.
- Neutralize all meridians by rotating scope in vertical, horizontal and other meridians by basic principal of neutralization.
- Note the power of neutralizing lenses and recheck the movement.

Note

In majority of these cases even after dilatation, retinoscopy is not easy and results are variable even in an expert's hand.

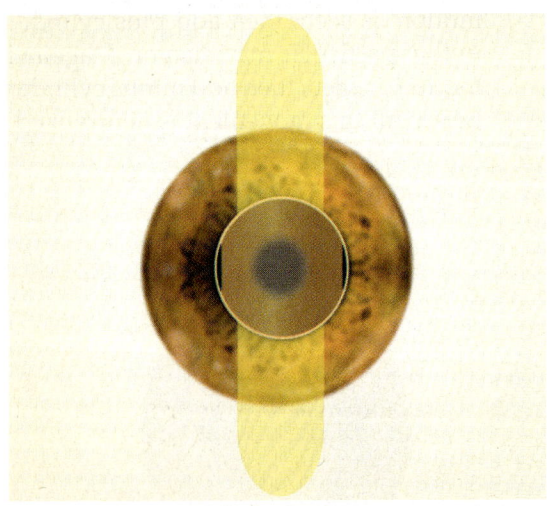

Fig. 2.44: Centrally dark retinal reflex

Retinoscopy after Refractive Surgery

Retinoscopy method remained constant since day of its origin, however; important advances have been achieved in refractive surgery field.

These new techniques have resulted in new challenges by producing various kinds of new retinal reflexes postoperatively. Development of newer corneal procedures generated the possible need to re-evaluate the routine retinoscopy techniques. Many a times, after corneal refractive surgery, ambiguous retinoscopic reflexes are seen depending on the patient selection, type of procedure, and complications arising after surgery (radial keratotomy, photorefractive keratotomy, penetrating keratoplasty, etc.)

Nowadays, LASIK surgery is the most commonly performed procedure for correction of refractive errors. Depending on various factors like use of different types of lasers, surgical techniques and instruments and patient's cornea, LASIK surgery can produce its own set of unique reflexes.

The optical zone of cornea (laser treated area) may differ in the geographic location and size. Moreover, the position of optical zone may not align with the visual axis of eyes. Due to all these variations, a number of possible reflexes may be seen in postoperative period. In early postoperative period (say first week) all these variables vary in nature. Continuous change of variables gives challenges to ophthalmologist and makes their job much more exciting as well as frustrating.

Refraction in post-LASIK patients is mainly discussed, however, these principles can be applied on other refractive surgery also done on the cornea.

- Usually in first few days after procedure, the good retinoscopic reflex of any type is not seen and also no directional indications are seen.
- Moving the retinoscope forward or backward will give no result, however, sometimes examiner may see two or three distinct areas of retinal reflexes. Out of these reflexes which one to be used for neutralization will be a dilemma for the examiner.
- By experience one will know that whenever in doubt always concentrate on the

reflex in the center of the pupil; a principal specifically used after corneal surgery.

- When central reflex is identified and point of neutralization is reached in the center of pupil, examiner may get confused by seeing 'with or against' reflexes in the surrounding cornea.
- Make sure to concentrate on the point of neutralization or neutrality reflex in the pupillary center because if examiner over refract this point an odd reflex will be seen which differs from "scissors" movement.
- This odd reflex becomes wider in one meridian and becomes narrower in the other meridian; and to some observers will appear as a "Guillotine effect".
- Hence observe very carefully in the center and judge neutrality when central retinal reflex is still having a little 'with motion'.

Rarely, surface reflections or glare from the flat treated cornea may interfere in the interpretation of fundus reflex and produces difficulty in assessing the type of reflex. When this becomes problematic, just move the streak of retinoscope to sideways. This method will decentre the retinal reflections from the centre of pupil as shown in Fig. 2.45.

First post-operative month after LASIK appears to be most challenging and it is better to wait till this situation subsides because as the corneal edema disappears, the retinal

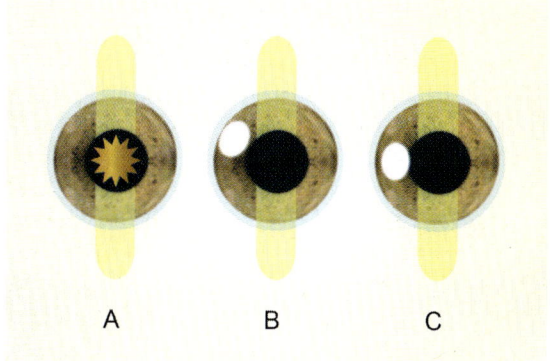

Fig. 2.45: Refractor reflections (A) Glare seen when centered on axis. (B) High reflex on lens indicates that too high. (C) Ideal situation in which reflex is beside pupil

> **Note**
>
> Sometimes dim reflex can be neutralized by starting with addition of high plus spherical lenses, especially in cases where adding quite high power minus spherical lenses are unable to produce a clearer with motion.

reflexes become sharper and one can easily interpret them.

Summary of Retinoscopy

Any type of refractive error can be neutralized via these six cardinal steps of neutralization.

Step 1: Use spheres
- Keep sleeve of retinoscope in up position, i.e. plane mirror effect, and observe reflexes in all the meridians to find 'with motion'.
- Then place appropriate power spheres to get 'with motion' in all meridians at your working distance.
- Now neutralize the spherical meridian or meridians (first, weakest or least with motion) by adding plus spheres or reducing minus spheres.

Step 2: Estimation of cylindrical axis and power
- Observe the remaining with meridian by making retinoscope sleeve down, which causes enhancement:
  - If no enhancement of reflex means cylindrical power is low, i.e. less than 1 D
  - If enhancement of reflex seen means cylindrical power is high, i.e. more than 1 D, means need to see the width of intercept to estimate the cylindrical power.
- With sleeve position either up or down (showing enhancement of reflex) observe the four axis characteristics as
  - Break
  - Thickness in high cylindrical powers
  - Intensity
  - Skew in low cylindrical powers
- Pin point the axis on the trial frame marking by moving sleeve down for enhancing the retinal reflex.

Step 3: Place cylinder on axis

An estimated power cylinder is placed at an approximate axis (the remaining with meridian).

Step 4: Refining of cylindrical axis

Cylindrical axis is refined by straddling method, i.e. move the sleeve up and then lean forward, now gradually recede in straddling meridians. Turn the cylindrical axis as per guidelines.

Step 5: Refining cylindrical power

Move the retinoscope sleeve in up position and lean forward; now recede gradually comparing the reflex in principal meridians. Gradually adjust the plus cylindrical powers until these meridians appear equally filled at same distance.

Step 6: Refine spheres

Check the working distance and gradually adjust the spherical powers (if needed) to get neutralization at 66 cm distance.

 Note

Once the retinal reflexes are neutralized, a subjective verification of retinoscopy findings are necessary and a subjective refraction is performed.

Objective and Subjective Refraction

OBJECTIVE REFRACTION

With this enormous theoretical knowledge of retinoscopy one can start retinoscopy on the patient practically as follows

- A fixation target is presented to the patient and a trial frame is placed, keeping both the eyes open.
- Advice the patient to fixate on the target with his/her right eye, while examiner scope the left eye of patient as shown in Fig. 3.1A.
- Study the reflexes and make them 'with motion'.
- Neutralize the retinal reflexes by using six cardinal steps.
- Now scope the right eye while patient is fixating the target with his/her left eye as shown in Fig. 3.1B.
- Repeat the same procedure to neutralize, as in right eye.
- Note the gross retinoscopy values in both the meridians.

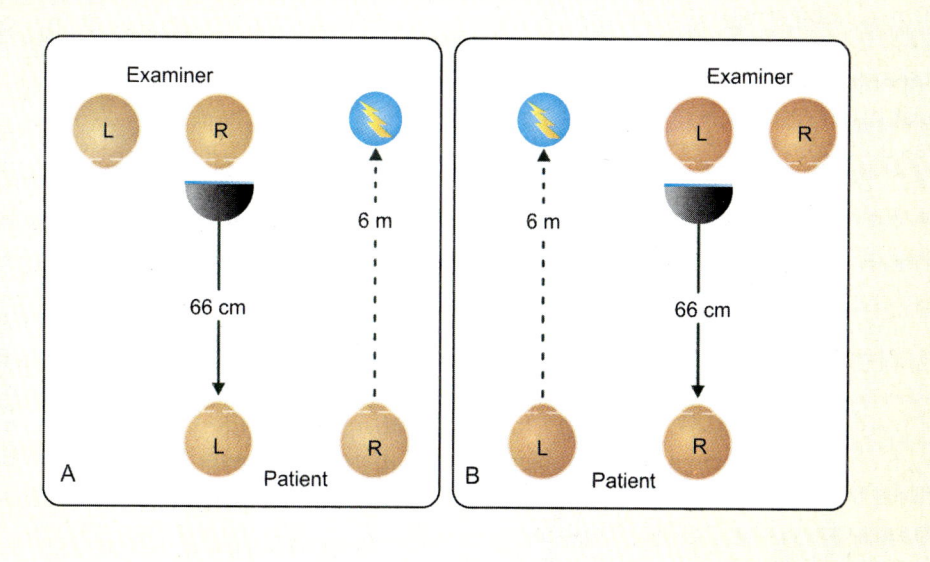

Fig. 3.1: Retinoscopy method: A. For patient's left eye; B. For patient's right eye

SUBJECTIVE REFRACTION

Once an estimate of refractive error is obtained by objective retinoscopy as described above, a subjective verification is done. This is less time consuming and not very cumbersome, however, when objective refraction is impossible in conditions like media opacities or dense hazy media, examiners are dependent only on this subjective refraction for improvement in visual acuity.

Here, the patient is asked that which lens help him/her to see the visual acuity chart best. In subjective refraction, more complex phenomenon involved like quality of retinal image, photoreceptors integrity, visual pathway up to hindbrain and lastly the occipital cortex response. All these factors decide the response of the patient about the better visualization of the target. Along with these factors intelligence, emotions, and fatigues of patient will also influence the test result. Hence in young children and incoherent patients it is difficult to perform a subjective refraction so in these cases glasses are prescribed only on the basis of objective retinoscopy values.

If a cycloplegic drug had been used to perform retinoscopy, then post-mydriatic test (PMT) or a subjective refraction should be done after some interval, e.g. if homatropine or cyclopentolate has been used for refraction, then post-mydriatic test is done 4–5 days later, whereas if atropine has been used, then PMT is done 2–3 weeks later.

Subjective refraction is performed on the following guidelines
- Adjustment of refraction
- Refinement of refraction
- Binocular balancing

Adjustment of Refraction

Although one can perform a totally subjective refraction but it is always better to do an objective refraction prior to subjective refraction which not only saves the time but also gives an idea where to start.

Patient is made to sit at six meters distance from Snellen's chart and a trial frame is placed, visual acuity of both the eyes is tested separately and noted. Place the lenses of power obtained from objective refraction in front of the each eye accordingly. Now a subjective verification and adjustment of spherical and cylindrical lenses can be done by either of two techniques
- Trial and error technique
- Fogging or astigmatic dial technique

Trial and Error Technique

Different spherical and cylindrical lenses are tried to get the best corrected visual acuity as follows.

Spherical Lenses
- Spherical lenses are adjusted first and the patient is asked that with the help of which lens he/she is able to see clearly and comfortably. Strongest plus lens and weakest minus lens which provides the best corrected visual acuity is noted in case of a hypermetrope and myope, respectively.
- In myopic patients record the power of that weakest minus lens which makes the letters of Snellen's chart clear not that one which make them darker and smaller.

Cylindrical Lenses

Cylinders need adjustment both in terms of axis and power and by the rule axis must be adjusted first followed by the power.
- *Axis verification:* Simply rotate the axis of cylinder at a step of 5° in either direction and ask the patient whether visual acuity improves or detoriate. Although, with small cylindrical powers patient may not be able to appreciate the difference in visual acuity, then high power cylinders can be used to verify the axis.
- *Cylindrical power verification:* Once axis is confirmed power of cylinder can be adjusted simply by changing the cylindrical

lenses of various powers in the trial frame and asking patient at every step about the improvement in clarity of visual acuity.

Fogging or Astigmatic Dials Technique

Astigmatic dial is a chart having radial lines drawn at 30 degree intervals. Before starting test it is necessary to make the patient artificially myopic (fogged) by adding a plus (convex) sphere (+0.50 D) before the eye so that all meridians are focused in front of the retina, thus the fogging of the eye eliminates the natural accommodation response and artificially increases blurring of vision as naturally seen in myopia.

Test Method

- The spherical powers are placed in front of test eye (e.g. right eye) and the other eye is occluded, i.e. to obtain a state of compound myopic astigmatism the right eye is fogged by placing sufficient plus spheres in front of it in the trial frame. This brings forward all hyperopic meridians, i.e. simple, compound or mixed to get focused in front of the retina as shown in Fig. 3.2.
- Because of fogging the accommodation will blur the lines more than normal, hence patient tries to relax his/her accommodation to prevent the further blurring of lines. In Fig. 3.2 vertical line (V) on dial (appearing darkest), is focusing in front of the horizontal line (H) on dial (appearing broken) inside the eye.

- After fogging the eye, now patient is instructed to look at the astigmatic dial. He/she is asked to identify the darkest and sharpest line (V) seen on the dial say at 6–12 o' clock position or at 90° axis in our example as seen in Fig. 3.3.
- Once patient identifies the axis showing darkest line, i.e. 90° (V) in our example, now gradually add increasing power minus cylinders at an axis perpendicular to it (i.e. 180° in our example) till all the lines appear equally dark or blur to the patient as shown in Fig. 3.4.
- As shown in Fig. 3.4, addition of minus cylinder moves the vertical focal line (V) to a backward position where horizontal line (H) is present, hence the interval of Strum's conoid collapsed and a focal line becomes a point focus (C).
- To calculate the axis of correcting minus cylinder a 'rule of 30' can be applied. Multiply 30 to the lower number of clock hour showing the darkest line, i.e. 6–12 o'

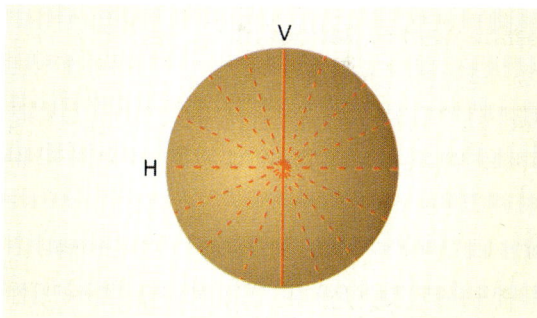

Fig. 3.3: Astigmatic dial showing darkest line V

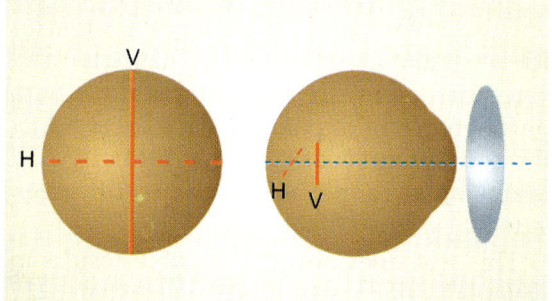

Fig. 3.2: State of compound myopic astigmatism induced by high plus spherical lens

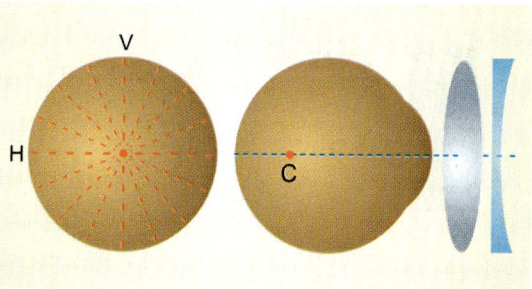

Fig. 3.4: Addition of minus cylinder focuses both line V and H at point C

clock in our example. Hence in our example the axis of minus cylinder is 6 × 30 = 180°. If darkest line is at 3–9 o' clock position, then minus cylinders will be applied at 3 × 30 = 90° axis. Similarly if this darkest line is seen between one clock hour, say 2 and 3 o' clock; then to get axis of minus cylinder, multiplication is done with lower number plus half, i.e. 2.5 × 30 = 75°.

- Now all the lines on astigmatic dial appear equally dark but none of them are clearly focused, because of the fogging of the eye.
- Change the fixation of patient to a Snellen's chart and gradually reduce the plus spherical power either by removing the plus or adding minus spheres until patient is able to read the chart clearly (Fig. 3.5).

> **Note**
>
> After performing a subjective verification of refraction either by trial and error method or by fogging or astigmatic dial method; always refine the refraction subjectively. Like retinoscopy first refine the spheres and then cylindrical axis and power.

Refinement of Refraction

Refining Spheres

Snellen's distance vision chart is used to refine the spherical powers along with help of Duo chrome test and/or pinhole test.

Snellen's Chart for Refining of Spheres

- Simple method to refine the spherical power is that once the cylindrical axis and

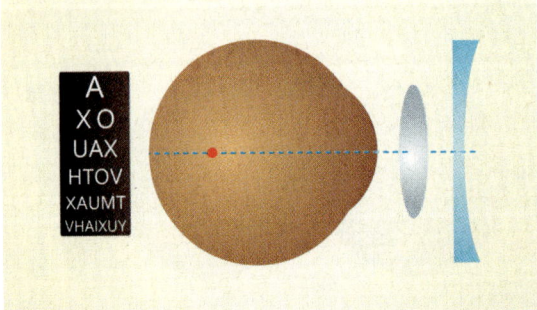

Fig. 3.5: Final adjustments done in astigmatic dial technique

power had been established by fogging method, then gradually defog by decreasing the spherical power at steps of 0.25 D and ask the patient to read the Snellen's chart after every step.

- Once patient reads 6/6 line comfortably, stop the changing of spherical power, however, near the end point there may be some confusion because patient will comfortably read at certain point even if examiner defog for another 0.25 D power.
- Accurate assessment of end point is a little difficult because patient may not be able to read 6/5 line with increasing or decreasing spherical power to 0.25 D range, this can best be assessed by help of duo chrome test.

Duo Chrome Test

Principle: Basic principle of test depends on the phenomenon of chromatic aberration. When a target of letters having red and green background are presented to an emmetropic person then he/she sees these letters equally sharp and bright because green light rays focuses slight anteriorly to the retina, whereas red light rays focuses slight posteriorly to the retina (wavelength of green light is shorter than red light thus green light waves are refracted more than red light waves).

For example, if during subjective refraction more minus power lenses are added, then patient will see the green portion clearer (Fig. 3.6A) while if too much plus power lenses are added then patient will see red letters more clear as shown in Fig. 3.6B.

This test is simple and reproducible, but the only disadvantage is that it does not relaxes the accommodation of patient, hence to relax accommodation slight fogging is done with plus spheres until patient is able to see only the red letters clearly. Now gradually add minus spheres in a 0.25 D steps, till green letters also becomes clearer.

This test does not give reliable results in patients having visual acuity worse than 6/12 because a difference of more than 0.5 D power gives difficulty in distinguishing the letters.

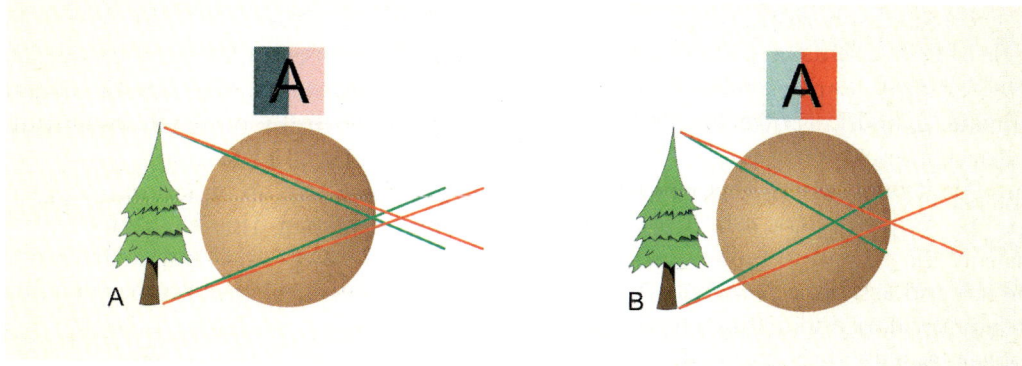

Fig. 3.6: Duo chrome test. A. Too much minus power green is clearer; B. Too much plus power red is clearer

Pinhole Test

Accuracy of optical power correction is confirmed by pinhole testing (Fig. 3.7).

Test method: After placing the entire optical correction in the trial frame the patient is instructed to look through the pinhole, if he/ she reports no improvement in the visual acuity, it means the total correction given is correct.

Suppose if, the patient reports further improvement in the visual acuity with pinhole, then it means that total correction given is incorrect. So reconsider the refraction and try to improve the optical correction till the patient gives no improvement with pinhole testing.

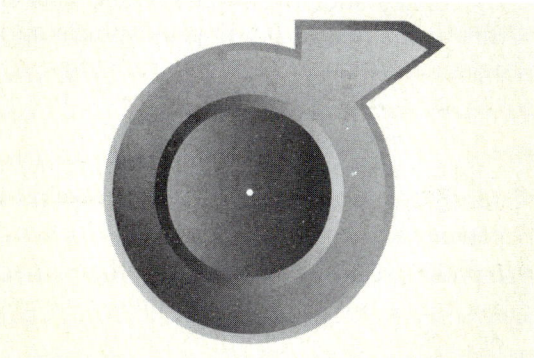

Fig. 3.7: Pinhole

Refining the Cylinders

Most common employed methods to refine the cylinders are

• Astigmatic fan and block method
• Jackson's cross cylinder method

Astigmatic Fan and Block Method

This is an old method to assess the axis of astigmatic error and is also called Maddox V test. This consists of two components; a fan and a block. Fan is nothing but a series of 100 angled radiating lines appears as the rays from a rising sun. Whereas block is a centrally placed panel having a letter 'V' along with two sets of mutually perpendicular lines. For testing

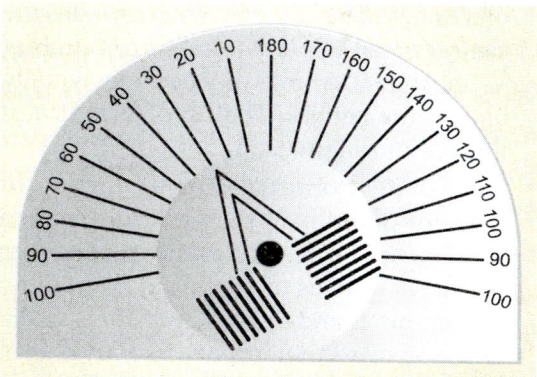

Fig. 3.8: Astigmatic fan

purposes this central panel having V and block lines can be rotated up to 100° on either side against the dialing fan (Fig. 3.8).

Test procedure

• Best corrected visual acuity is obtained by using only spheres; considering the fact that best corrected spherical powers brings the circle of least confusion on the retina.

- Then add plus spherical equivalent of estimated cylindrical power (spherical power half of cylindrical power is called as spherical equivalent to cylinder); this will make the eye in a simple myopic astigmatic state.

- Instruct the patient to look at the lines on the fan and ask him/her whether all lines are equally dark and distinct. If all the lines appears equally dark or equally blur; then either there is no astigmatic error or the eye is fogged in the excess.

- For confirmation of simple myopic state at this juncture add 0.5 D plus sphere and again ask the patient whether there is any change in the darkness on group of lines. If yes, then state of simple myopic astigmatism is present and if answer is no, then add another plus sphere at 0.5 D steps, till patient sees a change in the darkness of lines.

- If patient sees some lines darker than other, ask him/her which group of lines is clearer or darker.

- Now instruct the patient to focus on the Maddox V and ask which limb of V is blurring. Then examiner slowly rotates the central panel towards the blurred limb of V, until both the limbs of V becomes equally blur to the patient. The tip of V indicates the axis of astigmatism.

- Once patient observes equal blurring of limbs of Maddox V then ask him/her to focus on the blocks of lines and ask him/her which set of lines or block is darker. Now add minus cylinders in 0.25 D steps at the direction of axis determined as above; until lines in both the blocks appear equally dark.

- To confirm this, add plus 0.5 D sphere and patient should see the lines in both the blocks equally blur. If dark lines are changed to other block which was originally blur, then we had overcorrected the cylinders and if the originally darker block lines become more darker then initially added spherical power was not correct.

Jackson's Cross Cylinder Method

Jackson's cross cylinder

In the year 1887, Dr Edward Jackson discovered the cross cylinder which is essentially a spherocylindrical lens having plus power in one meridian and an equal minus power in the other meridian. This is used to refine both the axis and power of cylindrical lens and also can be used to check the accuracy of spherical power.

Jackson's cross cylinder is effectively a lens having two cylinders of equal power with opposite signs placed 90° to each other, which is mounted on a handle at 45° angles to these meridians as shown in Fig. 3.9. In routine ophthalmic practice cross cylinders of power 0.25 D or 0.5 D are most commonly used. Plus meridian is marked by black/white line and minus meridian by red line. This cylinder is flipped by rotation of handle, which shows two blur images to the patient, then ask the patient to compare on which side the image is more blurred. When both the images become equally blur that is the endpoint of testing.

Test procedure

This test is performed for refinement of cylindrical axis and power, and it is recommended that always refine the axis of

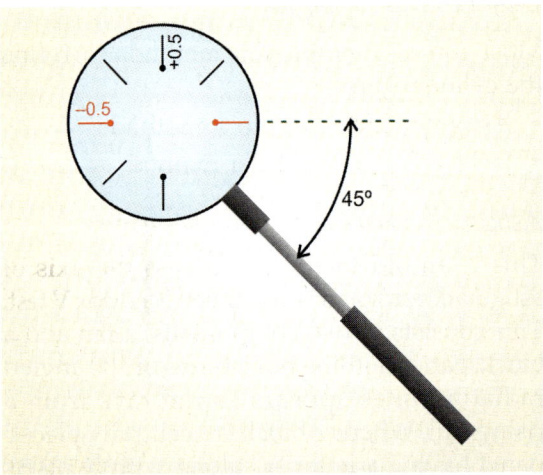

Fig. 3.9: Jackson cross cylinder

cylinder before the power, because correct power cannot be found in the absence of correct axis.

Refining the cylindrical axis

After placing the entire optical correction in the trial frame cylindrical axis is verified uniocularly.

- Align the handle of cross cylinder with the axis of astigmatic error X (Fig. 3.10A); hence the plus meridian of cross cylinder will lie at 45° off on one side of astigmatic axis.
- Now flip the cross cylinder by rotation of handle so that plus meridian will lie on other side of astigmatic axis (Fig. 3.10B).
- Ask the patient to compare the two images in these two positions of cross cylinder.
- If both images are equally blur, then astigmatic axis placed in the trial frame is accurate.
- When refining the plus cylinder and suppose if in any one position of two plus meridians the image appears clearer to the patient then rotate the plus cylinder axis toward that plus direction.

- Similarly, when refining the minus cylinder then rotate the correcting minus cylinder axis in the direction of clearer image towards minus meridian.
- Repeat this procedure at steps of 5° rotation of correcting cylinder until both the images appear equally blur after flipping the cross cylinder.

Refining cylindrical power

After placing the entire optical correction in the trial frame and verifying cylindrical axis, verify the power of correcting cylinder uniocularly.

- Align the handle of cross cylinder so that it lies at 45° angles with the astigmatic axis 'X' and plus meridian of cross cylinder align with the astigmatic axis as shown in Fig. 3.11A.
- Now when examiner flips the cross cylinder, there is an alternate alignment of plus and minus power with the astigmatic axis of correcting cylinder as shown in Fig. 3.11B.
- Ask the patient in which position of cross cylinder the image is clearer.
- Suppose if the image is clearer with alignment of plus meridian, then we increase the power of plus correcting cylinder, because when we place plus meridian over the astigmatic axis we are increasing its power.

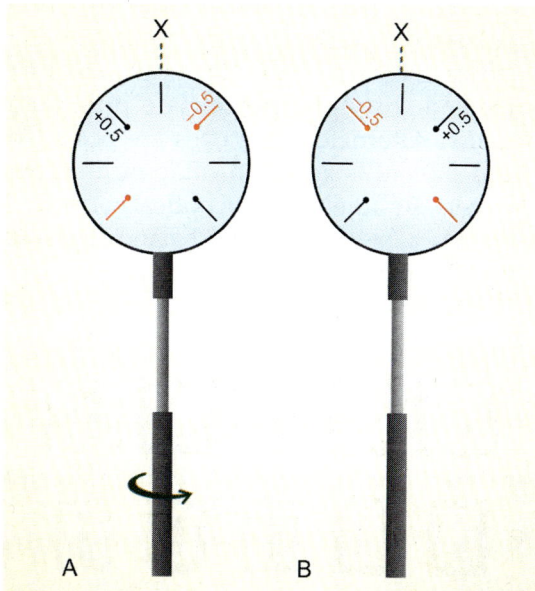

Fig. 3.10: Refining the cylindrical axis. A. Alignment of cross cylinder handle with astigmatic axis X; B. Flip position of cross cylinder

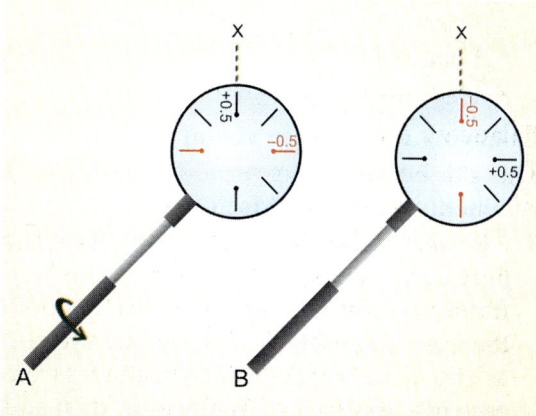

Fig. 3.11: Refining power of cylinder. A. Alignment of cross cylinder handle at 45° with astigmatic axis X; B. Flip position of cross cylinder

- On contrary, if image is getting clearer with alignment of minus meridian, then we decrease the power of plus correcting cylinder or increase the power of minus correcting cylinder, because when we place minus meridian over the astigmatic axis we are decreasing its power.
- End point of test is when both the images get equally blur.

Binocular Balancing

Once the refractive status and best visual acuity has been confirmed uniocularly, then to confirm the optical correction or balance of vision under binocular conditions, a binocular balancing is needed. This can also be termed an equalization of visual or accommodative efforts. Binocular balancing provides a ground to focus a simultaneous retinal image in both the eyes because an imbalance in images will give rise to asthenopic symptoms.

Binocular balancing is done for both distance and near vision and many studies were done in past to achieve the accommodation balance for distance and near vision after refraction. Basic mechanism require to perform balancing is done by masking certain portions of the visual stimulus from either eye and this can be achieved by

- Alternate occlusion with fogging
- Complementary colors
- Prismatic doubling
- Polarization
- Haploscopic presentation

Balancing for distance vision

This can be done by several methods. Most commonly used methods are explained here

- *Alternate occlusion with fogging:* Place the best corrected optical lenses in the trial frame and add + 1D sphere in front of both the eyes. Alternately, occlude one eye and ask the patient to compare the images from each eye. If both are equally blur, then add –0.25 D sphere in front of one eye and again alternately occlude one eye. Now ask patient to compare the images from each

eye. He/she will report a clear image from the eye in front of which a –0.25 D sphere was added. Suppose patient says no, then add or subtract spherical power in a 0.25 D steps till balancing or image clarity becomes equal in both eyes.

- *Turville binocular balance technique:* In the year 1930, Turville proposed an infinity balance technique for binocular balance of refraction. Principle of this method is that a septum is positioned at the junction point of two diagonals from each eyes, which were connecting the nodal points and foveal targets. Various foveal targets or test objects shown in original test method are shown in Fig. 3.12A. This septum occludes one of the two foveal targets and hence only one retinal image from either eye is formed when both the eyes remain open. In case of binocular balancing the images will be seen as shown in Fig. 3.12B.
- *Bichromatic binocular technique:* Cowen modified binocular unit in an instrument which projects the ring targets (Verhoeff) in opposition to two halves of red and green duchrome background, which are cross polarized. After placing the best correcting lenses in the trial frame, the ring targets are viewed through appropriate polarized filters. Alternately, the eyes are occluded and patient is asked to compare the ring targets. By adjustment of optical correction we can achieve binocular balancing using these duchrome charts.

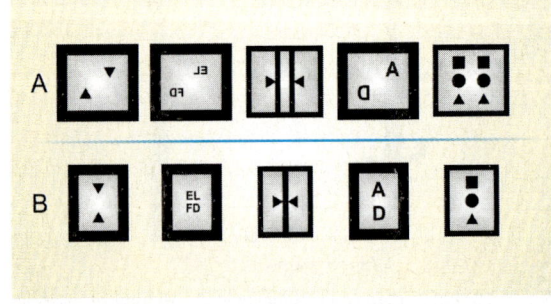

Fig. 3.12: Turville infinity binocular balance test. A. Test objects; B. Normal results

- *Prism dissociation method:* It is most commonly used and is the most sensitive method to test binocular balancing. Minimum amount of binocularity is a prerequisite to perform this method. This method is not useful in presence of severe amblyopia or high anisometropia.

Test method
- Place the best corrected optical lenses in the trial frame and perform uniocular acuity.
- Project a single row of letters on Snellen's chart of 6/9 (preferably a line better than weaker eye). Now place a vertical prism of 4–5Δ in front of one eye in the trial fame. (This will dissociate the images of two eyes).
- With both the eyes open ask the patient to read the letters of Snellen's chart. Now add plus 0.25 D sphere in front of one eye and then alternate it with other eye.
- If refractive correction in both the eyes is balanced, then patient will see blurring of letters from the eye having additional plus 0.25 D sphere.
- Once balance is achieved in both the eyes prism is removed and the patient is defogged until maximum acuity is reached, either with a maximum plus power or with minimum minus power.
- *Fogging with Duo chrome test:* In this method of binocular balancing of refraction, testing of corrective power by duo chrome chart is done along with fogging of one eye.
Test method
- Best corrected optical power lenses are placed in the trial frame and patient is asked to see the red green bars present on a vision chart.
- Fog one eye with a plus 2 D sphere and ask the patient to observe the red green bar with the other unfogged eye.
- Patient is asked which bar either red or green, he/she sees clearly.
- If both the color bars are equally clear then binocular balance is present and no correction in optical powers is needed.

- If both the bars are not seen equally clear, then adjust the spheres in front of the observing eye, until they become equal.
- Repeat the same with fogging the other eye.

Near vision

Once the patient is fully corrected for distance vision then test for near vision may also be required if patient age is over 40 years, or hyperopic, or has any difficulty in reading. In appropriate illumination in room, ask the patient to read the near vision chart preferably at 35–40 cm distance after wearing of full optical correction for distance vision. Always check with both the eyes open, do not occlude either eye.

Examiner asks the patient whether he/she can read the smallest line with ease or not. If not, then add plus spherical powers in front of both eyes together, according to the age or by assuming till which line patient can read comfortably as shown in Table 3.1.

If patient is unable to read the smallest letter line, then add the power as per chart and increase gradually in 0.25 D steps till patient is able to read comfortably. Difference in spherical powers for near and distance is calculated and recorded as 'Add' for near vision.

For example, if power of distance vision is plus 1.0 D and near vision is plus 2.5 D then 'Add' for both the eyes is plus 1.5 D. Similarly, in myopes if distance power is minus 1.0 D and near power is plus 2.0 D then 'Add' in both eyes will be plus 3.0 D.

Table 3.1: Average addition required by emmetropes at 35–40 cm reading distance

Age in years	Plus addition in dioptres
40–45	0.75
46–50	1.25
51–55	1.75
56–60	2.00
60–70	2.50
71 and above	3.00

Binocular balancing for near vision refraction is done by several methods such as

- Near vision balance with Bisurface reflectors
- Freeman near vision unit
- Rodenstock near vision unit
- Osterberg-Bino near vision unit

Near vision testing by bisurface reflectors

In this instrument an angled bisurface mirror is used to separate the right and left eye fields, whereas in original Turville method a septum was used. One area has figured target and other area has undifferentiated targets, however, patient can compare both images by rapid alteration of bifixation of either views.

Freeman near vision unit

This unit consists of bichromatic polarized modified ring targets (Verhoeff types) along with two cross-polarized letter charts (Fig. 3.13).

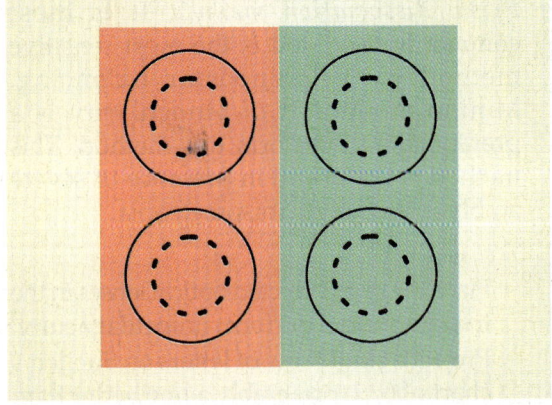

Fig. 3.13: Freeman bichromatic polarized modified ring targets

> **Note** _____
>
> These near vision units have similar kind of purpose. Binocular bichromatic balancing method is better than simple duo chromatic principle as it assesses the balancing of monocular accommodation efforts.

Rodenstock near vision unit

Here balancing of accommodation is done by presenting a duo chrome target having letters and double Verhoeff rings. For balancing of near vision two cross-polarized letter charts are also present in testing unit.

Osterberg-Bino near vision unit

This consists of a non-polarized duo chrome reducing number chart along with two cross-polarized charts, which are separated vertically.

Prescription Writing for Glasses

Retinoscopy Representation

Universal method of representation of retinoscopy values are in the form of a cross as shown in Fig. 4.1.

Here, X and Y represent the two principal meridians, i.e. 90° and 180°, respectively. If the neutralization meridians are not at these angles then they can be represented accordingly, for example a 40° meridian and 140° meridian, which will be represented as shown in Fig. 4.2.

Similarly, the gross retinoscopy values are represented along the axis of neutralization.

For example,

- If both vertical and horizontal meridians get neutralized by plus 5 D power, when retinoscopy is done at 66 cm distance with atropine as cycloplegic drug, then value of 1.5 D for distance and 1 D for atropine drug is reduced from gross retinoscopy and net value of retinoscopy will be represented as shown in Fig. 4.3.
- If vertical meridian is neutralized by plus 5 D power and horizontal meridian by plus 7 D when retinoscopy is done at 66 cm distance with atropine drug then the gross and net retinoscopy will be represented as shown in Fig. 4.4.
- Similarly if neutralization occurs by –4 D power in both the principal meridians

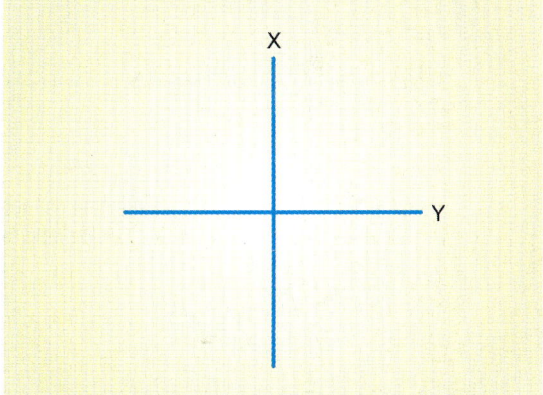

Fig. 4.1: Retinoscopy representation (*see* text)

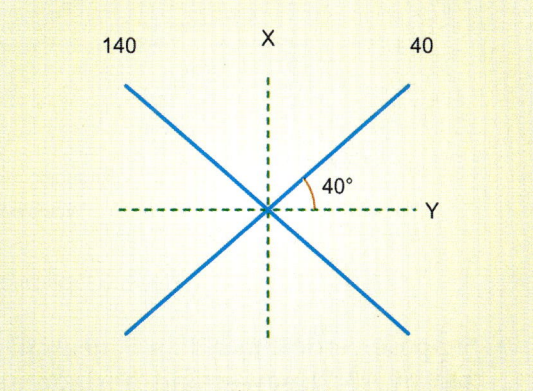

Fig. 4.2: Retinoscopy representation (*see* text)

when retinoscopy is done at 66 cm distance with atropine, then gross and net retinoscopy is represented as in Fig. 4.5.

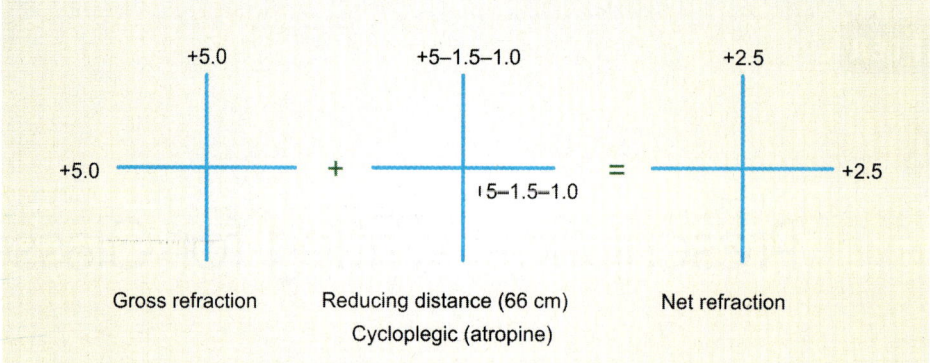

Fig. 4.3: Optical cross in simple hypermetropia

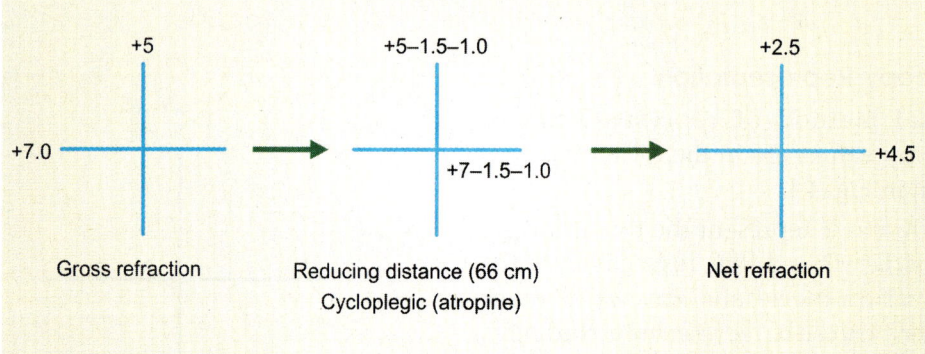

Fig. 4.4: Optical cross in compound hypermetropia

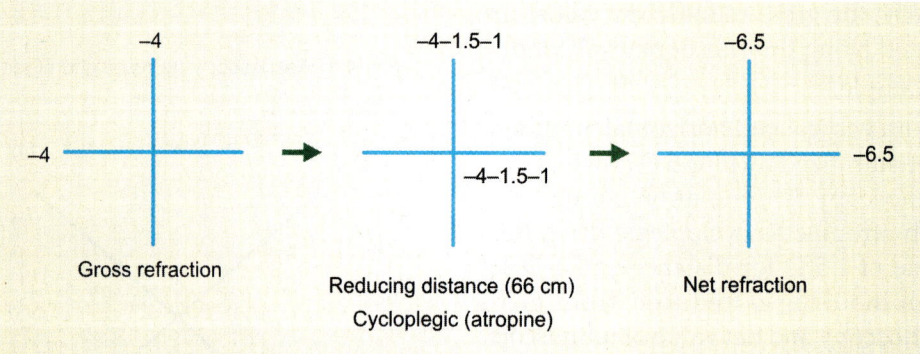

Fig. 4.5: Optical cross in simple myopia

- Suppose vertical meridian is neutralized by –3 D power and horizontal meridian by minus 5 D, when retinoscopy done at 66 cm distance with atropine drug then gross and net retinoscopy will be represented as shown in Fig. 4.6.

- In case of oblique astigmatism when neutralization is at 30° meridian and 120° meridian say with +2 D power and +4 D power, respectively and retinoscopy is done at 66 cm distance with atropine then gross and net retinoscopy will be represented as shown in Fig. 4.7.

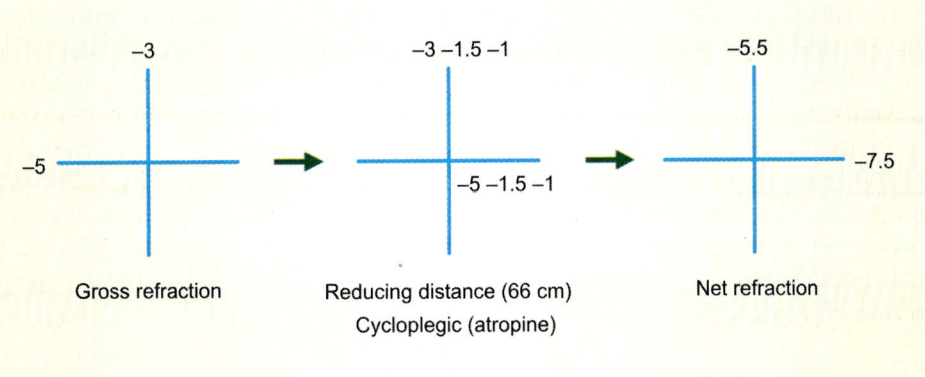

Fig. 4.6: Optical cross in compound myopia

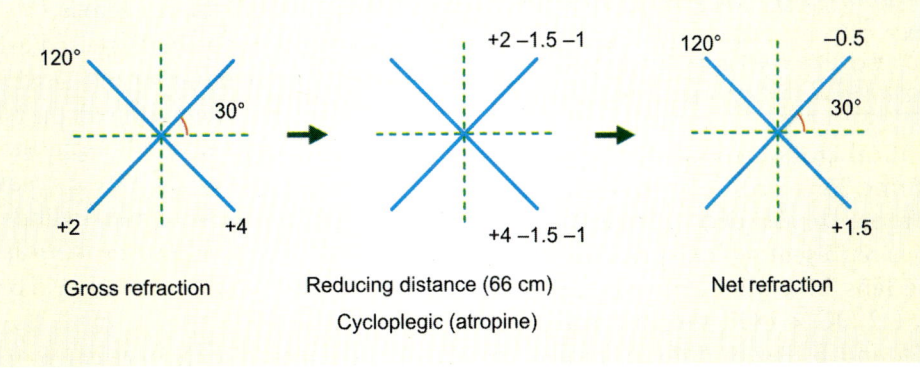

Fig. 4.7: Optical cross in oblique astigmatism

Prescription Writing

In an ophthalmic lens prescription, spherical lens power is written first, followed by cylindrical lens power and then cylindrical lens axis. These values are represented with the help of net retinoscopy representation.

For example, the above net retinoscopy findings will be written as

- Figure 4.3: + 2.5 DS
- Figure 4.4: + 2.5 DS/+ 2 DC × 90°
- Figure 4.5: – 6.5 DS
- Figure 4.6: – 5.5 DS/–2 DC × 90°
- Figure 4.7: – 0.5 DS/+2 DC × 30°

Plus versus minus cylinder form

These plus or minus cylinder forms represent the toric surface and may be grounded either on the front or back surface of the optical lens,

hence these prescriptions for an optical lens can be written either as plus-cylinder form or minus-cylinder form. If the front surface of a lens is grounded it forms a plus cylinder and if the back surface of a lens is grounded then it forms a minus cylinder.

For example,

$$- 5.5 \text{ DS}/–2 \text{ DC} × 90°$$

This above prescription is written in a minus cylinder form but suppose the cylinder needs to be grounded on the front surface of lens then the same prescription will be written as

$$–7.5 \text{ DS}/+2 \text{ DC} × 180°$$

THE OPTICAL CROSS

Optical cross is a graphical representation which explains the relationship between spherical and cylindrical components of an ophthalmic lens, also known as power diagrams. To understand power diagrams three crosses are drawn; one will represent the spherical component where power is same in both the principal meridians. Second cross will represent the cylindrical component where maximum power of the cylinder is specified in a meridian, while the power in remaining meridian is zero (since the power is zero in axis meridian of a cylindrical lens).

> **Note**
>
> The power of cylindrical lens is represented at an axis perpendicular to the one written in net prescription, means when cylindrical axis is written as 90° in the prescription, then the power in the optical cross will be taken at horizontal or 180° and vice versa.

The optical crosses shown in Fig. 4.8A is representing lens prescription in a minus cylinder form, i.e. –5.5 DS/–2 DC × 90° while Fig. 4.8B is representing lens prescription for the same lens in a plus cylinder form, i.e. –7.5 DS/+ 2 DC × 180°. We can observe in Fig. 4.87A and B that in both examples, the optical crosses for total power in the vertical meridian is –5.5 D, whereas in the horizontal meridian it is –7.5 D. Furthermore, for a minus cylinder form the total power of the least minus meridian is selected as spherical power while for a plus-cylinder form the total power in most minus meridian is selected as spherical power.

There is another way to write a net power figure in a prescription form as follows: Consider any meridian power as spherical power, say vertical or horizontal. Now just subtract the spherical meridian power from the other meridian power mathematically and get the cylindrical power with spherical meridian axis as cylindrical axis.

If we consider above discussed example:

If horizontal meridian is considered as spherical power (–7.5 D), then subtract the horizontal meridian power, i.e. –7.5 D from the vertical meridian power, i.e. –5.5 D and resultant is –5.5 – (–7.5) = +2.0, i.e. plus cylinder at 180° (horizontal/spherical power meridian)

Hence, the final prescription will be –7.5 DS × +2 DC × 180°

Alternately, when vertical meridian is considered as spherical power (–5.5 D), then subtract the vertical meridian power, i.e.

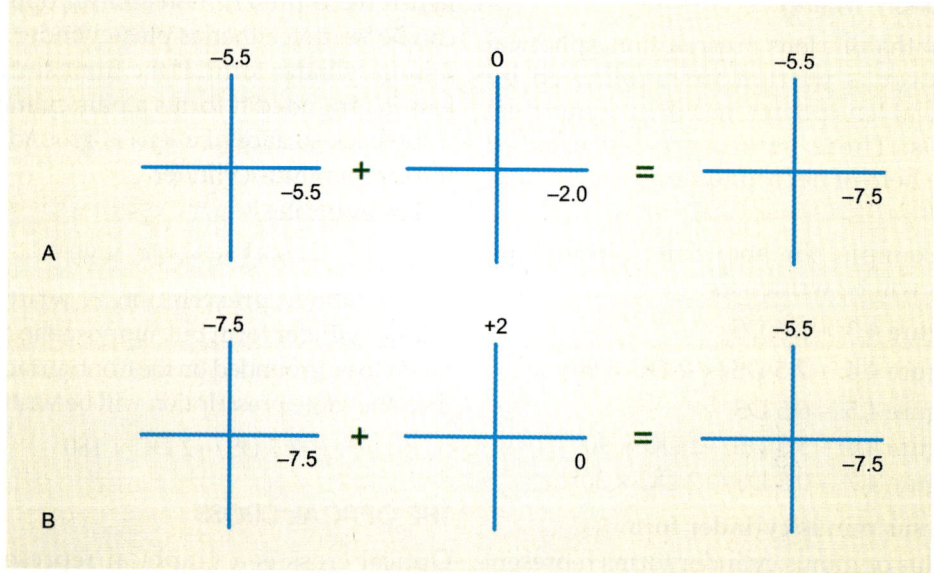

Fig. 4.8: Optical cross representations of same prescription in various cylindrical forms. A. Minus cylinder form; B. Plus cylinder form

–5.5 D from the horizontal meridian power, i.e. –7.5 D and resultant is –7.5 – (–5.5) = –2.0, i.e. minus cylinder at 90° (vertical/spherical power meridian)

Hence, the final prescription will be –5.5 DS × –2 DC × 90°

So in a nutshell we can consider any meridian power as spherical power and to get final prescription just follow this simple rule:

"Always spherical powers are deducted from cylindrical powers mathematically and the resultant power becomes cylindrical power, whereas for cylindrical axis use the same axis of spherical power".

Transposition of Prescription

Transposition of a spherocylindrical percep-tion is necessary for a laboratory when they need to manufacture a specific form of lens, i.e. either the front surface cylinder or back surface cylinder lens.

Three steps rule for transposition of prescription
This simple 3 steps rule is applied for transposition of a spherocylindrical prescrip-tion to convert plus (+) cylinder form into a minus (–) cylinder form or vice versa.

Step 1: Mathematically, add spherical power and cylinder power to get new spherical power.

Step 2: Reverse the sign of cylinder, i.e. from plus to minus and vice versa.

Step 3: Rotate the cylindrical axis by 90°.

Cross cylinder form: When a lens is grounded as plus cylinder on its front surface and as minus cylinder on its back surface, having axes of these two cylinders at 90° apart, is called as cross cylinder.

Note _____

In our example the total power of cross cylinder lens in the horizontal meridian is –0.5 D, while in the vertical meridian is +0.50 D.

An example of a cross cylindrical lens is + 0.50 DC × 180° combined with –0.5 DC × 90°. Optical cross representing this prescription is shown in Fig. 4.9.

In routine ophthalmic practice these cross cylinders are used to refine axis and power of patient's best cylindrical correction (Jackson's cross cylinder) and also can be used for near point testing (e.g. in determination of power of a bifocal addition).

A spherocylindrical prescription can be formed into a cross cylinder prescription by this simple two steps rule:

Step 1: First obtain both the plus cylinder and minus cylinder forms of the prescription.

Step 2: Now combine the two powers mathematically (connect extremes)

For example, if a spherocylindrical lens prescription is written in a plus cylinder form and then in a minus cylinder form, i.e. –0.5 DS/+1.0 DC × 90° and +0.5 DS/–1.0 DC × 180°, now if we connect the powers, the

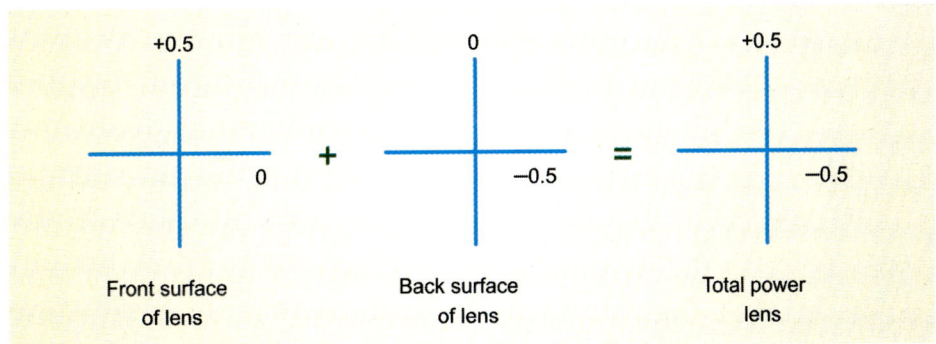

Fig. 4.9: Cross cylinder form representation

resultant prescription will be +0.50 DC × 90° combined with –0.5 DC × 180°.

Similarly, a crossed-cylinder prescription can be converted into a spherocylindrical prescription by this simple three steps rule

Step 1: Consider the first encountered cylindrical power as the spherical power.

Step 2: To get cylindrical power, reverse the sign of this new spherical power and then mathematically add it with second cylinder power.

Step 3: To get the cylinder axis use the same axis that of second cylinder.

Continuing to the same example of cross cylinder as above mentioned, the lens prescription is + 0.50 DC × 90° combined with –0.5 DC × 180° and by applying this three step

 Note _____

Spherocylindrical prescriptions are same in both the methods of transposition of cross cylinder. Since routinely in our ophthalmic practice we encounter transposition between minus cylinder and plus cylinder forms, hence readers are advised to memorize the original three steps rule for conversion of spherocylindrical powers.

rule to get a spherocylindrical prescription, + 0.50 DC × 90° will become as

$$+0.50 \text{ DS}/{-1.0} \text{ DC} \times 180°$$

Now on applying the original three steps rule and this minus cylinder prescription can be transposed into a plus-cylinder prescription as follows:

$$-0.5 \text{ DS}/{+1.0} \text{ DC} \times 90°$$

Spectacles

Spectacles: An Overview

HISTORY AND EVENTS OF PROGRESS

Introduction

Art of glass making is much older than invention of spectacles. Glasses were used since ages for various purposes, however first time glass were used as a visual aid in the form of a simple magnifying glass called eyeglass. These eyeglasses were mounted on various materials like wood, metals, leather, animal horn, bone, etc. and with the help of a handle these mounted eyeglasses were held in front of eye to visualize the objects.

An optical device used for visual purpose by only one eye is known as an eyeglass, however, when two such devices are used for both the eyes together, are called a pair of eyeglasses or spectacles. Initially, only eyeglass was invented and used in front of one eye but with trial and error two such devices were hinged in a manner that one of eyeglasses lies in front of each eye together and this leads to a primitive pair of spectacles as shown in Fig. 5.1.

It is not exactly known who invented the spectacles, but several people had contributed in the process of invention to produce the present form of spectacles.

Events of progress

- Roger Bacon, a monk in his famous Opus Magnus (1267) first described that small

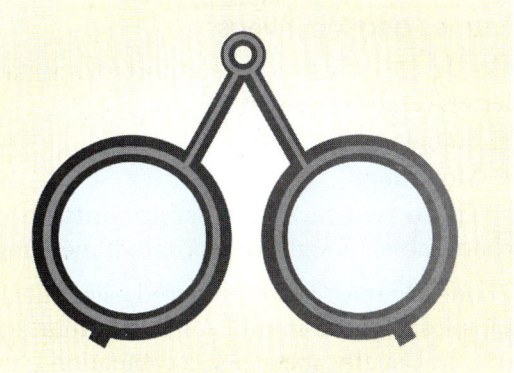

Fig. 5.1: Primitive spectacles

letters or objects can be magnified with help of a strong plano convex lens and he suggested that such device can be used in those people having poor vision. However, it is not exactly known whether he mounted these lenses in any frame or not.

- The first evidence about invention of spectacles has been found in a sermon (1305) written by the monk Giordano da Rivalto.
- Furthermore, other evidence about invention of glasses were found in a manuscript and an epitaph written by Alexandria de Spina and Salvino d'Armati of Florence.
- Primitive forms of spectacles because of their weight and assembly were difficult

to mount steadily in front of the eyes and thus were clamped to the nose which was uncomfortable for patient and often interfered with breathing. Subsequently, spectacle devices in the form of head bands were produced for better comfort.

- Around 17th century Spanish spectacle makers used loops of silk or cord which were attached with the outer edges of frames and then loop were extended to the ears.
- In the year 1730, Edward Scarlett (English optician) developed rigid side pieces (temples) of eyeglasses.

Frames and Mountings

The devices which act as support for spectacle lenses can be classified as

- Frames
- Mountings

These two terms are commonly interchangeable, though have different meanings.

Frames: Frames can be prepared using metals, plastics or combination of both metal and plastic. Usually, metal or a combination frame consists of an adjustable nose pads for better comfort, whereas plastic frames has fixed nose pads or no pads for adjustments as shown in Fig. 5.2.

Frame mainly consists of three parts

- Front: Encircles the lenses and hold them
- Bridge: Keeps the entire front together and rests on the nose
- Pair of temples: Rests on the ears and hold the front in alignment with eyes.

Mounting: A device which holds the two optical lenses in front of eyes without encircling them completely is called mountings as shown in Fig. 5.3. These mountings were classically manufactured with gold filled materials in past and were classified as either rimless or semi-rimless.

A typical rimless mounting has three parts

- Single bridge or center piece: Helps to hold the two spectacle lenses together towards nose (nasally).
- End pieces: Two in number which hinges the spectacle lenses with temples.
- Temples: Two in number, one on each side.

To fit lenses in a rimless frame, two holes are drilled in each lens, i.e. one hole nasally to fix the center piece and second hole temporally to fix the end piece. Center piece consists of two adjustable nose pads to be placed on the sides of nose, which carry the weight of entire mounting and lenses. Two temples are fixed with end pieces so that a rimless frame can be worn comfortably.

A typical semi-rimless frame also has three portions

- A front: Which has both bridge and two arms
- Two temples

In past, two commercial versions of semi-rimless mountings were manufactured

- American Optical Numount was the first version which attaches only to the nasal side of spectacle lens and requires only one hole per lens. Numount is a light weighted mounting and a tri-flex spring

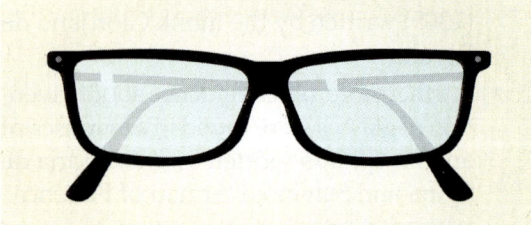

Fig. 5.2: Plastic frame

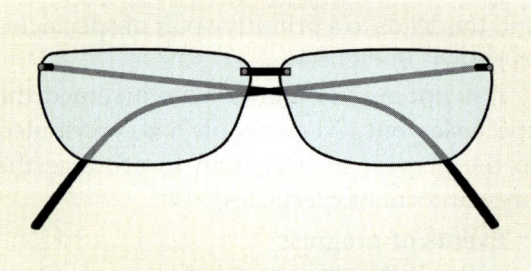

Fig. 5.3: Mounting

is present in mounting at the location where spectacle lens is attached with the mounting. Although in look, Numount mounting appears very delicate but presence of tri-flex spring prevents breaking of spectacle lenses during pressure and shocks (Fig. 5.4).

- Similarly, American Optical Rimway was second version of semi-rimless mountings which attaches to both the nasal and temporal sides of each spectacle lenses, thus require two holes per lens for fitting (Fig. 5.5). Although Rimway mountings were appearing tougher than Numount mounting but in reality temporal corner of this spectacle lens get easily breaks away on pressure application.

In addition to these abovementioned conventional frames or mountings which contain bridges and temples, the other devices were also available which hold either a pair of spectacle lenses or a single lens in front of the eye.

Pincenez or eyeglass was a term used for a pair of spectacle lenses, which were held in front of eyes by pinching the nose. These eyeglasses have no temples and lenses are fixed in a circular frame like structure as shown in Fig. 5.6.

Similarly, Lorgnette was spectacle which indicates that either a pair of spectacle lenses (usually) or a single spectacle lens (rarely), held in front of the eyes with the help of a handle as shown in Fig. 5.7.

Monocle which means a single lens, it appears similar to a trial case lens and was worn very often for special motive. The muscular pressure of facial and brow muscles hold this Monocle in front of one eye as shown in Fig. 5.8.

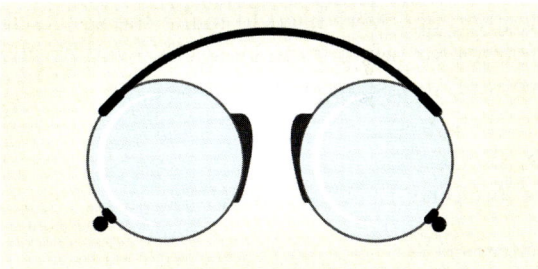

Fig. 5.6: Pincenez

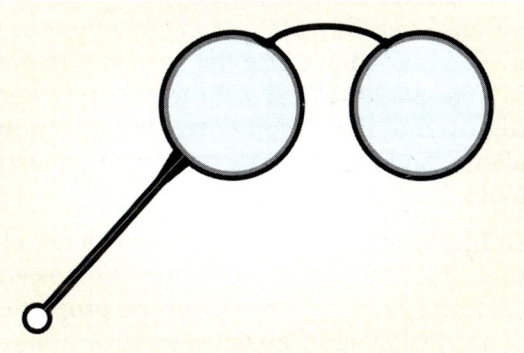

Fig. 5.7: Lorgnette

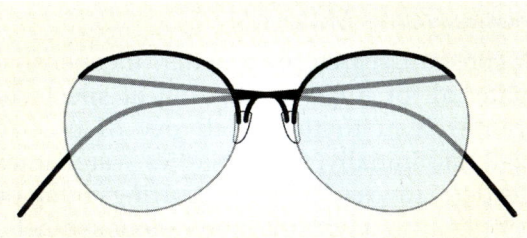

Fig. 5.4: Numount mounting

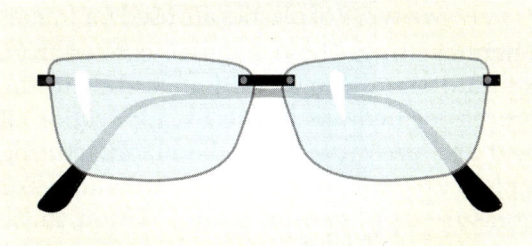

Fig. 5.5: Rimway mounting

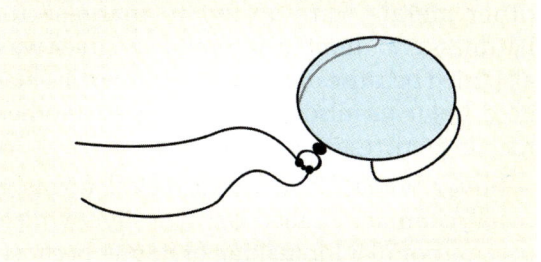

Fig. 5.8: Monocle

Materials of Frames and Mountings

Spectacle frames and mountings can be prepared by using various materials like natural substances or synthetics substances. Materials having following properties are considered ideal for manufacturing spectacles frames

- Non-corrosiveness
- Adjustability
- Light weighted
- Non-allergic
- Sturdiness
- Low cost

In older times, naturally available materials like wood, animal horns, tortoise shell and leather, etc. were used to make the spectacle frames for holding the lenses. Nowadays the commonly used materials are

- Metals
- Plastics
- Nylon

Metals

Most commonly and widely used material to manufacture the spectacles frames are metals; because use of metal was convenient and inexpensive to produce the spectacle frames in large quantity. Most of the metals used were highly moldable, non-corrosive and non-allergic and were durable with good cosmetic looks. Various metals used are

Gold and silver: Initially gold was extensively used for frames and mountings in western countries because it meets all the properties of an ideal material except cost. These frames were marked with content of gold percentage in terms of Karat. Pure gold was too soft, hence other metals were added to increase its hardness and durability. Similarly, silver was also tried because of its similar properties like gold, but it was also too soft and needed other metals to increase its utilization.

Silver when mixed with nickel forms a metal, commonly called German silver which became popular for making of frames because of its anti-corrosive property, however, the high percentage of contact allergy due to these metals discouraged its wide usage in population.

Later on, gold was layered over this German silver by electroplating process, which not only eliminated its allergic nature but also maintained the properties like adjustability and durability. These gold frames remain popular till date because of their cosmetic reasons, non-allergic nature and anti-corrosiveness; still the only hurdle is cost.

Stainless steel: This came as an inexpensive alternative to gold and silver in large-scale manufacturing of frames. Steel meet nearly all the qualities of an ideal material being very stable, adjustable, non-corrosiveness, non-allergic and light in weight, and can easily be manufactured in mass productions.

Aluminium: Like steel, aluminium is also inexpensive, noncorrosive, light-weighted material and thus can also be easily used in large-scale frame manufacturing. Aluminium metal also has an advantage over steel that the frames of aluminium can be dyed easily with different colors which improved its cosmetic appearance and sale value.

Plastic Frame Materials

A constant search for a better, inexpensive material for huge production of spectacle frames lead to the discovery of plastic material. Initially, these plastics were either the derivatives of natural occurring cotton or petroleum, but with the time various synthetic materials were developed in laboratories to produce plastics.

Mainly two types of plastics are used for frames **Thermosetting:** These materials convert from a liquid state into a solid state during the process of manufacturing by application of heat and pressure. Once the manufacturing had occurred, then even high temperatures or pressure application cannot soften these materials and in these circumstances they basically decompose. For example, melanines used for Melmac dishes, phenolics (Bakelite), polyesters used for clothing and allyls used in CR-39 material (very popular as plastic lens material, however, rarely used for manufacturing spectacle frames).

Optyl: Optyl is an epoxy resin containing thermosetting plastic material. To manufacture frames from optyl, the liquid of it at high temperature is poured into a mould followed by a curing process. After moulding different parts of the formed frame can easily be dyed using different colors. The optyl material on heating becomes soft and flexible and thus can be shaped in any desired form easily.

Advantages of optyl frames are
- Hardness
- Dimensional stability
- Good shine
- Non-inflammability
- Light in weight.

Disadvantages of optyl frames are that they need higher temperatures compare to their counterpart materials to work on; and if any attempt is made to adjust them in cold, frames will break.

Thermoplastic: These materials get soft on heating and hard on cooling and even basic structure of these material is not altered even on repeated exposure to this process.

Hence, these materials are widely used for large-scale production of inexpensive and durable spectacle frames. Various thermoplastics commonly used to manufacture spectacle frames are

Acrylics: Acrylics are the most common name for the family of thermoplastic materials, which include polymethyl methacrylate (mainly used in the manufacturing of hard contact lenses and occasionally used for spectacle frames). Various acrylics used commercially for spectacle frame manufacturing are
- PMMA
- Plexiglas
- Perspex
- Lucite

Most advantageous features of acrylics are dimensional stability, surface hardness, good wear resistance, clarity, color fastness, light weight, and non-flammable. Disadvantages of acrylics are brittleness and low impact resistance; due to which these materials are not preferably used for spectacle frames.

Polycarbonate: This thermoplastic material was used widely in past for manufacturing of spectacle frames. Only disadvantage was that it was too hard to work on, so gradually its use declined over a period of time.

Presently, mainly two materials are used for the mass manufacture of spectacle frames, cellulose nitrate and cellulose acetate. Although both are similar in appearance, but when used for spectacle frames they exhibit different properties.

Cellulose nitrate: This is also called xylonite and is commonly known as celluloid in the film industry. Camphor is added as a plasticizer during manufacturing of cellulose nitrate, hence when a cellulose nitrate frame is rubbed vigorously with a cloth, an odour of camphor may be noticed. Due to its hard nature it retains its shape even in hot climate.

Cellulose acetate: Most commonly used plastic material to manufacture spectacle frames is cellulose acetate because of its less inflammable nature and hardness.

Both cellulose nitrate and cellulose acetate are produced by cotton lint and are soluble in various ketones such as acetone; although neither of them is soluble in alcohol. Hence, acetone is often used as a polishing or repairing substance for the frames made up of cellulose material.

Comparison of cellulose nitrate and cellulose acetate

Cellulose nitrate is superior to cellulose acetate because
- Cellulose nitrate can be easily stretched by heat and also shrinks minimally when

cooled, so moulding of these frames is comparatively easier than acetate frames.

- Harder surface of nitrate frames is an advantage for better polish and trouble-free maintenance.
- Much thinner frames can be made by nitrate because it is tougher than cellulose acetate.
- Nitrates softening point is higher than that of cellulose acetate; and its water absorption is lower, hence better dimensional stability is seen in warm and clammy environments.

Conversely, cellulose acetate is superior to cellulose nitrate because

- Less production time as compared to cellulose nitrate.
- Frames made are more colorfast compared to cellulose nitrate.
- Cellulose acetate frames are much less flammable compared to cellulose nitrate.

Cellulose propionate: It is also an ester of cellulose family. Several properties of propionate resembled the optyl material including the manufacturing by moulding process. Frames prepared by cellulose propionate are quite tough and light in weight, so can easily be made into various styles and sculpturing effects. However, use of cellulose propionate frames has decreased in recent years.

Nylon: Polyamides are a generic class of thermoplastic polymers which are commonly known as nylon. Nylon material is very costly when manufactured in the form of sheet, hence an injection moulding technique is used to decrease the cost of manufacturing. Nylon is very tough and hard in nature but its brittleness, poor color acceptance, high water absorption and less transparency has limited its usefulness in competitive spectacle frame

---

Note _____

Although several materials have been used for the manufacture of plastic frames; but great majority spectacle frames are currently made of thermoplastic material, cellulose acetate.

market. Nylon spectacle frames are currently available in market, but are less preferred as compared to the cellulose material frames.

Bridges and Temples

Following types of bridges and temples can be used in plastic spectacle frames

Bridges: Usually in metallic frames and/or rimless or semi-rimless mounting, bridges make no direct contact with nose; rather contact is made with the help of adjustable nose pads (Fig. 5.9).

However, in plastic frame there is a direct contact of bridge with the sides of nose. Plastic frame's bridges are either saddle type bridges or keyhole type bridges or occasionally modifications of either type.

A saddle bridge directly rests on the crest of nose like a horse back and distributes the weight of spectacles evenly on the top and sides of the nose (Fig. 5.10). It has no nose pads for contact to the sides of nose, hence suitable for those persons who compliant of sensitivity due to nose pads. For proper fitting of this kind of bridge, the saddle shape must be a

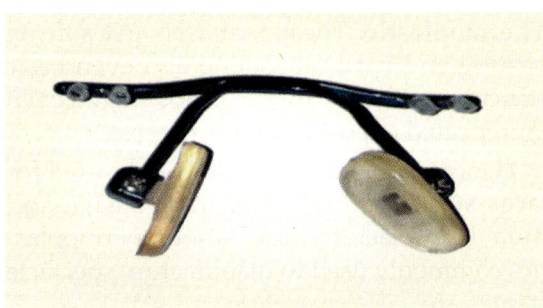

Fig. 5.9: Adjustable nose pad

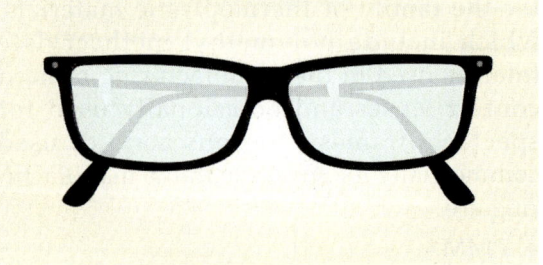

Fig. 5.10: Saddle bridge

perfect fit with contour of the nose. Various modified saddle bridges have also been developed which include built-up areas on either side of bridge in such a way that the apparent length of nose looks short.

The keyhole bridges are useful for those persons who cannot tolerate pressure on the top of the nose because these types of bridges make direct contact only with the sides of nose, not the top (Fig. 5.11). Fixed, nonadjustable pads are made with the frame which make the contact with nose and are usually of the same material as that of frame. As compared to saddle bridge, wearing of keyhole bridge frames usually accentuate the length of the nose.

Some plastic spectacle frames also contain other type of bridges which compromise features between saddle and keyhole types and are effective in better nose fitting.

Bridge width: For all types of spectacle frames bridge width remain specified and it defines as the shortest distance between the two lenses or in a simpler term, as DBL, i.e. distance between the lenses, measured in millimeter unit (Fig. 5.12).

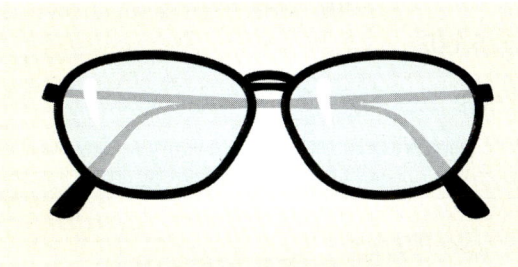

Fig. 5.11: Keyhole bridge

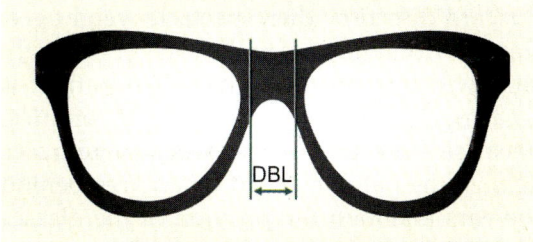

Fig. 5.12: Bridge width specification showing DBL

Temples: Temples are the part of spectacle which holds the front and rests on the ears of person. Common types of temples available are

- Skull temple
- Library temple
- Riding bow temple
- Comfort cable temple.

Skull temple is most commonly used temple designs for plastic spectacle frames. These types of temples remain bent downward behind the ear and follow the curve of the ear of person and shape of skull (hence are called skull temple). Advantage with skull temples is that they do not create excessive pressure on the mastoid process or ear lobe so are more comfortable for wearer. (Fig. 5.13A). Several modifications of skull temple have been done in terms of width which may vary in different frames from standard form of skull temple. Most of these modified skull temples, particular the thinner styles, contain a wire core to provide added strength.

Library or spatula temple does not have any curve like skull temple rather it lays straight back over the ear (Fig. 5.13D). Spectacle glasses remains in the position on the head due to pressure of temples which is exerted on the sides of skull by temple and this pressure is not seen with library temple, hence the fitting of these types of temples is difficult. The straight back design of temple helps the wearer to position the frame on and off the face very rapidly thus these temples are convenient for those who wear glasses irregularly and usually for a brief period of time.

Riding bow temple is the one which encloses the back and lower part of ear (Fig. 5.13B). Usually these are made up of plastic material having a central metallic core, mainly indicated for frames used in children and safety frames.

Comfort cable type of temple appears similar to riding bow temple; but the difference is that all and/or part of this type temple

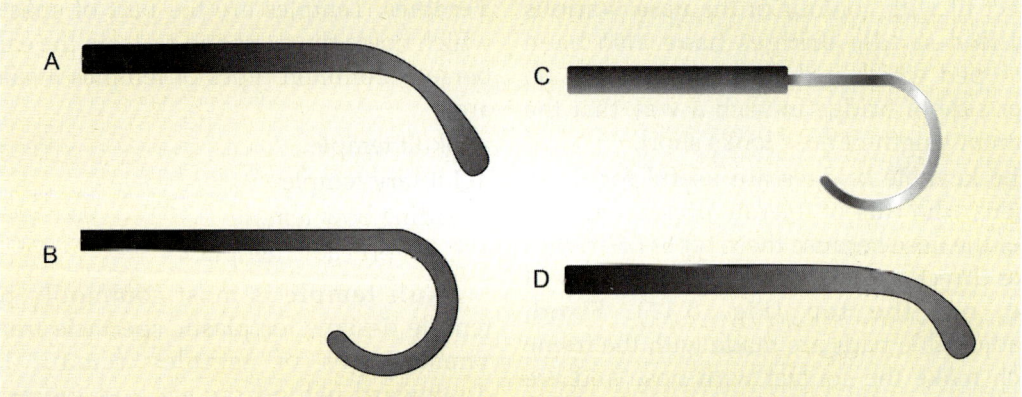

Fig. 5.13: Showing various types of temples. A. Skull type; B. Riding bow type; C. Comfort cable type; D. Library type

(specifically the part encircling the ear) is made up of a coiled metal cable instead of plastic (Fig. 5.13C).

Because of their identical appearance riding bow and comfort cable temples are used synonymously where a comfort cable temple is considered as a type of riding bow temple. Metal spectacle frames and mountings usually have comfort cable/riding bow temples. These types of temples because of their structure can hold a frame securely in place and thus commonly used for children's spectacles and in some occupation like by mechanics and electricians.

Temple length: Previously, temple length was calculated by either measurement from length to bend or overall length from front to tip of temple. Now usually temples are specified as overall length only. Previously it was measured in inches but now represented in millimeter unit.

Bridge Fitting

The bridge fitting is an important step during spectacle fitting because usually most of the weight of spectacles is carried on the nose of person holding head in erect position. However, different styles of frame and positions of head may affect the percentage amount of total weight of the spectacles which is carried by the nose. Ideally, bridge fitting should be in such a way that weight of the spectacle frame

remains distributed over a large area on the nose so that the irritation on the nose is reduced. It is essential to check bony angular configuration (i.e. frontal angle and transverse angle) of the nose by palpation of nose.

As shown in Fig. 5.14A, frontal angle of the nose is an angle formed between midline of nose and a vertical line passing through each sides of nose, whereas transverse or splay angle of nose is an angle formed between median sagital plane, i.e. an anterio-posterior plane passing through the midline of nose and line passing by the side of nose as shown in Fig. 5.14B.

> **Note**
>
> Nose pads are selected in such a way that they closely match both the frontal angle and transverse angle of nose.

Temple Fitting

Normally, majority of spectacle's weight is borne by the nose but if a person tilt head in forward direction, then spectacle weight gets transfer from the nose to the ears. This weight shift will possess difficulty when patient is wearing library or skull types of temples, because pressure of the sides of temples against the patient's head on an area behind the ears maintain the position of the glasses in these types of temple designs. On contrary, riding bow temples encircle the ears and hence

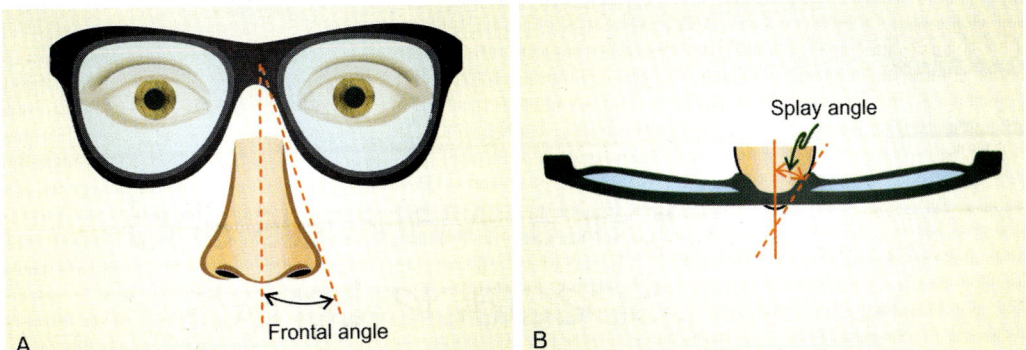

Fig. 5.14: Bridge fitting method. A. Frontal angle; B. Transverse or splay angle

secures the position of frame by making contact at the lower arc of the external ear.

Important features to remember while fitting the temples of spectacle frames are

- Relation of angle of external ear to sides of patient's head.
- Shape of mastoid process

Hence, it is important for ophthalmic personnel to inspect the top and back of ear along with mastoid process; before deciding upon the type of temple he/she is planning to dispense to the patient.

Optical Materials and Spectacle Lenses

OPTICAL GLASSES

History

- In the year 423 BC Aristophanes, a Greek play writer, mentioned the use of a convex lens as a burning glass in his play 'Comedy of the Cloud'.
- However, early forms of spectacles were invented in late 13th century and these primary lenses were utilized mainly for correction of presbyopia.
- With the invention of telescope in the year 1608 by Galileo, demand of high quality optical glasses rose abruptly.
- English scientist John Dolland developed an achromatic lens in the year 1757. These achromatic lenses were made up of compounds crown and flint.

Crown glass: Originally window glasses were called crown glass, pieces for these glasses were used to make lenses and were called crown lenses. Nowadays crown glasses are the one which have silica, soda or potash and lime as basic components.

Flint glass: In the year 1676, George Ravenscroft used ground flint as silica source and added lead as basic component to form brighter, clearer, softer and heavier glass which was called flint glass. Nowadays flint glass contains lead oxide primary component along with other crown glass components.

Events of progress

- In the year 1814 PL Guinand of Switzerland revealed that stirring of glass can increase its homogeneity.
- In the year 1827, Michael Faraday developed various methods for purification of glass substances. He designed a platinum melting pot for the purpose of purifying the glass substances, which was considerably resistant to the reaction of melted glass.
- In the year 1839, Chance brothers of England started manufacturing of wide range of optical glasses.
- Later on in the year 1876 Ernst Abbe and Otto Schott of Germany extended the use of chemical oxides in manufacturing of glass and produced an extensive range of all new glasses for optical purposes.
- Until 1880, optical glasses quality available was either crown or flint. In the year 1880, Abbe introduced a glass of high refractive index without any noticeable rise in its dispersive power.
- In the year 1915 Bausch and Lomb Optical Co. started producing an extensive quantity of glasses having very good optical quality. Nowadays Bausch and Lomb, Corning Glass Works, and Pittsburgh Plate Glass Company contribute as major optical glass manufacturers in the world.

Optical glasses have vital properties like

- Refraction index: This is identified at the wavelength (589 nm) for Fraunhofer D line and is denoted by symbol η.
- Dispersion: This is defined as the variation in refraction index with wavelength. This is quantified by Abbe number (v) and is called nu value.

Following characteristics in an optical glass are required to make them useful for ophthalmic purposes

- Physical and chemical stability of high grade
- Transparency of high degree
- Homogenecity in both physical state and chemical composition.
- Appropriate refraction index and chromatic dispersion values.
- Colorless

OPTICAL PLASTICS

Introduction

An organic polymeric material having large molecular weight which can be shaped by flow is referred as plastic material. Most of these plastics are synthetic materials produced by combination of organic and inorganic materials such as carbon, oxygen, nitrogen, hydrogen, chlorine, and sulphur. Commonly, plastic raw materials are derived from fossil-formed products such as oil, coal, and natural gas. Plastics used for optical purposes are very small fraction of total plastics. Materials used in fusion of bifocals should be physically stable; so that no stress occurs along the line of fusion.

Development of optical plastics: Different types of plastic materials were available since many years but use of plastics for production of lens increased primarily during and after World War II. Polymethyl methacrylate (PMMA), also known as Lucite or Plexiglas or Perspex, was one of the major plastic materials developed during World War II. It is a synthetic thermoplastic resin used for production of aircraft windshields. It is more durable than a non-tempered glass but also has a disadvantage of easy scratchability.

Another plastic material developed during World War II was allyl diglycol carbonate commonly called Columbian Resin 39 (CR- 39). A large series of 170 clear allylic materials were compounded when concentrated on a thermosetting in place of a thermoplastic material. The thirty-ninth compound among 170 were designated as CR-39, which was an allyl diglycol carbonate monomer. CR-39 was much more scratch resistant than PMMA.

- Robert Graham in 1947 made first ophthalmic lenses from CR-39.
- In the year 1957 GE Company developed a new plastic material, a polycarbonate resin called Lexan. This material has a great mechanical strength and high service temperature. In the year 1978, first ophthalmic lenses were produced from this material.
- In the year 1982, Corning Glass Works came up with a lens called Corlon. This was a two-layered glass lens where a very thin layer of polyurethane is bonded to the back surface of glass lens.

SPECTACLE LENS MATERIALS

Glass Lenses

As discussed above glass had been used since old ages to form a spectacle lens for correction of refractive anomalies. Main varieties of optical glasses are

- Crown glass
- Flint glass
- Barium crown glass

Crown glass: Glasses having nu value greater than 50 are called crown glasses. Basic components of an ophthalmic crown glass are 70% silica (sand), 14–15% sodium oxide (soda), 11–12% calcium oxide (lime), and small percentages of potassium, antimony, borax, and arsenic. These glasses are mainly used in single vision glass lenses, and also as distance portion in most of the glass bifocal and trifocal lenses. Its refraction index is 1.52 and nu value is 59.

Flint glass: Glasses having nu value less than 50 are called flint glasses. Basic components are 45–65% lead oxide, 25–45% silica, and nearly 10% mixture of soda and potassium oxide. These glasses have more refraction index from 1.58 (light flint) to 1.69 (dense flint) and higher chromatic dispersion with a nu value of 30–40. They are mainly used for near segments in bifocal and also as single vision lenses where thinner lenses are required due to high degree of refractive error.

Barium crown glass: Its basic components are 25–40% barium oxide, along with other crown glass compositions. These glasses have refraction index 1.54 to 1.61 with nu values from 59 to 55. Barium crown glasses are mainly used in near segments of fused bifocals (Nochrome series).

Plastic Lenses

PMMA lenses: Polymethyl methacrylate is a thermosetting plastic material mainly used to manufacture contact lenses, although spectacle lenses such as Igard lens were made in Great Britain by using PMMA material.

Lens properties
- Refraction index: 1.49
- nu value: 57.2
- Specific gravity: 1.19

Advantages of PMMA lenses are
- High order transparency
- Shatter proof
- Light weight
- Tintability
- Optical design versatility

Disadvantages of PMMA lenses are
- Easily scratchability
- Damage due to glazing
- Unsuitable in extremely hot environment

CR-39 Lenses: Ophthalmic lenses prepared from material allyl diglycol carbonate monomer, popularly called CR-39 (Columbia resin 39) were supplied as a yellowish viscous liquid from a single western manufacturer. Initially this manufacturer produced CR-39 lenses in a variety of forms, powers and sizes. Some manufacturers added substances like UV absorbers, anti-yellowing agents and mould releasers to change the properties of lenses for better clinical usage.

Lens properties
- Refraction index: 1.498
- nu value: 58
- Specific gravity: 1.32

Advantages of CR-39 lenses are
- CR-39 lenses are chemically inert to majority of commonly used solvents such as benzene, acetone and gasoline.
- These lenses are highly resistant to impact.
- CR-39 lenses resist pitting from scatter particles especially from welding or grinding machines.
- Fogging due to sudden change in temperatures is less common than glass lenses because of lower thermal conductivity of CR-39 material.
- Other properties like tintability, light weightedness and optical design versatility are similar to PMMA lenses.

Disadvantages of CR-39 lenses are
- Increased lens thickness compared to glass lens due to lower refraction index.
- CR-39 lenses have relative lower resistance than glass lenses for surface aberrations.
- Significant damage to lens surface due to glazing.
- CR-39 lenses loses its photochromatic property in very less duration, hence are not used widely as photochromic lenses.

Polycarbonate Lenses: Polycarbonate is a thermoplastic material exist in solid state which is melted at about 320°C temperature and then injected in a mould to form a lens. A device then squeezes the lens to prevent shrinkage and to ensure the optical accuracy of surfaces. Polycarbonate lenses need a hard coating of surface to increase scratch resistance and chemical protection.

Lens properties
- Refraction index: 1.586
- nu value: 30
- Specific gravity: 1.20

Main advantages are high resistance to impact and higher refraction index, so very thin durable non-breakable lenses can be formed from polycarbonate material. Disadvantages are difficulty in surface molding, lens glazing/fitting and easily scratchability.

Absorptive Lenses

Absorptive lenses have been developed with the purpose to decrease the amount of light transmission or radiant energy, i.e. lens works as a filter. The light absorption may be uniform (absorbs all wavelengths of light) or selective (absorbs some wavelengths). These lenses are not colorless, so they are also called tinted lenses.

Mainly following types of absorptive lenses are routinely manufactured for optical purposes
- Tinted glass lenses
- Tinted plastic lenses
- Glass lenses with surface coatings
- Photochromic lenses
- Younger PLS filter lenses
- Polaroid lenses

Tinted glass lenses: Tinted glass lenses can be produced during manufacturing of crown glass (mixture of silica, soda, lime with small amounts of potassium, aluminium and/or barium oxides) by adding one or more metals or their oxides which results in the formation of different types of tinted color lenses as shown in Table 6.1.

Absorptive lenses have several advantages and disadvantages.

Table 6.1: Metallic oxides and respective tinted color lenses

Metallic oxides	Lens color
Iron	Green
Cobalt	Blue
Manganese	Pink
Cerium	Pinkish brown
Uranium	Yellow
Chromium	Green
Nickel	Brown
Gold	Red
Silver	Yellow
Vanadium	Pale green
Didymium	Pink

Advantages
- Low cost of manufacturing
- Little surface scratching
- Absence of reflection
- No special equipment needed for surfacing and lens finishing

Disadvantages
- Color tint of lenses is permanent in nature.
- High power tinted lenses had variations in transmission of light from central portion to peripheral portion of lens.
- Similarly, in patients having high degree of anisometropia the transmission of light in one eye is variable from fellow eye.

Tinted plastic lenses: Surface of plastic lenses cannot be coated by method of evaporation as there are chances of distortion of lens due to exposure to high temperature. Thus, these lenses are tinted by dropping them in a solution having desired organic dye. Resulting color density of tinted lens depends on two factors: Organic nature of the dye and immersion time.

To achieve a particular type of tint and/ or light transmission; these plastic lens may be immersed into several kinds of tinted solutions. The variation in thickness of lens from center to periphery does not affect the density of tinted lens as penetration of dye in the surface of lens is up to a uniform depth.

Hence, lenses of uniform density are formed. For any reason, if required, the tint color of lens can be changed by dipping the lens in bleaching solution.

Glass lenses with surface coatings: Surface of a glass lens can be tinted by coating it with a layer of metallic oxide by evaporation process under high temperatures in vacuum conditions. As discussed above plastic lenses are unsuitable for this process due to high temperatures. Refraction index of metallic oxide is higher than the glass, hence the amount of light reflecting from absorptive surface is more than that of uncoated surface of glass lens. To prevent this phenomenon of higher light reflection an anti-reflection coating of magnesium fluoride is done over and above the metallic oxide coating.

Photochromic glass lenses: In the year 1964, Corning Glass Works company begins the manufacturing of glass lenses having photochromatic properties, means these lenses become dark in sunlight and converts back to clarity when sunlight exposure is seized.

These lenses are composed with silver halide microscopic crystals. Sunlight (ultraviolet radiation) decomposes these microscopic crystals into silver and halide ions. These ions cluster together and when these clusters get larger they become darker. Hence the lens color appears darker in the presence of sunlight, whereas in the absence of sunlight these silver and halide ions again converted into crystal form. Lens color fades and becomes clear in the absence of sunlight.

Rate of darkening of lens depends on the temperature, faster and deeper degree of darkening occurs in low temperature.

Degree of darkening of lens depends on
- Intensity of the radiation
- Length of exposure
- Surrounding temperature

Similarly, rate of fading of photochromic lenses depends on
- Glass composition

- Thermal bleaching (higher temperature, faster fading)
- Optical bleaching means exposure to a longer wavelength than that used for darkening

Photochromic plastic lenses: Photosensitive plastic for formation of ophthalmic lenses was introduced by American Optical Company (1982) and named the plastic photochromic lens as Photolite. These lenses were manufactured by the process of chemical impregnation rather than a usual dye pot process.

Properties of Photolite lenses are
- It shows about 90% transmittance of light in the faded state and about 45% transmission in dark state.
- Within 2 minutes time lens become darker to 45% out of total darkened state.
- Similar to other photochromic materials, less is the temperature of surrounding more will be the darkening of lens.
- Normally Photolite (fully activated) lens turns into blue color however, it can also be tinted to different colors.
- Life expectancy of Photolite lenses is nearly 2 years.

Younger PLS filter lenses: In the year 1984 Younger optics introduced a series of CR-39 lenses, called as Protective Lens Series (PLS). These lenses were design to protect the eyes by using selective filters for invisible ultraviolet and visible blue radiation. PLS lenses are neither photochromic nor tinted, rather are manufactured in a specific manner. Protective additives are added throughout the lens material uniformly so that these additives cannot be bleached or removed.

A specific wavelength is nominated to these PLS filter lenses as product code; below this wavelength these lenses literally block all of the ultraviolet and blue visible radiations.

A few specific product code lenses are summarized in Table 6.2.

Product code	Natural color of PLS filter lens	Wavelength designated	UV and blue radiation blockage (%)
PLS 400 lens	Pale yellow color	<400 nm	Approx. 100
PLS 530 lens	Orange-amber color	530 nm	95–97
PLS 540 lens	Brown color lens	540 nm	95–97
PLS 550 lens	Red color lens	550 nm	95–97

Table 6.2: Various PLS filter lenses and their properties

> **Note**
>
> Using standard methods for cosmetic tint, the natural color of any of these PLS filter lenses can be changed without disturbing the lens performance.

Uses

- PLS lenses are advised to be used for protection against ultraviolet and visible blue radiations, because many researchers concluded that short wavelength radiations such as ultraviolet and blue radiations are harmful for eyes.
- These lenses are successfully used for protection in patients having ocular conditions like cataracts, corneal dystrophies, macular degeneration, and retinitis pigmentosa.

Polaroid lenses: As discussed in Chapter 1 and as shown in Fig. 6.1 normally light beam is circularly symmetrical and unpolarized (Fig. 6.1A) but when it passes through crystals like quartz or calcite it becomes polarized (Fig. 6.1C), however, in between some light rays may also emit as partially polarized rays (Fig. 6.1B).

To manufacture polaroid filters, a thin sheet of polyvinyl alcohol is heated and then stretched so that it becomes about four times of its original length. Due to effect of stretching the molecular structure of polyvinyl alcohol get aligns in the form of long chain in the direction parallel to the stretching. The thin sheet of polyvinyl alcohol is then passed through a solution of weak iodine so that iodine molecules diffuse into layers of polyvinyl and gets attached to chains of long polyvinyl alcohol molecules. Hence, a thin

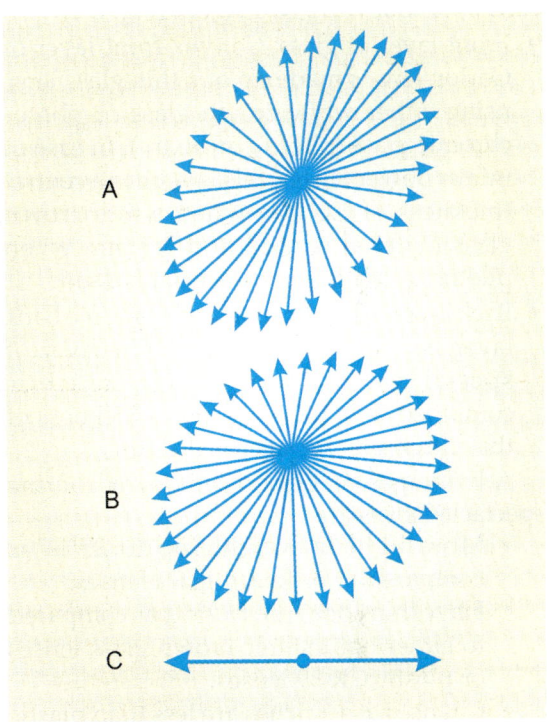

Fig. 6.1: Polarization of light. A. Unpolarized rays; B. Partially polarized rays; C. Linear polarized ray

sheet of polarizing filter is formed which is then laminated between two layers of coated cellulose acetate butyrate. These laminated sheets can be pressed into the desired curvature to form a lens. To create polarized glass lenses from thin sheet of polarizing material, the thin sheet is laminated between two layers of glass which then tinted and surfaced with power according to choice. In standard polarized sunglasses lenses, the tinted layer over lens has a uniform thickness, thus density of the lenses is uniform from center to periphery of lens. Sometimes, to increase the absorptive power of lens for ultraviolet radiations, special additives can be added in tint coating.

The Corlon lens: Corning manufacturers (1982) introduced a new specialized type of spectacle lens known as Corlon or bonded lenses because this lens was manufactured using both glass and plastic materials. Corlon lenses consist of following two layers (Fig. 6.2)

- Front layer of glass: Convex front layer of Corlon lens is made up of a thin glass lens, using either white crown glass or photochromic glass (photo grey extra). In case of minus power lenses, this layer has a central thickness of 1.3 mm when white crown glass material is used and 1.5 mm when photochromatic glass material is used.
- Back layer of plastic material: Concave back layer is made up of a very thin layer of special polyurethane plastic which is combined with the glass lens. Thickness of this polyurethane layer is 0.4 mm.

Advantages of Corlon lens over routine spectacle lenses are

- More light in weight (up to 25%) as compared to ordinary glass lenses.
- Have thin edges (up to 25%) as compared to either ophthalmic crown glass lenses or plastic CR-39 lenses.
- Chances of scratches are less than plastic lenses because front surface is made up of glass.

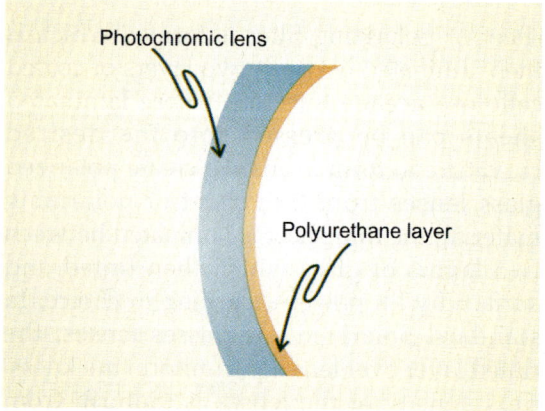

Fig. 6.2: Corlon lens

- More resistant to shock caused by impacting object because of its two-layer construction. Impact of an object can break the front glass layer but polyurethane layer remains intact which protects the eyes from injuries due to glass particles.
- Its unique construction design eliminate the need for tempering because Corlon lens is more resistant from back surface infiltration as compared to both white crown glass and CR-39 plastic lenses.
- Its photochromic layer is thinner compared to a regular photogray lens so Corlon lenses darken less than regular lens.
- Polyurethane layer of the Corlon lens can easily be tinted by technicians in desired solid colors or gradient tints by using special types of water based dyes for better cosmetic looks.

SPECTACLE LENSES

Spectacle Lens Design

Spherical Lens Design

- Most primitive ophthalmic spherical lenses were of biconvex type, however, biconcave ophthalmic lenses were also produced in later years. Both types of lenses were easy to manufacture but these lenses had very weak surface powers and having same curvatures on both the sides.
- In subsequent years, with development of more manufacturing techniques flat ophthalmic lenses (flat plus lens with flat back surface, minus flat lens with flat front surface) were also produced.
- Later on, in the year 1804, meniscus (convex –concave or moon-shaped) form of lens was introduced by William Wollaston, and named them 'periscopic lenses' because of their property to provide a wider field of vision.
- Nietzsche and Gunther (German company) in 1867 developed uniform surface lenses of 1.25 D and termed them 'periscopic lens'. The plus lenses were having –1.25 D back surface and minus lenses were having a

+1.25 D front surface. They also introduced 6.00 D base curve lens where plus spherical lenses had the back surface power of –6 D and a minus spherical lens had front surface power of +6.00 D.

- Tscherning (1904–1908) first identified the importance of center of rotation of the eye as a reference point in the lens design. He proposed that an oblique astigmatism might be eliminated by using two forms of bent lenses, i.e. deeper and shallower form.
- Moritz von Rohr (1908) worked on spectacle lenses with the aim to eliminate the oblique astigmatism and made following conclusions
  - Each lens has a specific thickness.
  - Distance between center of rotation of eye and back pole of lens was 25 mm.
  - Viewing angle for plus lenses was 35° and for minus lenses was 30° and viewing distance was infinity.
  - Sphero-cylindrical lenses can be manu-factured in plus toric form.
  - He also described the back vertex system
- Subsequently, in the year 1913, Zeiss Optical Company started production of lens based on von Rohr's lens design as Punktal (point-forming) lens.
- In the year 1919, Edgar Tillyer designed lenses which were flatter than Punktal lenses. He considered both oblique astigmatism and curvature of image factors in his design. In the year 1923, American Optical Company commercially made these lenses available under the trade name Tillyer.
- In the year 1920, Kurova corrected curve lenses were developed by Continental Optical Company which were later on redesigned by FE Duckwall in 1925. These lenses were having 39 base curves ranging from +2.5 to +12.5 D powers.
- Wilbur Rayton designed Orthogon lenses with the aim to correct oblique astigmatism like Punktal lens. However, correction of curvature of image was not included in this design. These lenses were slightly steeper as compared to Tillyer lenses. In the year

1928, Bausch and Lomb Optical Company initiated production of Orthogon lenses.

- On the basis of 14 base curves, Shuron Optical Company designed Widesite lenses which all were made in a positive toric form.
- In the year 1950, famous Normalsite correc-ted curve lens series (designed by Foster Klingaman) was developed by Titmus Optical Company. These Normalsite lenses were flatter as compared to other lenses.
- In early 1964, Univis Lens Company introduced the Best-form lenses which were negative toric lenses designed by EW Bechtold.
- In the year 1966, Shuron-Continental Company developed a negative toric lens series called Kurova Shursite. The bending curvatures of the Shursite negative toric lenses were similar to those of Shuron Continental Kurova positive toric lenses.

Spherocylindrical Lens Design

Astigmatic lenses designed for correction of astigmatism consist of a spherical surface on one side and a toric surface on the other side with two principal meridians. One meridian of lens has minimum power and other meridian has maximum power. The total sum of powers of two surfaces in each principal meridian remains fixed so that an image of the lens/eye system is aligned with axial vision. As these lens design have two powers so when light ray from a point object situated on the optical axis of the eye falls on a sphero-cylindrical lens, it results in formation of an astigmatic pencil after refraction, which in succession pass through two focal lines.

Negative and positive toric lenses: Previously, all corrected- curve spherocylindrical lenses were developed as positive toric lenses but many researchers have redesigned them as negative toric lenses also. Advantages of negative toric lenses are that

- Most of the multifocal lenses are negative toric lenses where bifocal addition is given on the front surface.

- Negative toric lenses play an important role in the spectacle magnification factors. In positive toric lenses two front surface powers and two back surface powers are present, whereas in negative toric lenses front surface power is the same for both meridians. Hence, front surface powers contribute in a spectacle magnification difference between two surfaces in positive toric lenses and not in negative toric lenses.

Design of High Plus Lenses

It has been seen that by using ophthalmic lenses with spherical surfaces an oblique astigmatism in the range of –23 D to +7 D can be eliminated, however, beyond this range it was impossible to remove oblique astigmatism. In regular clinical practice, patients having refractive error more than –23 D are rarely seen, however, aphakic patients usually require more than +10 D power of optical correction. Though, contact lenses are good alternative to spectacles but many of these patients being old are not comfortable with contact lens. These persons who required more than +4D to + 6D correction of oblique astigmatism in lens can be prescribed aspherical surface lens design instead of a routine spherical surface. Aspheric surfaces are the one where power of lens gradually decreases toward its periphery. In other words, an aspheric surface is the one which is axially symmetrical and is formed by the rotation of a portion of an ellipse, a parabola, or a hyperbola. David Volk (1958) developed aspheric spectacle glass lenses known as Conoid lenses. Production cost of aspheric lenses has decreased greatly due to wide acceptance of CR-39 plastic lens material because these lenses could easily be manufactured by a molding process instead of routinely used grinding process.

Terminologies in Spectacle Lenses

To understand the details of above type of lenses we need to know these terminologies related to lenses.

Blanks

Zero powered roughly finished slabs of glass are called blanks. Commonly, these glass slabs are available in different diameter sizes of 50 mm, 55 mm, 60 mm and 65 mm, however, very large size blank, say 70 mm or 75 mm are also available for specific indications. Thickness of these blanks range from 4 to 14 mm at 2 mm steps.

All ophthalmic blanks have following two refractive surfaces with a resultant zero power

- Base curve
- Combining surface

Base Curve

It is a standard fixed power curve of a blank. Available base curves are with a standard power of zero D, 1.25 D, 2 D, 4 D and 6 D, however, best form lenses have a base curve of either 1.25 D or 6 D power.

Combining Surface

This is the other surface of blank on which desired power is grounded. Net power of the lens is produced by grinding the respective combining surface of a blank provided by manufactures. To get a net plus power lens, a blank having minus base curve is used and to get a minus power lens, a plus base curve blank is used.

For example, in Fig. 6.3A, to get a lens of +2 D, –6 D base curve blank is used and a +8 D power is grinded on combining surface of the blank to produce a net +2 D power lens. Similarly, as shown in Fig. 6.3B, to produce a –2 D lens, a +6 D base curve blank is used and a –8 D power is grinded on combining surface of the blank to produce a final –2 D power lens.

Lens Power

Refracting power of an ophthalmic lens can be expressed in several ways like

- Approximate power which is also called nominal power when the power of an ophthalmic lens is expressed in terms of its

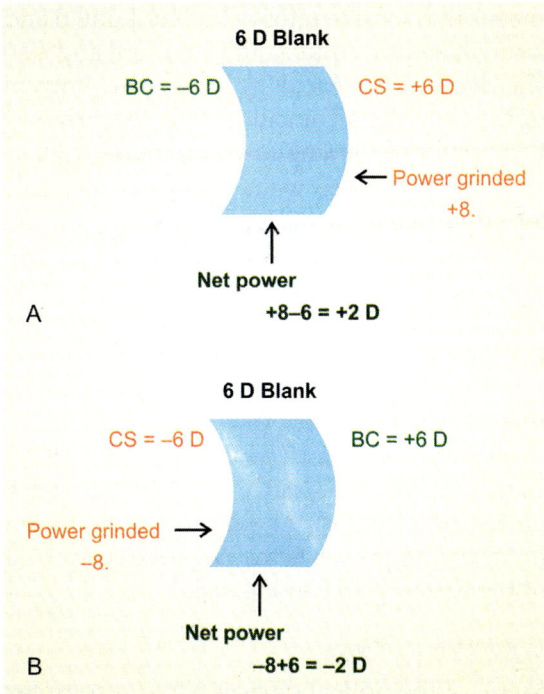

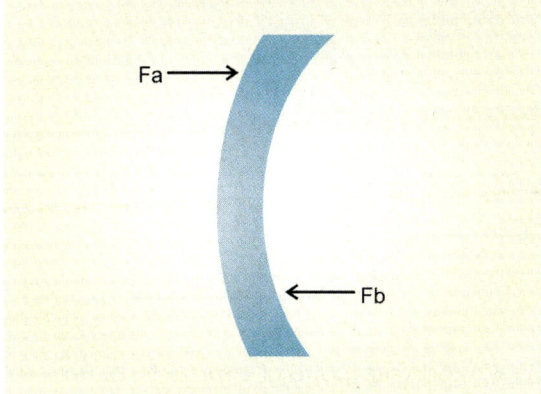

Fig. 6.4: Front (Fa) and back (Fb) powers of lens

Fig. 6.3: 6 D Blanks. BC: Base curve having fixed 6 D power CS: combination surface, used to grind power. A. Minus 6 D blank; B. Plus 6 D blank

In this formula for power calculation, thickness of lens is not considered as it is presumed that a lens has zero thickness. However, in reality most of the ophthalmic lenses cannot be considered to be markedly thin, thus we need a more accurate expression for calculation of lens power which includes back vertex power, front vertex power, and equivalent power.

front and back surface powers irrespective of lens thickness.

- Back vertex power and front vertex power when ophthalmic lens power is considered in terms of refracting power for emergent rays from its back surface or front surface.
- Equivalent power when power of a thick ophthalmic lens or optical system is equated as power of a single thin lens.
- Effective power: Here the power of an ophthalmic lens is dependent upon its distance from the wearer's eye.

Approximate Power

Approximate power of an ophthalmic lens is calculated by

$$P = Fa + Fb$$

Here Fa and Fb represents the powers of front and back surface, respectively (Fig. 6.4) and can be measured by lens measure or lens clock.

> **Note**
>
> Among all these expressions of power specification, practically only back vertex power is used by optical laboratories and practitioners to specify an ophthalmic lens power.

Back Vertex Power

This is expressed as the reciprocal of the back focal length [i.e. distance from the back pole (vertex) of lens (L2) to the second focal point (F′)]. The second focal point is the actual distance divided by the refractive index of ophthalmic lens media. In this Fig. 6.5, back vertex power of lens (F′v) in air is expressed as the reciprocal of the distance L2 to F′.

Back vertex power is considered important parameter to indicate the power of an ophthalmic lens because

- As discussed above to measure back vertex power, two points, i.e. back vertex of lens and second focal point are

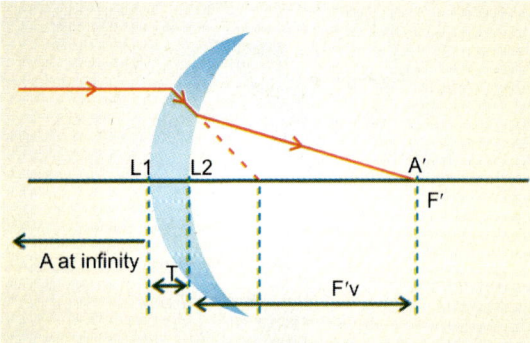

Fig. 6.5: Back vertex power of lens in air. L1, L2: Front and back refractive surfaces of ophthalmic lens respectively. F': Secondary focal point. T: Thickness of lens

considered. If we select such a power of lens at which the second focal point of the lens is placed at far point of the eye then lens can easily be placed at any position in front of the eye. Hence, an ophthalmic lens if placed either in a spectacle plane or on the cornea (contact lens) we can still be able to specify its back vertex power to get the expected optical effect.

- Back vertex power permits an indefinite utilization in terms of lens form like bend or cross section shape of ophthalmic lenses. We can use any form of ophthalmic lens either for examination purpose or fitting process in clinical practice. What we have to do is just to ensure that secondary focal point of our ophthalmic lens coincide with the far point of eye.

Note

Back vertex power can be measured by an instrument lensometer or vertometer.

Front vertex power or neutralizing power: The power of an unknown ophthalmic lens can be measured by neutralizing it with trial lens of known power. When these two lenses are positioned in close contact, these lenses are considered to neutralize the power of each other when their measured total refracting power becomes zero. The neutralization

means that focal lengths of both unknown and known lens are equivalent in amount and also the secondary focal point of the known ophthalmic lens coincides with the primary focal point of the unknown ophthalmic lens.

Routinely, when we neutralize a spectacle lens by placing the back pole of a trial lens on the front pole of the spectacle lens then we are measuring the front vertex power of spectacle lens. Hence, front vertex power is defined as the negative reciprocal of the reduced distance from the front pole (L1) of the lens to its primary focal point (F).

An expression for front vertex power (Fv) can be derived in a similar way as that for back vertex power (F'v). As per above definition neutralizing power is the negative reciprocal of the distance L1F in Fig. 6.6.

Equivalent Power

Many of the optical devices act as a complex optical system as they contain a series of lenses which remain separated either by air or by media of different refractive indices. Sometimes, it is suitable to consider this complex system of lens as an imaginary single thin lens (equivalent lens) so that it becomes easy to find out object–image relationship of equivalent lens. It is assumed that this imaginary single lens will produce the image of a distant object

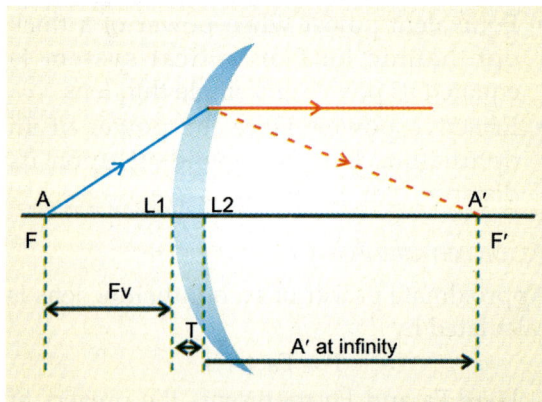

Fig. 6.6: Front vertex power of lens in air. L1, L2: Front and back refractive surfaces of ophthalmic lens respectively. F: Primary focal point. T: Thickness of lens

of same size and at same position as produced by series of lenses of optical system. The focal length of this imaginary single lens (equivalent lens) at which image of same size and at the same position produced similar to those by optical system is known as equivalent focal length. The reciprocal of this equivalent focal length (meters) is called the equivalent power.

Position of this thin equivalent lens with respect to the system is determined by locating the principal planes of the optical system. In symmetrical optical systems only a single pair of planes is present; which poses the property of positive unity (+1) magnification (means the object and its image are of same size and image is erect). These pairs of planes are called principal planes and the points of intersection of optical axis with these planes are principal points of optical system.

- Principal plane associated with the object space is termed primary principal plane and plane with the image space is secondary principal plane.
- The distance from the primary principal point (P1) to primary focal point (F) is called primary equivalent focal length (Fe) as shown in Fig. 6.7.
- Similarly, the distance from secondary principal point (P2) to the secondary focal point (F') is called secondary equivalent focal length (Fe'). The reciprocal of the secondary equivalent focal length is the equivalent power of an optical system.

Effective Power

An ability of a lens to focus parallel light rays at a specified plane is termed effective power of that lens. The term effective power is mainly considered to define the requirement of change in the power of lens when the lens is moved from one position to another position in front of the eye.

Practically we consider that plus lenses are more effective because when these lenses are moved farther away from the eyes they produce more change in vergence than required. While minus lenses are considered as less effective because when these lenses are moved farther away from the eyes, they produce less change in vergence than required.

Classification of Spectacle Lenses

Spectacle lens classification is summarized in Table 6.3. The specific features of each type of lens in relation to spectacle fitting purposes have also been explained.

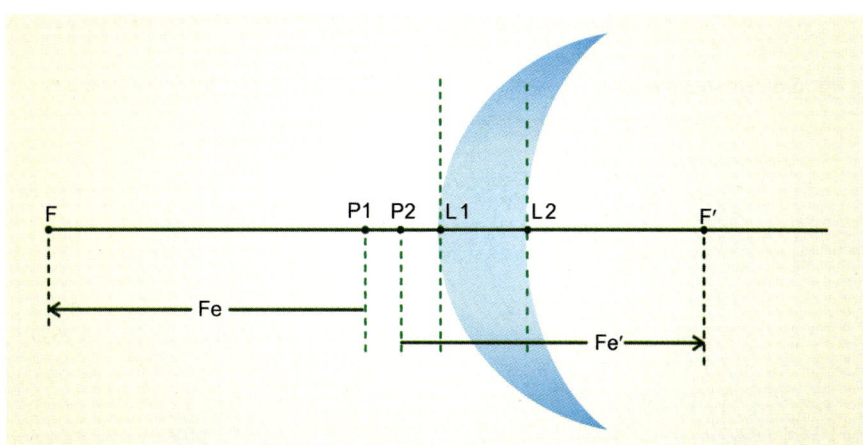

Fig. 6.7: Primary and secondary equivalent focal length. L1, L2: Front and back refractive surfaces of ophthalmic lens respectively. F: Primary focal point; F': Secondary focal point, P1: Primary principle plane, P2: Secondary principle plane, Fe: Primary equivalent focal length, Fe': Secondary equivalent focal length

Table 6.3: Classification of spectacle lenses	
Based on lens form	*Based on corrective power*
Symmetrical	Monofocal lenses
Asymmetrical	Plano focal lenses
Plano	Multiple focal lenses
Periscopic	• Bifocal lenses
Deep meniscus	• Tritocal lenses
Lenticular	• Varifocal or progressive lenses
Aspheric	

Various Lens Forms

Symmetrical lenses: When curvatures of both the surfaces of lenses are same, they are called symmetrical lenses as shown in Fig. 6.8.

Asymmetrical lenses: Ophthalmic lenses having different curvatures of both the surfaces are called asymmetrical lenses as shown in Fig. 6.9.

Plano lenses: In these types of lenses one surface has zero power or plane, whereas other surface has curvature. For example, Plano convex or plano concave as shown in Fig. 6.10.

Periscopic lenses: These lenses are considered as best form lens having a base curve of 1.25 as shown in Fig. 6.11 and on combined surface

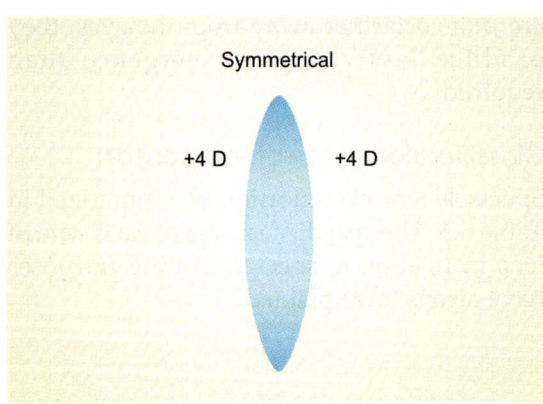

Fig. 6.8: Symmetrical lens

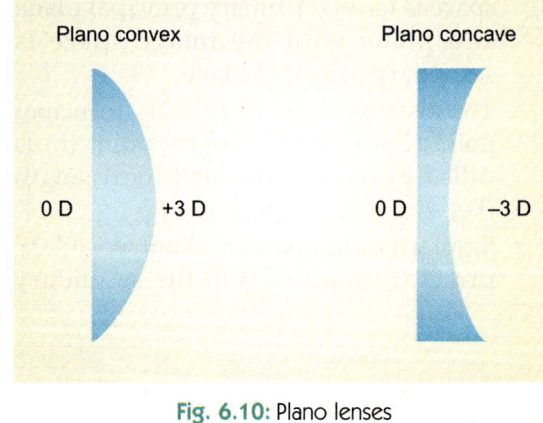

Fig. 6.10: Plano lenses

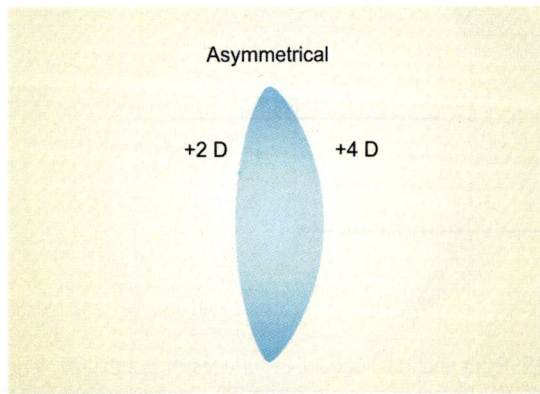

Fig. 6.9: Asymmetrical lenses

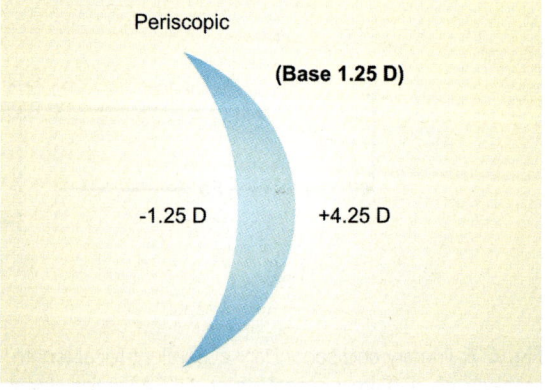

Fig. 6.11: Periscopic lens

(+4.25 D in our example) power for final lens is grinded.

Deep meniscus lenses: These lenses are also a type of best form lens where base curve is of 6 D as shown in Fig. 6.12 and on its combined surface (+11 D in our example) power for final lens is grinded.

Lenticular lenses: These lenticular lenses were designed by Obrig (1933) for correction of high degree myopia and named them Myo-disc. A small concave disc was grinded on the back surface of a Plano lens for formation of this thin and light weight Myo-disc lens as shown in Fig. 6.13. Most of the lenticular lenses which were manufactured later on were almost similar to this original Myo-disc lens in their designing.

Most of the lenticular lenses contain a powered central portion (optical zone) called as aperture which is about 30–40 mm in diameter. This aperture is surrounded by a carrier lens, having Plano or low plus power. Initially, these lenses were prepared with the aim to reduce the thickness of lens, hence in past for many years majority of the glass aphakic lenses were made in lenticular form with some minor percentage of plastic lenses.

Various types of lenticular lenses are

- **Solid state lenticular lenses:** Here the carrier is cut in a convex shape from the base lens as shown in Fig. 6.14 and this design is mainly used for plastic lenses.
- **Fused lenticular lenses:** Here aperture is fused on back surface of plus power lens under high temperatures and then desired power is grounded on the front surface (Fig. 6.15). These types of lenses are mainly used for glass lenses.

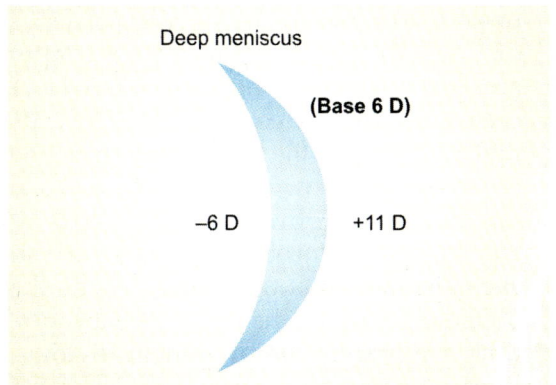

Fig. 6.12: Deep meniscus lens

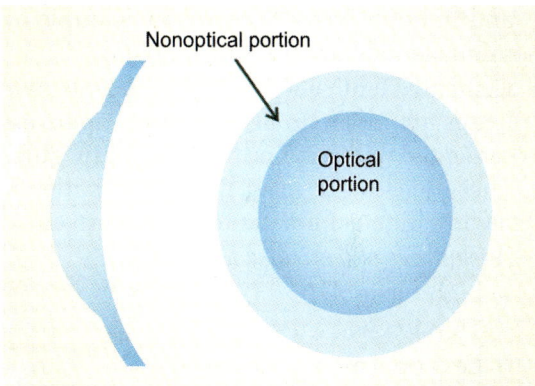

Fig. 6.14: Solid state one piece lenticular lenses

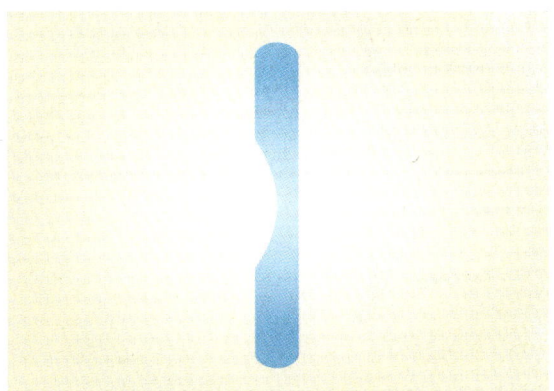

Fig. 6.13: Original Myo-disc lens designs

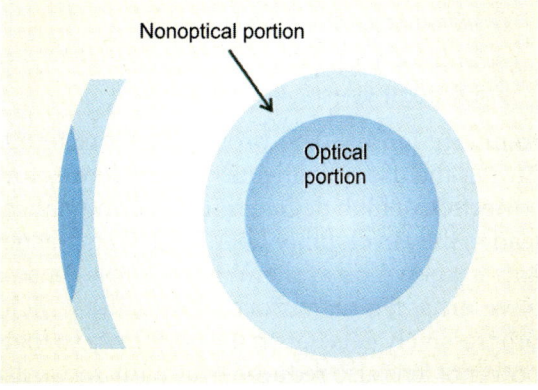

Fig. 6.15: Fused lenticular lenses

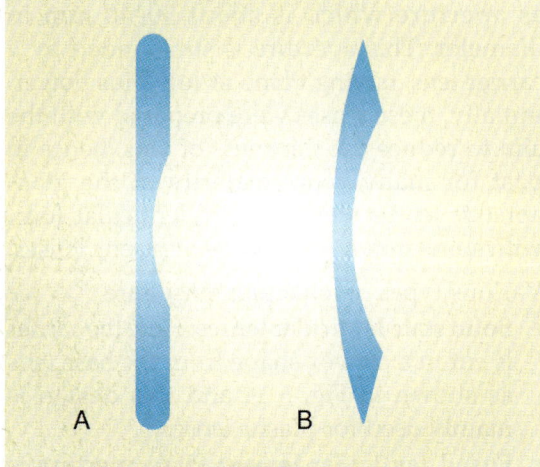

Fig. 6.16: Plano lenticular lenses. A. Concave aperture; B. Convex aperture

- **Plano lenticular lenses:** These lenses have either a convex or concave surface aperture and a plane surface carrier as shown in Fig. 6.16A and B. Initial Myo-discs are an example of minus lenticular lenses of these types.
- **Cemented lenticular lenses:** These lenticular lenses are made up of a spherical aperture cemented with a cylindrical carrier by glue. These lenses are used mainly in patients having high astigmatic refractive errors.

Advantages of lenticular lenses
- Light weight
- Thin lenses
- Less optical aberrations
- Less spectacle magnification
- Correct high refractive errors

Disadvantages of lenticular lenses
- Bull's eye or fried egg appearance
- Difficult spectacle fitting

Aspheric lenses: The problem encountered during the use of lenticular design lenses for correction of high degree refractive anomalies lead to the development of new design plastic lenses known as aspheric lens. These lenses have an aspheric surface (ellipsoid) which progressively gets flat on the periphery so that power of lens also reduced gradually towards the periphery, thus especially useful in aphakic patients. In addition, aspheric lenses also pose the advantages of lenticular form lenses, i.e. reduced aberrations of lenses along with reduced thickness and weight. To prepare ophthalmic aspheric lens design mostly conicoid (ellipse, parabola, or hyperbola) surfaces were used.

Presently to form aspheric surface for an ophthalmic lens, two manufacturing approaches are used

- American Optical Fulvue manufactures aspherical lenses which have a continuous aspheric surface. The curvature of continuous aspheric lens decreases constantly from its central portion toward the periphery as shown in Fig. 6.17. Hence, there is a continuous reduction in refractive power towards the edge or periphery due to reduction in curvature of the lens.
- Annular pattern arrangement aspheric lens designs: The lens surface consists of series of different zones (spherical in shape) around the center. The surface power of each zone progressively decreases towards periphery, means the farthest zone from the center has least power and the nearest zone has maximum power. The tangents to curves of adjacent zones are arranged in such a manner that they coincide with the boundary between the two adjacent zones; thus eliminating the prominent dividing lines on aspheric surface. The junctions

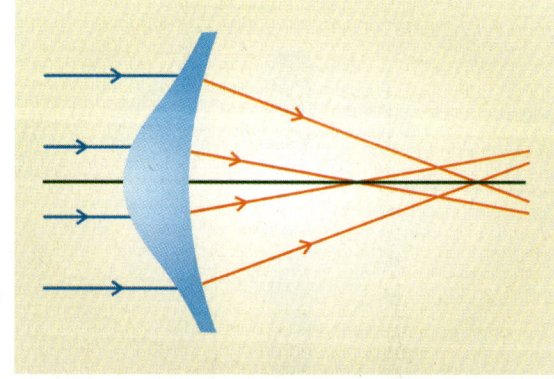

Fig. 6.17: Continuous aspheric lens design showing reduced surface focusing light rays nearer

present between two adjacent zones are made smooth by polishing the surface with flexible pads. Armorlite multi-drop lens formerly called Welsh four drop lens is one of the examples of aspheric design lens.

Monofocal Lenses

These are the lenses used to correct either distance vision or near vision problems, hence are also called single vision glasses. These lenses are either spherical or spherocylindrical in nature. Entire surface of these lenses has the same corrective power, hence are used to correct refractive anomalies such as myopia, hypermetropia, and astigmatism with presbyopia. Various designs of these types of lenses had already been discussed above.

Plano focal lenses: These lenses are similar to bifocal lenses in the shapes and designs but the upper portion of the lens is used for distance vision correction, has no optical power or plane, whereas the near segment has an appropriate power to correct presbyopia. These types of lenses are very useful in patient's having only presbyopic errors who perform continuous near work, if they use single vision glasses they need to remove the glasses very frequently to see the distance objects clearly.

Bifocal Lenses

- Invention of the bifocal lens was done by the scientist Benjamin Franklin in the year 1785, to avoid discomfort due to wearing of two separate spectacles for distance and near vision; he cuts both the glasses into halves and fixed them in a single spectacle frame as shown in Fig. 6.18. The bifocal lens designed by Franklin has looks similar to executive single piece bifocal (available nowadays) with a dividing line on the lens.

  Although these bifocals showed excellent optical property, but the dividing line across the lens produced reflections and had a tendency to collect dust, causing discomfort to wearer. The structural

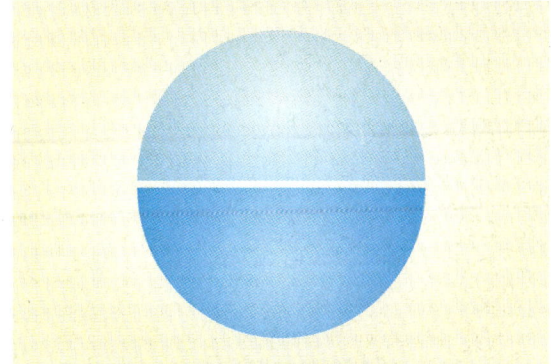

Fig. 6.18: Original Benjamin Franklin lens design

strength of lens was poor as both portions of lens were kept in positions with the help of eye wire of the frame.

- In the year 1838, Isaac Schnaitmann developed a type of bifocal lens called solid up-curve bifocal and it was first one-piece bifocal lens which gained popularity. This lens was having good structural strength, invisible dividing line, less chances of chromatic aberration and provided wide field of view for reading than Franklin lens. However, in the distance portion of lens significant amount of aberrations were noticed, hence restricted the field of vision for distance. Moreover, a strong base down prismatic effect was seen in the distance part of lens.

- August Morck (1888) developed modified form of Franklin bifocal and named it perfection bifocal lenses. Perfection bifocal contained a curved dividing line. Each glass piece of lens had beveled edge which led to more stabilization of lens in the spectacle frame as shown in Fig. 6.19. Morck also invented cemented bifocal design in the year 1888.

- John Borsch (1889) took another step in bifocal invention and developed cemented Kryptok bifocal lenses.

- In the year 1915, Henry Courmettes further improved the design of fused bifocals; by fusing a button (segment) into the major lens, which was made up of two types of glasses.

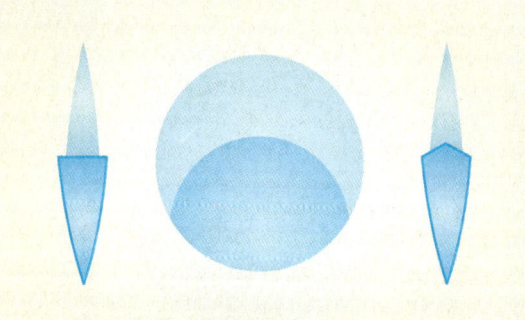

Fig. 6.19: Perfection bifocal lens design

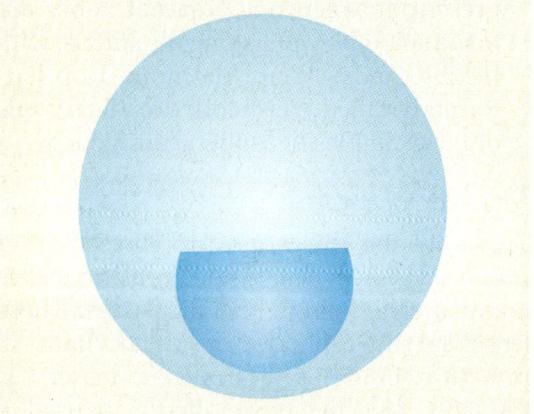

Fig. 6.21: Bifocal 'D' segment lens design

- Charles Conner (in 1910) produced a bifocal lens which was grounded from a single piece of glass, having a uniform refraction index. He called this lens Ultex bifocal.
- American Optical Company (in 1954) took the next step for the development and manufacturing of one-piece bifocal known as executive bifocal.

Bifocal lenses are broadly classified as summarized in Table 6.4.

Single Segment Bifocals

Cemented bifocals: In the year 1888, Morck invented the cemented bifocal lens. To produce cemented bifocal lens, a piece of thin glass (having refractive index similar to major lens) was cemented/glued on the back surface of the major lens as shown in Fig. 6.22. Morck used Canada balsam as cementing or glued

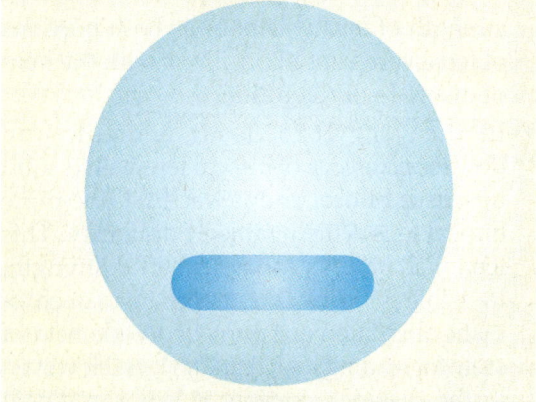

Fig. 6.20: Bifocal 'B' or bar segment lens design

- Subsequently, in the year 1931, Watson and Culver designed and also patented the bifocal "B" or bar segment bifocal lens (straight top) as shown in Fig. 6.20.

    Almost during the same period four inventors filed identical patent applications for the "D" style segment (looks like a letter D, lying on its back) as shown in Fig. 6.21. Finally, in the year 1933, NH Stanley got the patent, for this D style segment.
- Silverman (1932) developed the "R" or ribbon segment and patented R-compensated series of lenses; which contain 7 segments (R4 to R10) designed to compensate for vertical prismatic effects in the near vision.
- Hammon and Price modified the 'D' style design called as Panoptik (having rounded corners) and Widesite (having curved-top version).

Table 6.4: Classification of bifocal lenses	
Single segment bifocals	Double segment bifocals
Cemented bifocals	Fused double D segment bifocals
Fused bifocals	Double segment executive bifocals
One piece bifocals	Mixed double segment bifocals
Special type bifocals • Minus add bifocals • Golfers' bifocals	

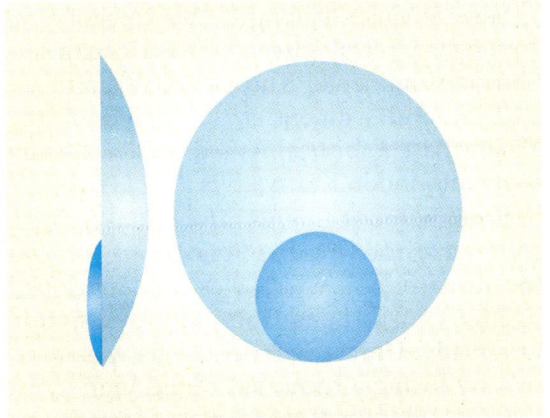

Fig. 6.22: Cemented bifocal lens design

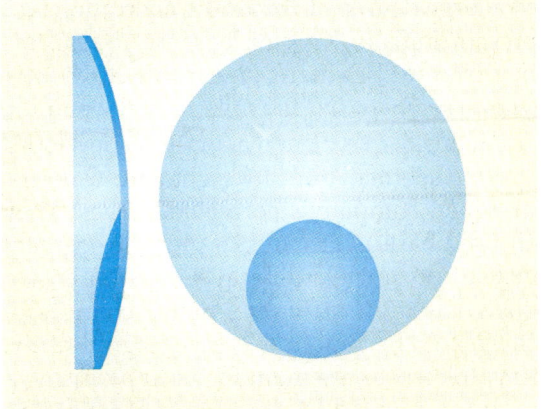

Fig. 6.23: Kryptok lens design popularly called KT

material because the refractive index of Canada balsam was equal to glass. The curvature of both, i.e. front surface of glass piece and the back surface of the major lens were equal hence no change in refractive power had occurred between these two surfaces. Power of addition was simply the difference between the powers of back surfaces of major lens and glass piece; as the back surface of glass piece was kept less concave as compared to the back surface of major lens.

Advantages
- Optically acceptable.
- Cosmetically widely accepted, hence was used nearly for a century.

Disadvantages
- Chances of dust collection on shoulder around the dividing line.
- Temperature changes were affecting the adherence property of the glass piece.
- Glass piece had a propensity to fall off easily with long usage.
- Cement was getting darken with use and time.

In the year 1889, Borsch developed Kryptok (means hidden) cemented bifocal lens. He created a countersink curve, like a depression on the front surface of major lens. Then a wafer or glass piece (flint glass) of refractive index 1.67 was cemented into this countersink area.

Finally, the surface of entire lens was covered with a thin meniscus of glass cemented in place (Fig. 6.23).

These were the first bifocal lens where refractive index of reading addition (near segment) material was higher (1.67) than the major lens.

> **Note**
>
> Occasionally, in some special conditions like low vision aid, temporary bifocals or for experimental purposes these cemented bifocals are still used and an Epoxy resin (Araldite) is used in place of Canada balsam as cementing material for better stability.

Disadvantages
- Difficult to manufacture because six surfaces needed to be grounded and polished.
- Lens covering of thin meniscus glass was very fragile.
- Darkening of cementing material.
- Chances of dislocation or separation of lens

Fused Bifocal Lenses: Most widely used bifocal lenses are fused types of bifocals and hence available in several segment styles like
- Round segments
- Straight top segments
- Modified straight top segments

Round segments bifocal lenses: Original Kryptok bifocal lenses were low in cost but made of flint glass (small nu value) segment so a large degree of chromatic aberration was present. Initially, Kryptok lenses were available in different segment sizes, but now only 22 mm segment size is available in the market.

Gradually, every lens manufacturer developed a round segment bifocal lens having a specific designed company's corrected curves. They all used barium crown glass for the segment instead of flint glass because barium crown glass has high nu value, hence chances of chromatic aberrations decreased significantly. Kryptok lenses are manufactured by fusing a round segment inside the groove of major lens as shown in Fig. 6.24.

Normally the segment size in the round fused bifocal lenses is of 22 mm in diameter, with the segment optical center located at 11 mm below the segment top in an uncut lens form (Fig. 6.25).

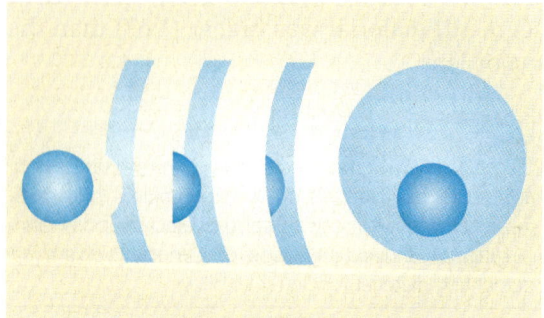

Fig. 6.24: Manufacturing process for round segment bifocal (Kryptok) lens

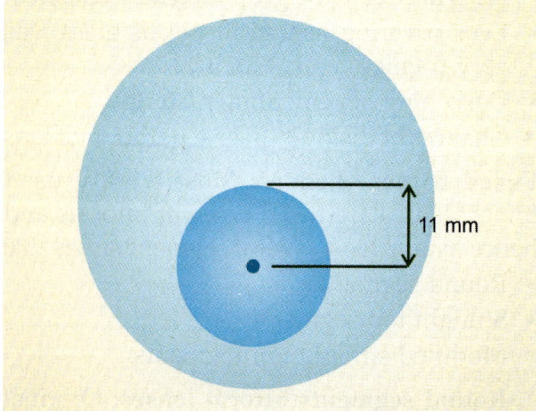

Fig. 6.25: Locations of segment and optical center in round segment bifocal lens

Several lenses belong to this category are American Optical Tillyer, Univis Unachrome, Shuron Continental Kurova and Vision Ease CRF. Round segment size in Univis R and Vision Ease R bifocal lenses is 22 × 14 mm segments and in Kurova B is 28 × 14 mm.

Straight top segments bifocal lenses: Most commonly used types of bifocal are straight top fused bifocal which was first developed by the Univis Lens Company of Dayton. Originally, Univis Sentinel D lens was made first by fusing a truncated round high index segment with small crown glass segment and then fusing this entire segment into a counter-sink area of major lens as shown in Fig. 6.26.

Once the patent of Univis got expired, straight top bifocal lenses were produced by many other lens manufacturers like American Optical Tillyer D, Masterpiece S, Shuron Continental Kurova D, and Vision Ease D. All of these lenses are available in various segment sizes as 22 × 16 mm, 25 × 17.5 mm, and 28 × 19 mm. Tillyer Masterpiece S bifocal lens is also available in a 20 × 15.5 mm segment and Vision Ease D in a 35 × 22.5 mm segment.

Courmettes fusing process of 'D' bifocal lens manufacturing involves usage of a button made up of two different types of glasses. This button is fused in a countersink area present in the major lens and a finally finished lens is manufactured as shown in Fig. 6.27.

Initially upper edge of the straight top segment was located 6 mm above the optical centre but finally after fusing the resultant segment optical center came 5 mm below the

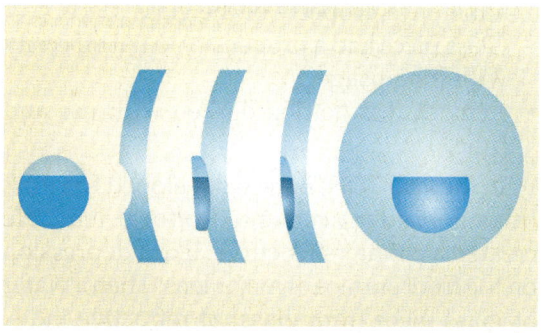

Fig. 6.26: Straight top bifocal lens manufacturing process

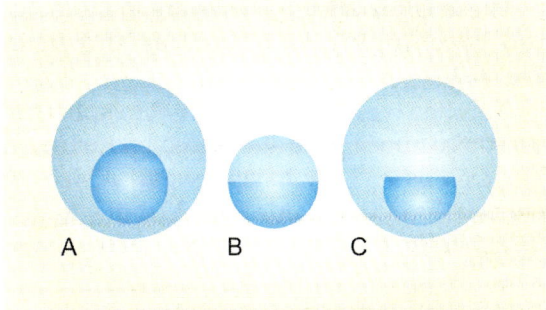

Fig. 6.27: Courmettes fusing process. A. Major lens with counter sink area; B. Button made up of two glasses; C. Finally fused bifocal 'D' lens

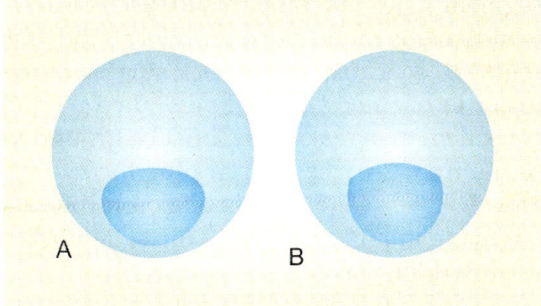

Fig. 6.29: Modified bifocal 'D' segment lens designs. A. Panoptic design with rounded edges; B. Widesite design with curved top

segment top margin (against 11 mm below top margin in round segment lenses) as shown in Fig. 6.28.

Modified straight top segment bifocal lenses: Enormous success of Univis straight top bifocal lenses encouraged other manufactures to develop modified forms of straight top bifocal. Panoptic design by Bausch and Lomb and Widesite lenses by Shuron were the earliest modified straight top segment bifocal lenses (Fig. 6.29).

Panoptic bifocal has a 23 × 15 mm segment with slightly rounded corners, whereas Widesite has a slightly curved top. Recently, Univis F and Vision Ease C bifocals were introduced having a similar shape as that of Panoptic while American Optical Tillyer Sovereign and Shuron Continental Kurova CT as that of Widesite.

Ribbon Segments bifocal lenses are essentially a modified type of straight top segment; here the lower part is cut off so that wearer can have distance vision from both below and above the segment as shown in Fig. 6.30.

In all designs of fused bifocal lenses, say round, straight top, modified straight top, or ribbon segments, the bifocal segment is located on the front surface of the major lens. As segment side of major lens should have a spherical surface for fusion process, in these fused bifocal lenses if a cylindrical correction is needed, then major lens must be made in a negative toric form.

One piece bifocal lenses: These lenses are available in both round and straight top

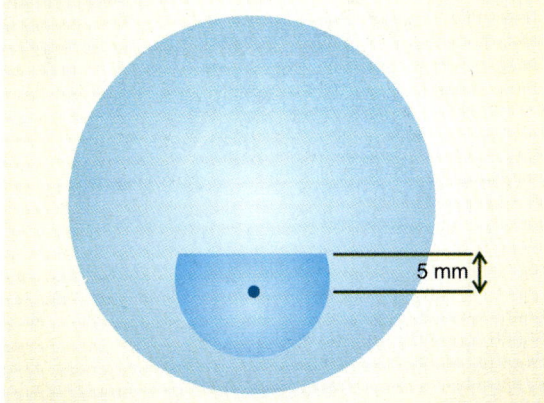

Fig. 6.28: Final 'D' bifocal lens showing 5 mm mark below top edge of segment

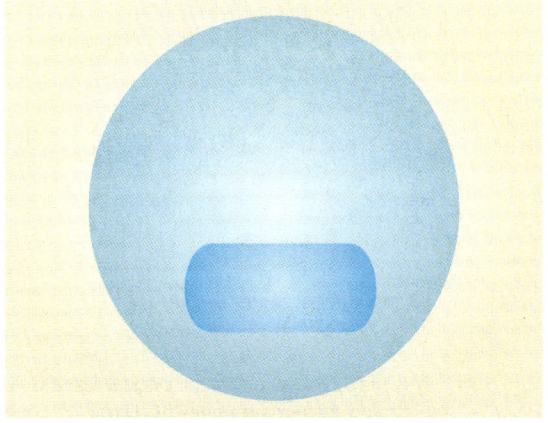

Fig. 6.30: Ribbon segment lens design

segment styles. As compared to fused bifocals in most of the round one piece bifocals the near segment is located on the back surface of the major lens. Hence, if a cylindrical correction is needed, then major lens must be grounded on its front surface or in a plus toric form. However, very few types of one piece bifocals are made in a negative toric form, similar to the fused bifocals.

One piece round segments bifocal lenses: Original Ultex A and AL type lenses have large round segments. The lower parts of the segment have been cut off, hence are also called hemispherical segments. Both Ultex A and AL lenses have segments having 38 mm diameter where in A type lens the segment is 19 mm high and in AL type lens it is 32 mm high in uncut lens form. Both forms of Ultex lenses have near segment on the back surface of the major lens as shown in Fig. 6.31.

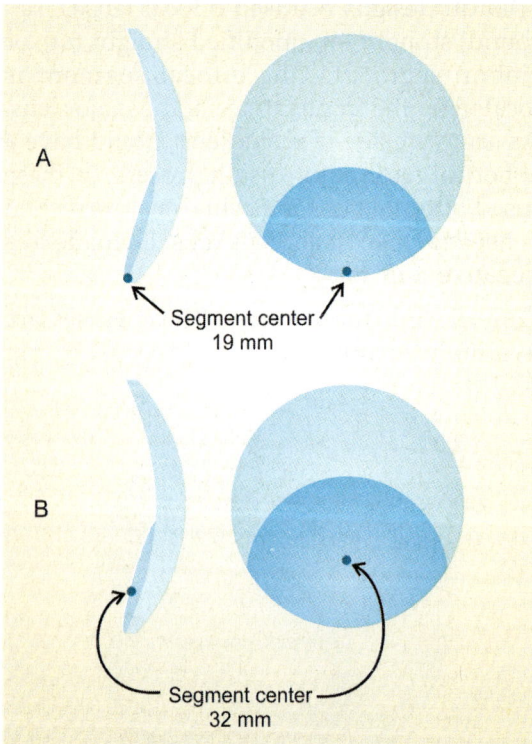

Fig. 6.31: One piece round segment bifocal lenses. A. Ultex A type having 19 mm segment; B. Ultex AL type having 32 mm segment

These Ultex design lenses are manufactured by chipping technique as shown in Fig. 6.32.

Another type of additional hemispherical one piece bifocal was developed by Robinson Houchin as Hydray having segment sizes of either a 40 × 20 mm or a 38 × 33 mm situated on either the front or back surface of the major lens.

Gross appearance of these lenses is like a Kryptok or any other round fused bifocal, however, a feeling in the change of curvature from major lens surface to near segment is present in one piece bifocals.

One piece straight-top segments bifocal lenses: Straight top one piece bifocal lenses are also called Executive bifocals and are produced by several manufactures under various names like Univis E, Kurova M, Vision Ease Bifield, and Hydray EX. In uncut lenses the standard height for near segments is 25 mm in all types (Fig. 6.33) except in Hydray lens where the segment is 29 mm high.

Manufacturing process of executive bifocal lens is simple and involves a rotating device over which the lenses are glued. Then another device create groove on this rotating drum as shown in Fig. 6.34.

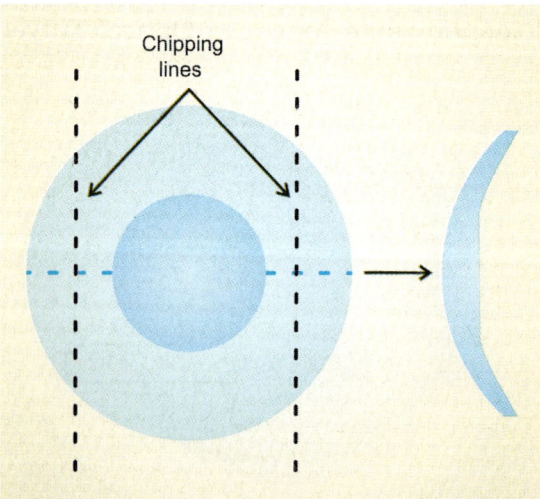

Fig. 6.32: Chipping technique for manufacturing of Ultex lenses

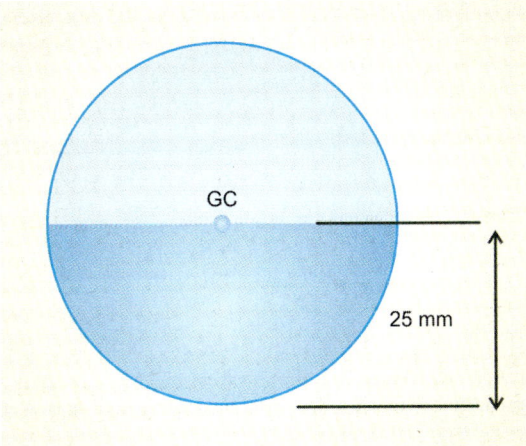

Fig. 6.33: Executive bifocal lens design

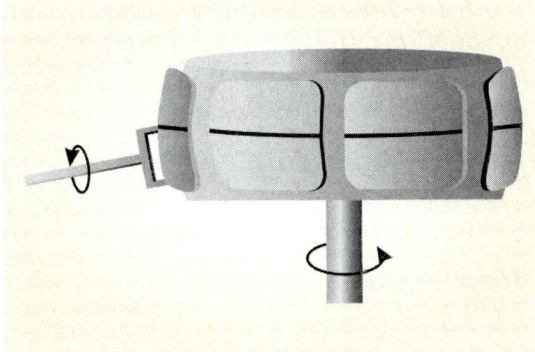

Fig. 6.34: Showing manufacturing of executive bifocal lenses

Special Types of Bifocal Lenses

Minus add bifocal: These minus add bifocal lenses were especially designed to perform near work having only a small distance window at top of the lens. These lenses are rarely used and are prescribed only for presbyopes in profession like barber or postal clerk, who need a larger near field to work.

Solid up curve bifocal lens were the first introduced minus add bifocal and currently an Ultex one piece form called Rede Rite bifocal is available in the market. Normally, in bifocal lenses the upper edge of the near segment is located at lower lid margin of wearer but in minus add lenses the edge of near segment is located above the center of pupil as shown in Fig. 6.35A.

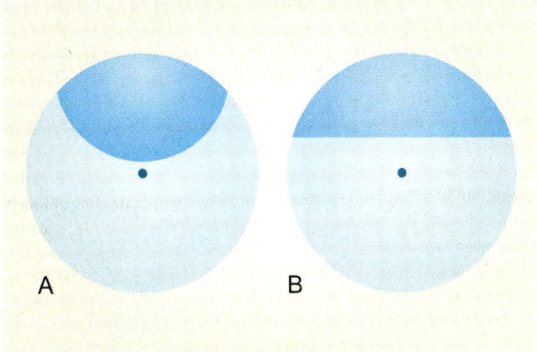

Fig. 6.35: Minus add bifocal lens designs. A. Solid up curve bifocal design; B. Straight top one piece design

Another way to obtain an unusually large reading field is by the use of a 28 mm high straight top one-piece executive style bifocal as shown in Fig. 6.35B. Even the standard executive style bifocal lens can be fitted as high as 25 mm, this will also bring add segment top, well above the center of wearer's pupil.

Golfers' bifocal lenses: A common multifocal lens can be changed into a special design lens on demand of specific occupation simply by changing its fitting position in the spectacle frame.

For example, a 50-year-old golfer regularly complain about the near segment of his/her multifocal lenses (even progressive lenses) that near segment obstruct the view of golf ball or when he/she tries to line up a hole. To solve this problem a special type of bifocal lens was developed called golfer's bifocal lens. Here the near segment usually of round shape is placed in the outer lower corner of just one lens of spectacle as shown in Fig. 6.36.

For a right hander Golfer this near segment is placed only on right side of the spectacle and for a left hander golfer in the left side of the spectacle frame. This peculiar position of the near segment remains completely out of the way, when person is playing however, enough near vision is present to read score card or menu card.

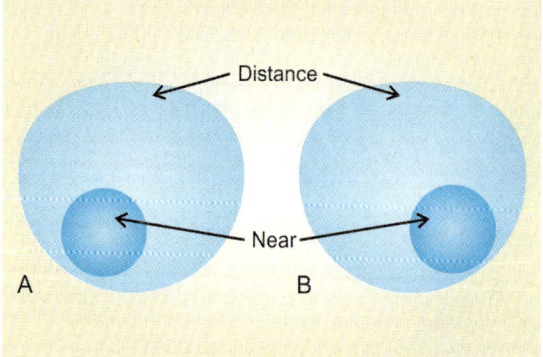

Fig. 6.36: Golfer's bifocal lens designs. A. For right eye; B. For left eye

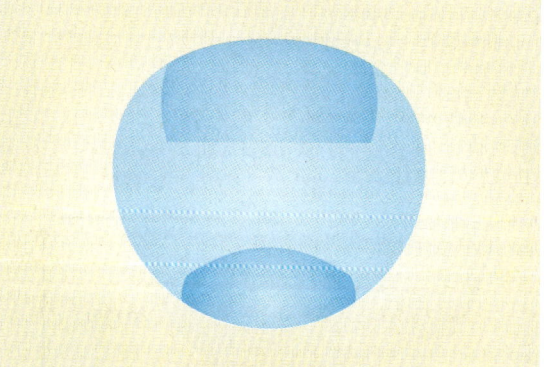

Fig. 6.38: Mixed double segment bifocal lens showing various types of segments

Double Segment Bifocals

Bifocal lenses having two addition segments, i.e. one below the level of pupillary margin and another above the level are called double segment bifocals. These are mainly used by electricians, painters, and by other professionals, who do close work above the level of the eye. Majority of these lenses are of straight top variety which are available in both fused and one-piece forms. Distance between upper and lower addition segments is 13 mm in almost all varieties of these types of lenses.

The first double segment bifocal lenses were introduced by Univis as fused double D (Fig. 6.37A) and is available in either 22 or 25 mm add segments widths. Tiyler double executive lens designs are also popular as shown in Fig. 6.37B.

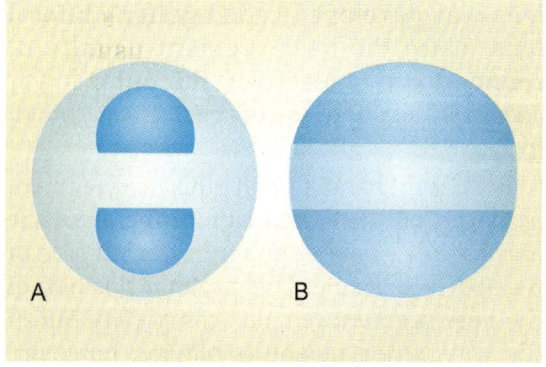

Fig. 6.37: Double segment lens designs. A. Round segments; B. Straight top segments

Several companies like Vision Ease, American Optical, Robinson Houchin and Shuron Continental make mixed double segment bifocals in various segment combinations as shown in Fig. 6.38.

> **Note**
>
> Double segment bifocal lenses are not trifocal lenses.

Trifocal Lenses

With bifocal lens many presbyopes, wearing +2 D or more optical correction feel difficulty to see an object situated at an intermediate distance (say 1–1.5 meters) either via distance or near segment of that bifocal lens. It happens because when the presbyope see the object at this distance through the distance portion of bifocal lens, his near point of accommodation lies beyond the object of interest, while when the object is seen by person through the near portion of bifocal lens, then the far point of accommodation lies too close for the object of interest. To eliminate this problem trifocal lens were introduced in which another intermediate segment having an additional intermediate power in lens was added. This intermediate segment is added just above the near segment of lens. Univis introduced trifocal lenses first time by name of Continuous Vision lenses. Originally, in Univis lenses the height of intermediate segment was kept 6.0 mm, which later on changed to 8.0 mm occupational segment, however, nowadays almost all trifocals have an intermediate segment height of 7.0 mm as shown in Fig. 6.39.

Trifocal lenses are available in various styles and combinations in both fused and one-piece forms. Univis, American Optical, Vision-Ease, and Shuron-Continental all these companies manufacture a straight top trifocal lens, whereas American Optical, Vision-Ease, and Robinson Houchin manufacture an Executive style one piece trifocal.

For occupations like computer operator, a special design of CRT trifocal lenses has been introduced having a 14 mm high intermediate segment as shown in Fig. 6.40. CRT lens is suitable for professions where high percentage of near work is needed at an intermediate distance.

Plastic multifocal lenses: Presently, demand of plastic multifocal lenses has increased. Almost all plastic multifocal lenses are one piece design where near segment is located on the front surface of lens. These lenses are produced in finished or semi-finished form.

Varifocal or Progressive Lenses

These lenses have corrective power for distance and near vision along with a progressive power zone or corridor which extend across the entire width of lens and connect distance and near portions of the lens.

Central portion of the progressive lens is the functional area of progressive power zone and is known as progressive corridor or zone (Fig. 6.41). Refractive power of varifocal lens increases progressively from the distance to the near portion along this progressive corridor. All powers lying in between the distance and near powers are present in this progressive corridor. No visible reading segment and/or no dividing lines are present in this corridor, hence practically there is no image jump.

The most important factors of a progressive lens are interconnected and include

- Size of distance and reading areas
- Types and intensity of aberrations
- Depth and functional width of corridor

Various types of progressive lens designs available differ in high image performance and the severity of aberrations. An inherent

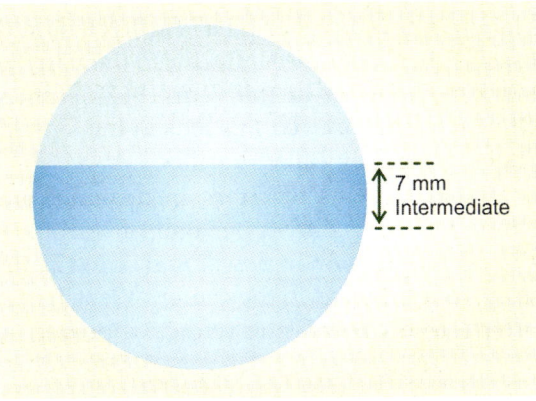

Fig. 6.39: Trifocal lens design

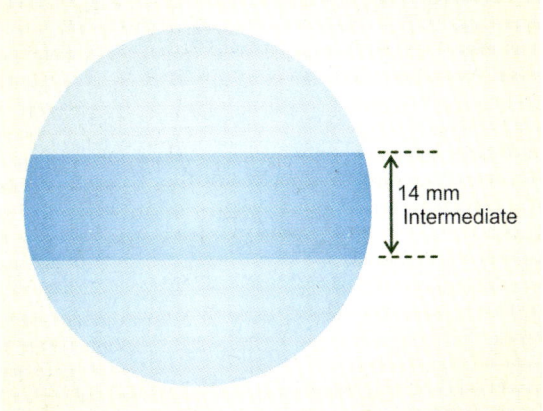

Fig. 6.40: CRT lens design having 14 mm segment

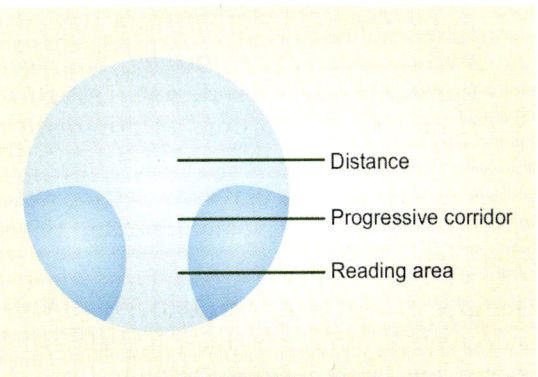

Fig. 6.41: Varifocal or progressive lens

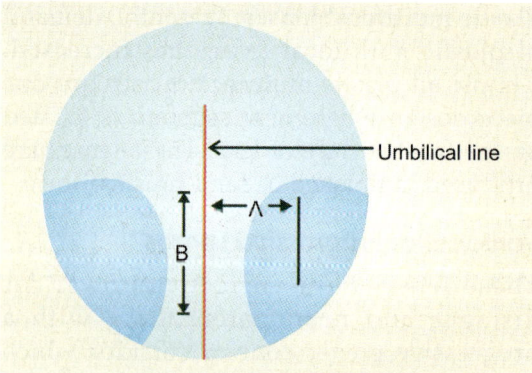

Fig. 6.42: Umbilical line and astigmatism in proportion to displacement. For same amount of astigmatism, vertical displacement B is twice the lateral displacement A

astigmatism may be produced either right or left of the umbilical line (A line at center of progressive corridor as shown in Fig. 6.42) during creation of an aspherical surface with variable radius of curvatures; this astigmatism is proportional to the rate of change in the curvature.

This designing principle of progressive lens developed two approaches of production of progressive lenses

- **Hard design:** Progressive lenses designed on this basis give a relatively larger area of high quality images in all areas of lens, i.e. distance portion, progressive corridor, and near portion. However, there is an associated high degree of astigmatism in lateral portions of progressive corridor.
- **Soft design:** Progressive lenses designed on this basis give a smaller area of high quality images in all areas, i.e. distance portion, progressive corridor, and near portion; but has a low degree of astigmatism in lateral portions of progressive corridor.

Several types of progressive lenses were produced till date and some important types of progressive lenses are

Omnifocal Lens: In the year 1961, David Volk and Joseph Weinberg introduced first successful progressive lens known as Omnifocal, which was manufactured by Robinson Houchin.

These lenses were made of glass and having aspherical or progressive front surface. Radius of curvature of aspheric surface of lens (front surface) progressively reduced in vertical meridian from top to the bottom, whereas in the horizontal meridian radius of curvature remained same.

The distance optical center of lens lies at a vertical distance of 25 mm from near optical center of lens. Total amount of plus power decreases upwards from distance optical center and increases downwards from distance optical center as shown in Fig. 6.43.

Omnifocal lens was an example of soft design because the progression of power is from top to bottom in entire front surface of lens. These lenses are now obsolete but mentioned due to its historical importance.

Varilux lens: In the year 1959, Bernard Maitenaz developed original Varilux lens and Essel Optical of France introduced them in the market. Later on in the year 1967, Titmus Optical Co introduced this lens in the United States, popularly called Varilux 1.

Varilux 1 was different in design from Omnifocal lens. The upper half of Varilux 1 had no progression in power and only 12 mm deep zone situated in the center of lens had a progressively increasing refractive power. A

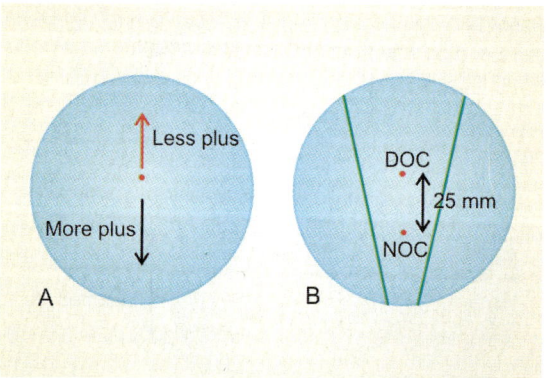

Fig. 6.43: Omnifocal lens designs. A. Plus power increases downwards from distance optical center and decreases upwards; B. Functional area of lens decreases gradually from top to bottom showing distance optical center (DOC) and near optical center (NOC)

zone of maximum addition with a constant power having a width of about 22 mm was situated below progressive corridor of lens as shown in Fig. 6.44. In original Varilux design lens, astigmatism free progressive corridor of 5 mm width was also present but on increasing the power of near addition, the functional width of the progressive corridor decreased.

Varilux lens is considered as a hard design lens because progressive front surface is limited to a 12 mm deep zone, rather than extending from top to bottom as in soft design lenses. Varilux lenses are manufactured differentially for the right and left eyes, because the line of symmetry is inclined nasally toward the bottom of lens as shown in Fig. 6.45. Original Varilux lens were available only in glass material.

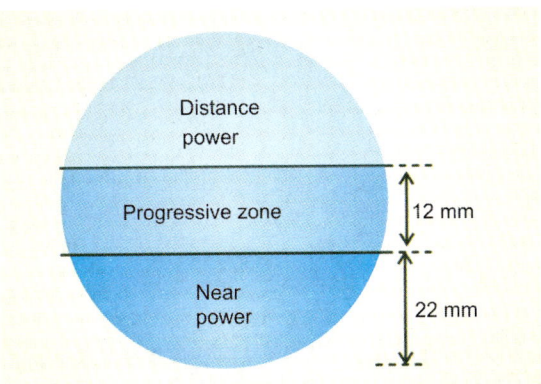

Fig. 6.44: Varilux lens design with central 12 mm progressive zone and constant power in distance and near zone

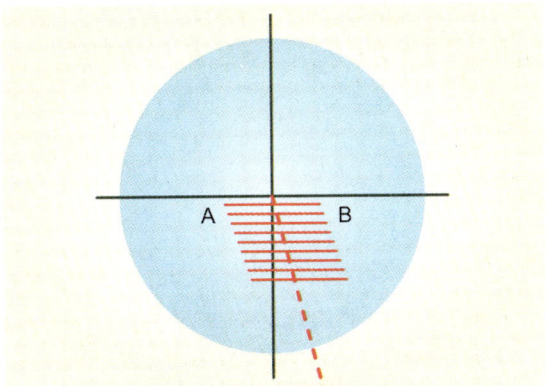

Fig. 6.45: Nasal inclination of progressive zone in right-sided Varilux lens

Later on after expire of patent of Varilux 1 progressive lens, the Varilux 2 lens was introduced by Essel. In this lens not only the progressive zone but also entire front surface of lens was of aspherical design. Hence, this lens was considered as soft design progressive lens. Lateral astigmatism was greatly reduced in Varilux 2 with improvised vision qualities.

Once the patent on original Varilux expired several manufactures introduced their own version of progressive lenses. For example,

- In the year 1973, American Optical introduced Ultravue CR-39 plastic lens. A 25 mm wide segment corridor was present in this lens, hence was renamed as Ultravue 25. In the year 1978, another lens with same design called Ultravue 28 was introduced with a 28 mm wide segment. Ultravue lens has an advantage of a well-defined distance portion, astigmatism-free surface and wide segment area, but at the cost of higher rate of progression. This lens was of hard design category.
- In the year 1978, Younger optics introduced Younger 10/30 CR-39 plastic lens. This lens has a 10 mm deep progressive corridor with 30 mm wide functional segment area, hence the name 10/30. This lens was in hard progressive lens design category.
- In the year 1980, Silor Optical started marketing Super NoLine lens. This improvised version of original NoLine progressive lens has a progressive corridor 12 mm deep. This lens has wide distance and segment area of about 25 mm width, hence designated in hard design category. NoLine lenses are available in CR-39 plastic, ophthalmic crown glass, and photochromic glass materials.

Many more companies came up with several types of progressive lenses, although list is exhaustive but a few examples are

- Cosmetic Parabolic Sphere (CPS) progressive lens by Younger Optics

- In the year 1982, American Optical introduced Truvision lens.
- Titmus Optical in the year 1983 started marketing NuVue 75 lens.
- In the year 1984, Coburn Optical Industries started marketing of Progressive R lens.
- Sola Optical in 1984 introduced a lens called VIP lens.
- In the year 1986, Seiko Optical Products introduced two progressive lenses called P-2 and P-3.
- Polarite in the year 1986 developed a plastic polarized progressive lens by the name of Progressive M. Most recently Varilux infinity (1988) and Varilux comfort (1993) progressive lens designs were developed to increase the comfort of wearer in advancing presbyopic age.

Spectacle Lens Fitting

SPECTACLE LENS FITTING METHOD

For an ideal fitting of a lens in the spectacle frame knowledge of these following components is essential

- Interpupillary distance
- Frame dimensions
- Frame specification
- Spectacle frame selection

Interpupillary Distance

Optical center or major reference point of the lens, these are two interchangeable terms which indicate a point on the lens, where maximum effect of a prescribed prism will be seen. Distance between these two points on two lenses of a spectacle lens is called inter-pupillary distance (IPD).

Measuring interpupillary distance: First step for accurate lens fitting in a spectacle frame is the measurement of interpupillary distance, commonly called IPD or PD and both the distance PD and near PD has to be measured. These measurements are defined as distance between two visual axes for distance and near vision, respectively at the level of spectacle plane.

As shown in Fig. 7.1 lines of sight are parallel for distance vision, hence inter-pupillary distance will be the same, whether measured at the level of center of rotation plane, corneal plane or spectacle plane.

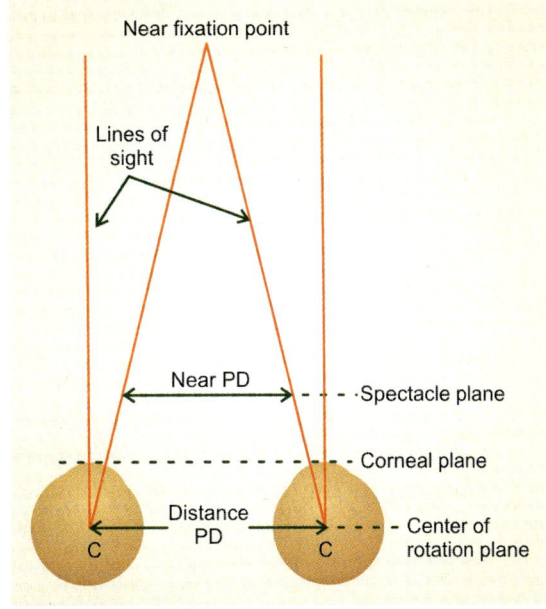

Fig. 7.1: Measuring interpupillary distance at various planes

However, in convergence condition for near fixation, eyes rotate about their center of rotation with simultaneous convergence of lines of sight, hence distance between them decrease from center of rotation plane to corneal plane and further at spectacle plane level as shown in Fig. 7.2.

Visual axes distance can be measured by using:

- Millimeter ruler
- Elissor pupillometer

99

- AO Grolman device
- Cal Coast PD ruler
- Bausch and Lomb PD gauge
- Topcon digital PD gauge
- Rodenstock interpupillary gauge

Similarly, pupil center and size can be measured by

- Antique Pulzone hardy rule
- Bishop Harman rule
- Fairbanks facial gauge
- Basic pupillometer

Simplest and most widely accepted method to measure both distance and near PD is by millimeter ruler method.

Test procedure for distance PD measurement (Fig. 7.2A)

- Examiner sits in front of the patient at a distance of about one and a half feet (16 inches), holding a millimeter ruler in one hand at the level of patient's spectacle plane.
- Then examiner instructs the patient to look in his/her left eye, simultaneously aligning the temporal edge of patient's right pupil with the zero mark on millimeter ruler.
- Then the patient is asked to look at examiner's right eye, so that examiner can record the reading on millimeter ruler which is aligned with nasal edge of patient's left pupil.

Note

Sometimes it is difficult to see the pupillary border especially in patients having very dark iris, then the alignment of millimeter ruler is done with the temporal limbus of right eye and nasal limbus of left eye.

Test procedure for near PD measurement (Fig. 7.2B)

- Examiner sits in front of the patient at a distance of about one and a half feet (16 inches), holding a millimeter ruler in one hand at the level of patient's spectacle plane.

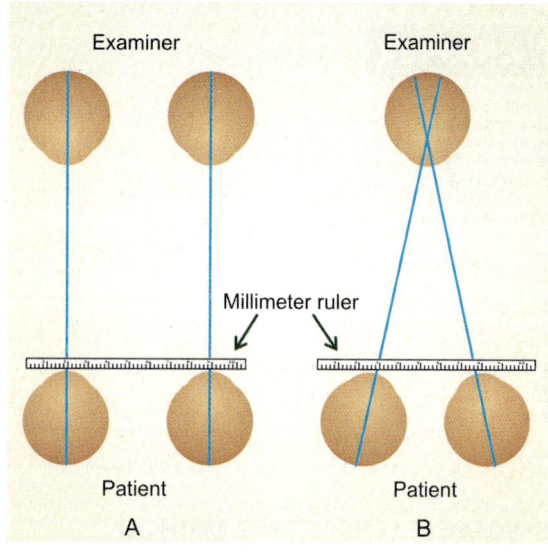

Fig. 7.2: Measurement of PD. A. Distance PD measurement; B. Near PD measurement

- Then examiner instructs the patient to fixate either his/her right or left eye, which is accordingly positioned on the patient's midline area by the examiner.
- Then examiner aligns the temporal edge of patients right eye pupil with zero mark on the millimeter scale, while note down reading corresponding to nasal edge of patient's left eye pupil.

Note

Normally at this measuring distance (16 inches) near PD is usually about 4–5 mm less than the distance PD.

Due to practical difficulties, it is probably advisable to measure the distance PD with accuracy and then find out the near PD by calculation with this formula.

For each eye, difference between distance PD and near PD (say d) is calculated by

$d/27 = \frac{1}{2}$ distance PD/427 or simply $d = 27$ ($\frac{1}{2}$ distance PD)/427

For example, suppose distance PD is 64 mm, then difference d for each eye, will be

$$d = 27 (32)/427$$
$$= 2.02$$

Hence near PD is 64–2 (2.02) = 59.96 mm

Following conditions can create problems while measuring the PD by using a millimeter rule

- Difference in patient's and examiner's PD can introduce a parallax.
- Anisocoria or pupil size difference in both eyes can alter dimensions.
- Asymmetry of the face
- Invisible pupil margins
- Vertical differences of the two eyes.
- Lateral head or ruler movement while measuring a PD.

To align the visual axis of eye and optical axis of spectacle lens sometimes we have to decenter the lens horizontally depending upon the frame dimensions and PD. To get the best possible visual results, it is necessary to align visual axis and optical center of spectacle lens. However, to get desired prismatic effect various types of lenses (spherical, plano-cylindrical or spherocylindrical lenses) can be decentered.

The lens decentration is done to control prismatic effects, means either to produce a prismatic effect or to avoid a prismatic effect.

Frame Dimensions

For measuring lenses, a system of reference points was established for spectacle frames and spectacle lenses which assist in accurate fitting of corresponding optical center and bifocal segments inside the spectacle frame. Two systems were developed to ease the lens fittings are Datum system and Boxing system.

Datum System

In the year 1935, Cole and Blackburn introduced Datum system (Fig. 7.3) for accurate fitting of lenses in spectacle frames. Various terminologies used in this system are

Datum line (AA): Placing the lens in a position as it should be fitted in a frame, the two horizontal tangents corresponding to highest (UU') and lowest (LL') edges of lens are drawn. A parallel line drawn midway between these two horizontal tangents is called datum line of reference.

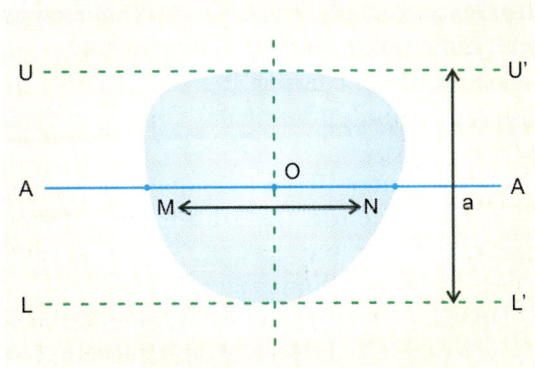

Fig. 7.3: Datum system

Datum length (MN): The peripheral portion of the lens which bound the datum line in horizontal plane is called datum length and it represents the horizontal dimensions of a lens.

Mid-datum depth (a): Vertical line joining upper and lower horizontal tangents from lens edges is called as mid-datum depth and it represents the vertical dimension of the lens.

Datum center (O): A cross section point present midway between the datum length and a vertical line from upper and lower lens edges is called datum center.

Application of datum system to the frame (Fig. 7.4) gives the frame dimensions and various additional terminologies are as follows

Frame difference: When there is a difference between vertical dimension and horizontal dimension of a frame, it is called frame

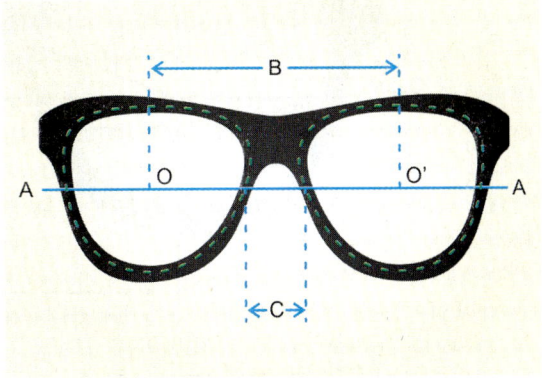

Fig. 7.4: Application of datum system on spectacle frame

difference. Usually it is a few millimeters, as both dimensions are also in millimeter.

Datum line of frame: It a continuous line joining Datum's line of both the spectacle lenses, i.e. AA.

Datum center distance (B): After fitting the two lenses inside the frame, a distance between datum centers (OO') of these two lenses is called datum center distance.

Distance between lenses (DBL): Distance between the nasal edges of lens measured at Datum line plane is called distance between lenses (C) and is a parameter used in various calculation of lens fitting.

Due to several technical difficulties this datum system was not used widely and a better measuring system known as boxing system was developed.

Boxing System

In the year 1961, American Optical Manufacturers Association introduced a universal system for measurement of lens and frames called boxing system. In this system the lens boxing was done by both horizontal (used in Datum system) and vertical lines (not used in Datum system). Hence, boxing system is considered as an improved version of datum

system. Boxing system uses bevel apex of the edged lens as a constant reference point for all measurements in millimeters, hence the chances error in prescription interpretation were reduced.

Boxed lens: Consider the front and cross section view of a lens as shown in Fig. 7.5. Suppose a square made by the horizontal and vertical tangent lines touching the lens edges is drawn, which completely surrounds the lens is called boxed lens. Various terminologies used (Fig. 7.6) in boxing system are:

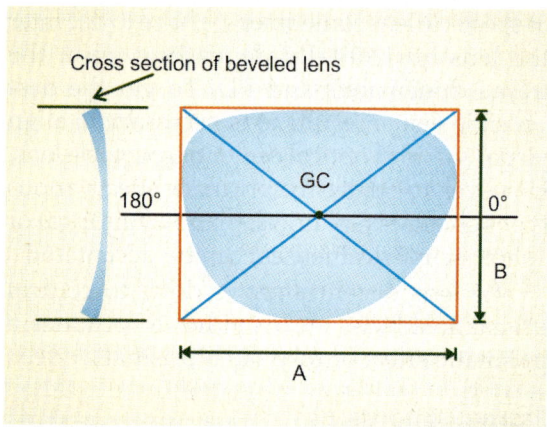

Fig. 7.5: Boxing of a spectacle lens, GC: Geometrical center

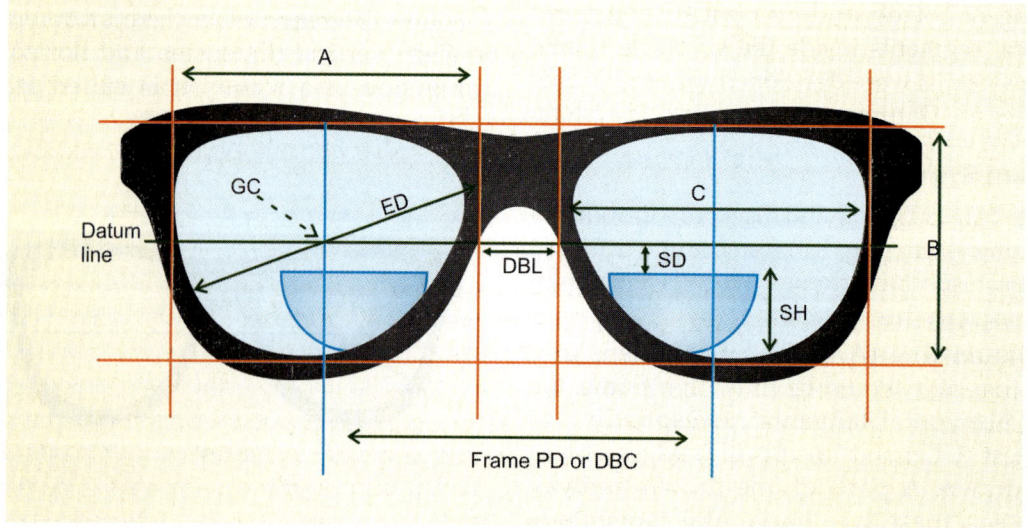

Fig. 7.6: Application of boxing system on spectacle frame

Eye size (Lens size): Horizontal measurement (A) of this box is called eye size for frames and lens size for lenses.

Frame depth: Vertical measurement (B) of this box represents the frame depth.

Box center: It is the point where two diagonals of box are intersecting with each other. It is also called the geometric center (GC) of the frame opening or aperture. It also represents the geometric center of a lens edges for a given frame.

Suppose both the right and left lenses have been boxed, as if they were inserted into the spectacle frame as shown in Fig. 7.6, then following parameters are also added in existing terminologies as

DBL: It is the minimum horizontal distance between two lenses mounted in a spectacle frame. The measuring points are the bevels of nasal side of two lenses; DBL also represents the bridge size of the frame.

Distance between centers (DBC): It is the distance between two geometrical centers of the frame (or lens) and is commonly called frame PD. This can be represented by the following formula

DBC = Eye size or lens size + DBL

Segment height (SH): Vertical distance between top edge of bifocal or trifocal segment and bottom edge of box is called segment height.

Segment drop (SD): Vertical distance between top edge of bifocal or trifocal segment and datum line is called segment drop.

Frame Specification

Size: Spectacle frames are typically marked for size, which help in calculating other dimensions of the frame. For example, marked as 50–22, where 50 represents the eye size or lens size and 22 represents the distance between lenses (DBL) or bridge size.

Effective diameter: Another important specification provided by manufacturer is effective diameter (ED) as shown in Fig. 7.7. It is defined as twice the distance from geometrical

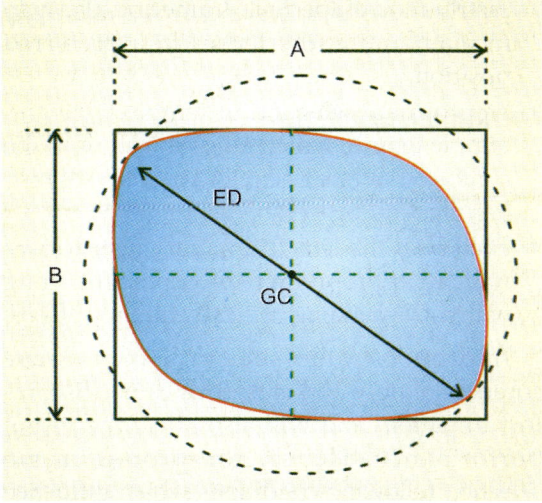

Fig. 7.7: Effective diameter (ED) and geometrical center (GC) of a lens

center of lens to the peak of beveled edge of lens situated farthest from geometrical center. Effective diameter is used to determine the minimum size of blank. This blank size is calculated by doubling the amount of decentration in millimeter and adding the resultant value with effective diameter of lens.

Minimum blank size = ED + 2 × Amount of decentration in millimeter

Spectacle Frame Selection

Primary function of a spectacle frame is to keep prescribed lenses in such a position that give an optimum visual efficiency. Also the frame should be comfortable in wearing and look attractive to fulfill the patient's expectation.

For Bifocals and Multifocal Lenses

To fulfill the requirement of optical performance and comfort expert ophthalmic personnel should take care of these facts about selection of a spectacle frame
- Thoroughly consider the factors related to prescribed lens such as refractive power, lens material, lens centration, base curve specification, multifocal type and glass tint.
- Appropriate selection of bridge design that remains stable, provide the proper weight

distribution of spectacle frame and also help in maintaining the lenses in a preferred position.

- Appropriate selection of temple style and temple length, which adjusts well with the contour of wearer's ear and to shape of his/her mastoid process.
- Facilitates the lens fitting very near to face with an appropriate pantoscopic tilt along with corresponding vertical centration of lens.

Improper frame selection may cause soreness of nose and ears, thus cause discomfort to patient and will also affect the visual performance. Hence, for proper frame selection following conditions which influence the frame selection should be assessed properly

- Type of lens, because multifocal or progressive lenses will need specified minimum vertical frame dimension for proper fitting.
- Probable size and exact lens power, because these factors will affect the thickness and weight of lenses
- Relationship between patient's PD and spectacle frame PD will affect the resultant appearance of centrality of patient's eyes and also decides that whether the prescribed lenses can be chipped out from the standard uncut blanks or not.
- To avoid the rejection of spectacles by patient always enquire about the purpose of wearing the spectacles, so that suitable type of frame can be selected.

For Progressive Lenses

For a proper and satisfactory dispensing of spectacle in case of progressive lenses fitting, the frame selection is an important step. Frame should have these specific features for proper fitting of progressive lenses.

- As shown in Fig. 7.8, for fitting of progressive lenses selected frame must have a total vertical measurement of minimum of 40 mm.

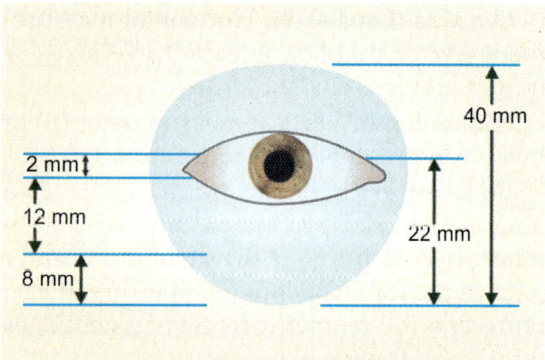

Fig. 7.8: Spectacle box vertical dimension, minimum of 40 mm

- Frame must offer a minimum vertical distance of 22 mm between the pupillary center of patient and the horizontal line tangent to bottom edge of spectacle lens, means in a Varifocal lens (having 12 mm progressive zone) this type of fitting will give reading area of 8 mm width, considering that progressive zone begins 2 mm below the pupillary center.

If the distance below pupillary center is less than 22 mm, then the remaining depth of maximum near power prescribed for reading will be very small.

- The selected frame should fit on patient's face very near (maximum 11–12 mm) to the back vertex distance, so that a wide lateral field of view and stable near vision area can be provided to the patient.
- Pantoscopic tilt of nearly 12–15° with slight amount of face forming will help in stabilization of near area and provide wider view of lateral visual field.
- Frames with an adjustable nose pads will permit flexibility in positioning the frame, while dispensing and also in follow-up.

Principles of Fitting

Once the accurate spectacle frame has been selected, the fitting of the lenses into this selected frame is an important step. For practical purposes proper alignment of spectacle frame is done by the manufacturer. The dispenser should confirm precise fitting of frame or lens on patients according to the following guidelines

- Pantoscopic tilt
- Temple angle
- Fitting triangle

Pantoscopic Tilt

Pantoscopic tilt or angle of a spectacle frame means that the bottom edge of the spectacle lens is tilted away from the vertical axis (5–8 degrees) in the inward direction (i.e. towards the cheeks of wearer) (Fig. 7.9). In other words, the upper edge of spectacle lens is more forward than bottom edge. The inward tilting of frame improves the cosmetic looks of the spectacles, provides a better protection from flying objects, increases the field of view of wearer and decreases effect of oblique astigmatism.

Change in pantoscopic angle or tilt helps in adjustment of spectacle frame. For example, if right-sided lens appears higher on patient's face as compared to the left-sided lens, then by increasing the pantoscopic angle for the left lens will make both the lenses in level or one can decrease the pantoscopic angle for the lens which is higher (right lens in our example).

Sometimes, to achieve a satisfactory fit on wearer's face we may need to tilt the frame, so that lower part of the lens tilted away from the wearers' face, this is called retroscopic tilt, used rarely when absolute indications are there.

Temple Angle

Temple angle is an angle formed between front and temple of the spectacle frame in the horizontal plane. Degree of temple angle is dependent on elements like front width of spectacle frame and patient's head width, but in majority of the cases, frame temples are bent outwards up to a few degrees (Fig. 7.10).

> **Note**
>
> Recently, very large size spectacle frames are also used and these frames generated a need to bend the temples slightly inwards.

Temple angle helps us to check the distance of two lenses from the patient's eyebrow (which should be equal on both sides) and this can be observed when patient bends his/her head in downward direction. If the temple angle on one side is too small, then the patient will feel an excessive pressure on that side of head, because the lens on that side extends outward as compared to fellow lens. The problem can be solved by increasing the

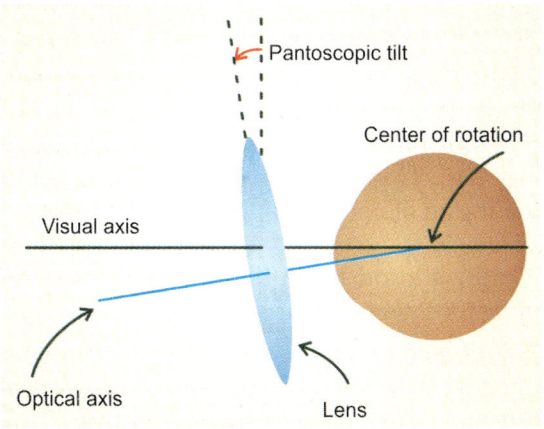

Fig. 7.9: Pantoscopic tilt

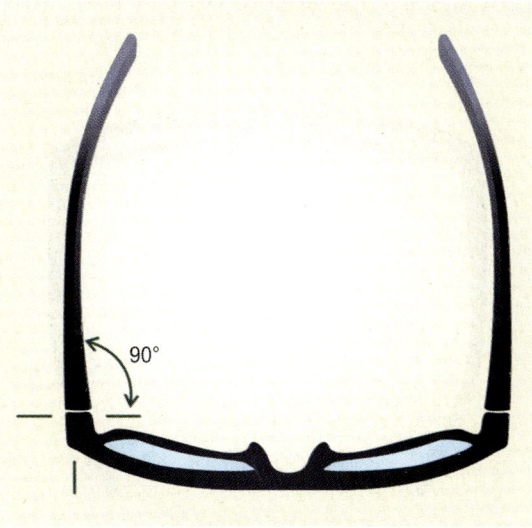

Fig. 7.10: Temple angle

temple angle on this side, however; in some cases reduction in temple angle on other side can also give good results.

Fitting Triangle

Spectacle frame or mounting may be compared with a triangle having three points of contact; one at the crest of the nose (A) and two on the apex of each ear (B, C) as shown in Fig. 7.11. Normally when head is kept in erect position, about 65% of total spectacle weight is taken up by the nose, whereas remaining (about 35%) of total weight is shared by the ears. However, on bending the head in downward direction, the majority of the spectacle weight gets transfer to the ears.

During routine work, mainly the weight of spectacles remains on the nose of individual, hence it becomes necessary to provide cushioning effect to the nose to tolerate the spectacle weight and to prevent pressure effects. It is done by prescribing spectacle frames having adjustable nose pads and the whole surface of these pads should make contact with the nose. Sometimes frames with large size nose pads (jumbo pads) can be used in those having sensitive nose skin. In case of plastic frames, as there is no adjustable pads so such a frame should be selected which provides a large area of contact with nose.

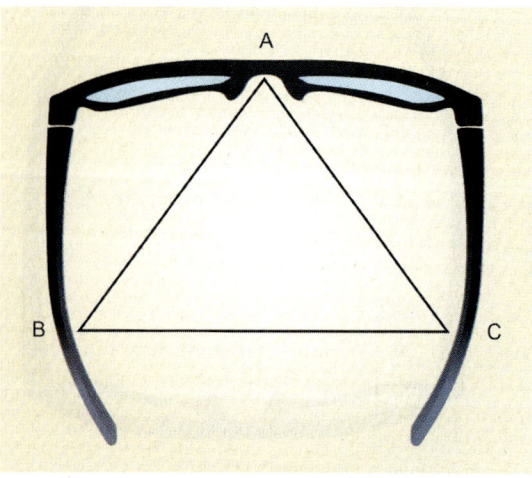

Fig. 7.11: Fitting triangle

Frame style having a saddle bridge is appropriate for patients who have a relatively wide, protruding, high nose crest. However, for patients having narrow and flat crest, a keyhole bridge is a better choice.

Fitting of bifocal lenses: Fitting of a bifocal lenses require knowledge of not only of the corrective powers of distance and near vision, but also the positions of optical center of the segment. This placement of optical center of segments is done in vertical and lateral positions of the bifocal lenses.

Vertical position of the segment: In bifocal lenses the vertical positioning of segment is decided by the following factors
- Optical center position of distance portion of lens.
- Optical center position of the near segment.
- Reading center which is a point in lens corresponding to the wearer's line of sight during reading or close work.

Optical center position of distance portion of lens: For best functioning of a lens, the optical axis of the lens should pass through the center of rotation of the eye. Level of distance optical center of a bifocal lens is decided on the basis of amount of pantoscopic tilt. To get 2° of pantoscopic tilt, distance optical center need to be lowered to 1 mm, and a tilt of 6° is usually cosmetically desired, hence a lowering of 3 mm of distance optical center as compared to center of pupil is done in a bifocal lens as shown in Fig. 7.12.

Optical center position of near segment: Similarly, position of optical center of various types of bifocal lens segments is shown in Fig. 7.13. This clearly gives us an idea about the fitting of various types of bifocal lenses in spectacle frames, so that the reading line of wearer should be in alignment with these optical centers of near segments.

Reading center: It is considered as a point on the spectacle lens through which the foveal line of sight passes during reading. It is situated about 11 mm below the center of

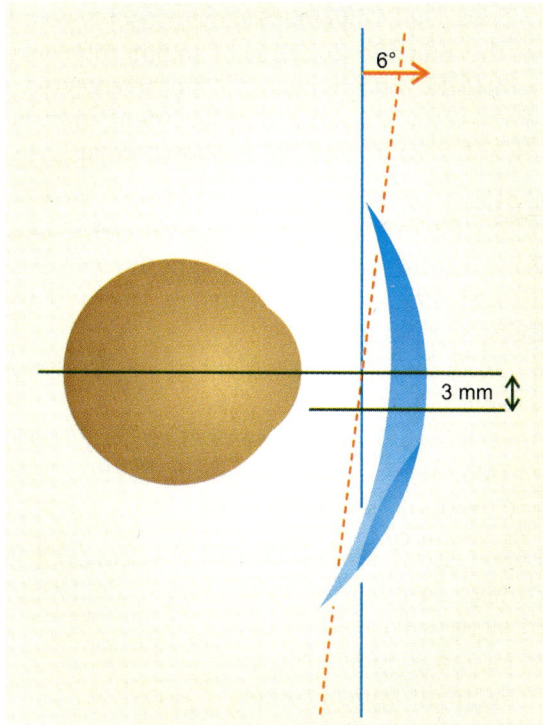

Fig. 7.12: Lowering (3 mm) of distance optical center to get a 6° pantoscopic tilt

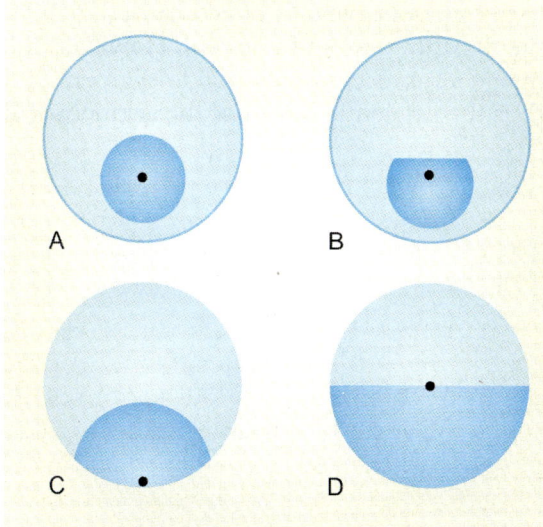

Fig. 7.13: Optical center for various bifocal lens designs from segment top. A. Fused round segment bifocal (11 mm below); B. Fused straight top bifocal (5 mm below); C. One piece bifocal (19 mm below); D. Executive bifocal (at segment top)

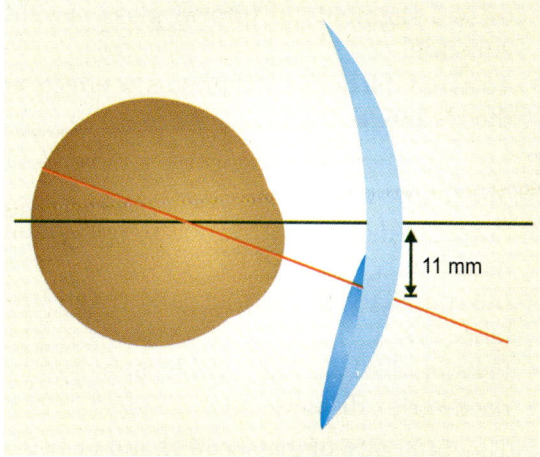

Fig. 7.14: Reading center in bifocal lens is usually 11 mm below pupillary center

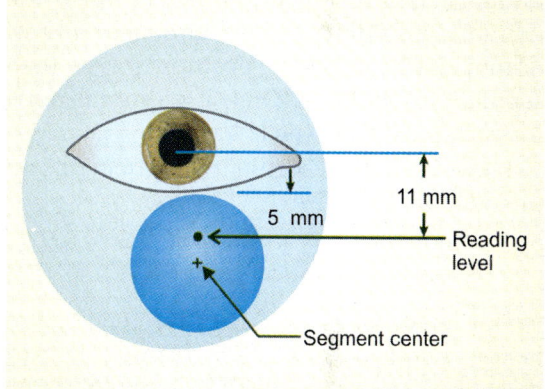

Fig. 7.15: Round segment fitting with reading level 11 mm below pupillary center

pupil (Fig. 7.14). As discussed above to get a pantoscopic tilt of 6° the bifocal distance optical center lies at 3 mm below the pupillary center, hence the reading center of segment is located 11–3 = 8 mm below. On this principle bifocal lenses are fitted as shown in Fig. 7.15, i.e. segment top is kept in alignment with the lower eyelid margin of wearer.

Lateral position of the segment: Normally segment optical centers are fitted in an inward position as compared to the distance optical points of bifocal lenses; this is known as segment inset. Purposes of segment inset are
• To make sure that when patient looks with both the eyes, then the field of view

of two segments of bifocal glass should coincide.

- To avoid the horizontal prismatic effects at the reading center.

Proper placement of segment inset is dependent on the following factors

- Power of distance correction in horizontal meridian.
- Interpupillary distance usually called distance PD.
- Fixation distance of bifocal lens.
- Back vertex distance.

The difference of distance PD and near PD is equally divided in each spectacle lens for nasal displacement. For example, suppose a patient has a distance PD of 66 mm in the primary position of eyes and near PD of 62 mm in the converging position of eyes, then segment inset of 66–62 = 4/2 = 2 mm is done for each bifocal spectacle lens.

However, a total segment inset depends on position of

- Major reference point (MRP)
- Geometrical optical center (GC)

Major reference point: Major reference point is the difference between frame PD and distance PD where frame PD is a sum of frame size and distance between lenses (DBL).

Total displacement of segment inset depends on the relative position of major reference point (MRP) and geometrical optical center (GC) of the lens and total displacement may be inward, zero or outward as shown in Fig. 7.16.

Optical performance of bifocal lenses: Evaluation of properly fitted bifocal lens is done by observing the optical performance of bifocal lens, which in turn is decided by following parameters

- Differential displacement at segment top called image jump.
- Differential displacement at reading level
- Total displacement at reading level
- Chromatic aberration

Differential displacement at segment top (Image Jump): The bifocal lens consists of three optical centers, i.e.

- Distance optical center
- Segment optical center
- Resultant optical center

The prismatic effect in bifocal lens also exists in the segment and this prismatic effect at any given point in the segment will be equal to the sum of prismatic effects caused by both the distance lens and segment. However, the image jump occurs only due to segment and thus the prismatic power of the segment will

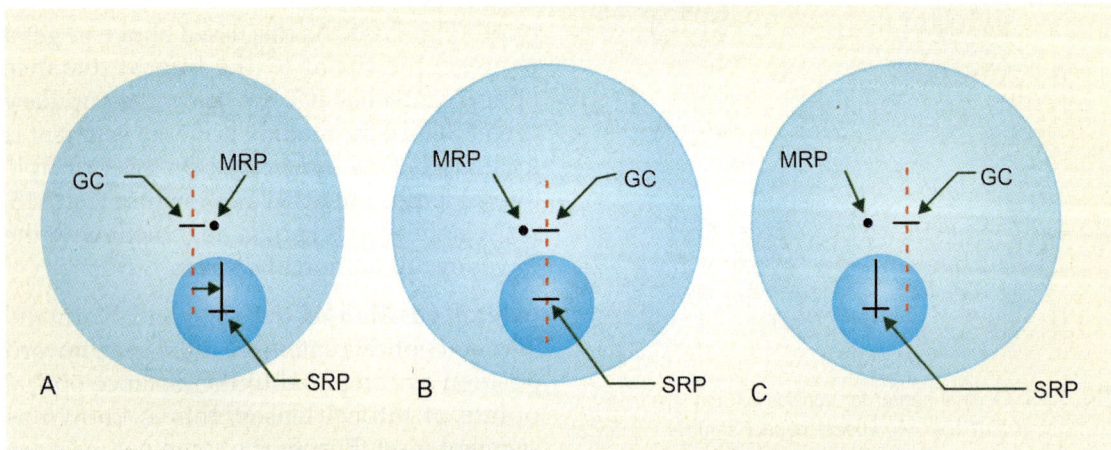

Fig. 7.16: Total displacement of segment reference point (SRP) in relation to geometrical center (GC) and major reference point (MRP). A. Inward, most common; B. Zero; C. Outward, least common

decide the amount of image jump. Although the image jump can occur at any point on the margin of segment but it is annoying when occur from top edge of segment which is considered as zone of confusion. When an attempt is made by a bifocal wearer to look at an object through the top edge of segment, he/she sees two images because a part of bundle of rays entering the bifocal wearers' pupil is passing through the distance lens and remaining part is passing through the segment. Images formed by these two bundles of rays will differ from each other in

- Direction, i.e. differential displacement.
- Focus, because of differences in refractive power of distance and near portion of bifocal lens.
- Size, because of differences in magnification of images formed by distance and near portion of bifocal lens.

Differential displacement at reading level: Relative position of reading level in different types of bifocal lenses is represented in Fig. 7.17. These relative positions of reading level and position of segment center (solid red line) of a bifocal lens determines the differential displacement at reading level in terms of prismatic effect. Various types of prismatic effects produced are as follows

- Reading level and segment center on the same line, then no prismatic effect produced. For example, straight top D bifocal lens as shown in Fig. 7.17A.
- Reading level is above the segment center, hence a base down prismatic effect is produced. For example, Ultex AL lens as shown in Fig. 7.17B.
- Reading level is below segment center produces a base up prismatic effect. For example, executive bifocal lens as shown in Fig. 7.17C.

Total displacement at reading level: Both the factors, i.e. image jump and the differential displacement at reading level, have no relation with the refractive power of the bifocal lens. However, the total displacement at reading

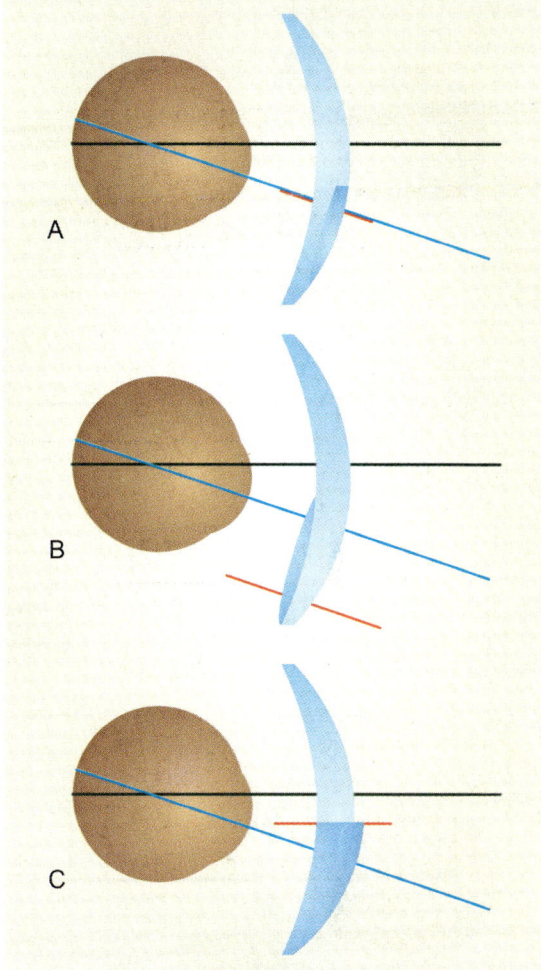

Fig. 7.17: Prismatic effects of various segment designs on reading level. A. No prismatic effect; B. Base down prismatic effect; C. Base up prismatic effect

level depends on the refractive power of the distance portion and addition power in the near segment of a bifocal lens.

In case where power of distance portion of the lens is plus, a base-up prismatic effect is added with near segment. However, in case where power of distance portion of the lens is minus, a base-down prismatic effect is added with near segment as shown in Fig. 7.18A and B.

Total displacement of object at reading level is determined by both the combined effect of power of the distance lens and near segment as shown in Fig. 7.19.

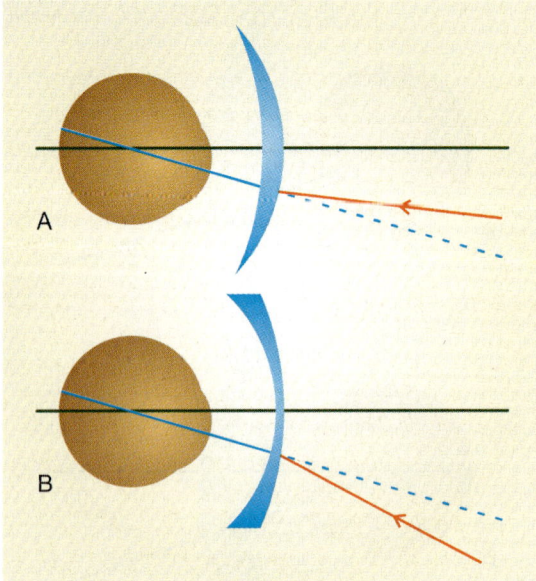

Fig. 7.18: Effect of power of distance portion of the lens. A. Plus power lens will add base up effect; B. Minus power lens will add base down effect

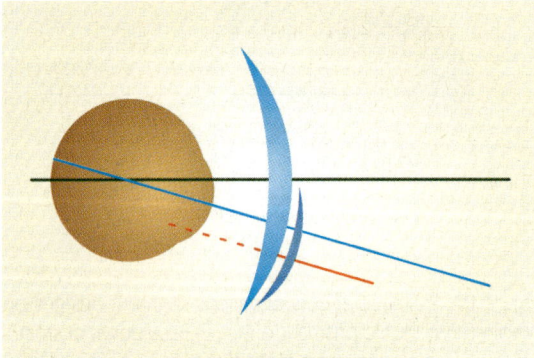

Fig. 7.19: Total displacement of reading level both by distance and near segment

Chromatic aberrations: There are mainly horizontal chromatic aberrations in high power lenses in the periphery because of difference in image sizes of red and blue images.

Selection of an ideal bifocal lens: An ideal bifocal segment selection criteria include following features

- *Elimination of image jump:* Bifocal segment should not have jump phenomenon. It can be achieved by selecting 'no jump' bifocals (e.g. executive style straight-top bifocal).

- *Elimination of differential displacement at reading level:* Straight top fused bifocal lenses fulfill this criterion, because these lenses have the segment pole at reading level.

- *Total displacement at reading level:* It should be zero or nearly zero and it can be achieved in bifocals where segment gives an opposite prismatic effect than that of distance lens. For example, a bifocal with minus distance power (means base down prismatic effect at reading) can be opposed by executive style segment having base-up prismatic effect; or a plus distance power bifocal needs base-down effect as in an Ultrex A segment, to oppose base-up prismatic effect by distance portion.

Factors required for selection of an ideal bifocal lens include: Segment size, segment height and segment shape.

Segment size or width: The size of segment of bifocal lenses has progressively increased in size as the size of spectacle frames has increased. Earlier available fused round segment bifocals had segment size of 17 mm, which has gradually increased up to 22 mm in recent years, however, segments of as wide as 35 mm are also available in special cases. Decision of segment width is made on the basis of patient requirement for near work; if more near work is requireds then a wider segment is needed.

Segment height: Initially, many practitioners thought that near segment should be placed as low as possible to avoid the interference in distance visions however, low placement of segment led to stiff neck problem in many patients. An ideal reference point for segment height is then decided as the lower lid margin. The top edge of segment is kept at level of lower lid margin or ciliary line in round top bifocals and 2–3 mm below ciliary line in straight top bifocals as shown in Fig. 7.20A and B.

Segment shape: Segment shapes are an important factor in deciding about the type of

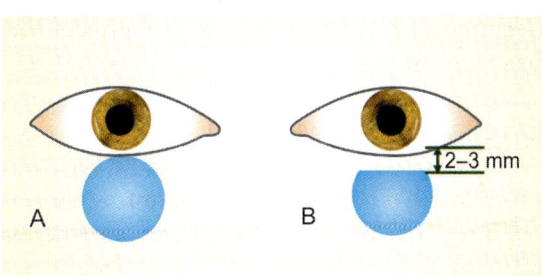

Fig. 7.20: Fitting of segment height. A. Round top segment at ciliary margin; B. Straight top segment 2–3 mm below ciliary margin

bifocal needed for various professions. Advantage of a round fused segment is that it is less visible than a straight top fused segment, hence for cosmetic reasons it is better preferred by the patients. Least visible segment is present in Nochrome round segment lens having a flesh color tint. For example, Softlite A or Cruxite A.

A very small fused round segment of about 12 mm diameter is called spot or button segment and was preferred by patients involved in profession related to distance vision. Similarly, in case of construction worker, the ribbon or bar segment bifocal lens designs with height of 9 mm was recommended because they do an occasional near work.

Lens Decentration

Lens decentration means displacement of the lens pole from its geometrical center, i.e. lens pole did not coincide with the geometric center of the rectangle of boxing system. For proper centration of the lens the geometrical center of the spectacle lens and the geometrical center of the rectangle surrounding the lens (boxing system) should correspond with each other. However, sometimes decentration is required to regulate the prismatic effects.

The prismatic effect can be added in the lens prescription by either ground the prismatic power on the lens surface or by decentering the spectacle lens. However, in a fully finished uncut lens whether prism has been grounded on the lens surface or a decentration is done to get the prism effect, the resultant prismatic

effect will be the the same. In a fully finished uncut spectacle lens decentring is generally more cost-effective as compared to grinding prism by surface procedure. Decentration is done when a small amount of prismatic effect is needed, or in high power lenses where small degree of decentration will produce desired prismatic effects. However, if prismatic effect is needed in great amount, then prism must be produced by grinding the lens surface.

Decentration of spherical lenses: Relationship between prismatic power and refractive power of the lens is represented by Prentice's rule. This rule states that on a spherical lens at any given point the prismatic effect is equal to the product of refractive power of lens and the distance of that given point from pole of the lens.

$$Ap = dP$$

Here,

Ap = Prismatic power (prism dioptre)

d = Distance from lens pole (centimeters)

P = Refracting power of lens (dioptres)

By mathematical calculation, the above formula can also be represented as

$$d = Ap/P \text{ or}$$

Decentration (d) = Prismatic power/Refracting power

The methods of decentration can be understood by this example

Consider that the spectacle lens prescription as, OD –5 DS/OS –5 DS distance PD = 66 mm, frame size = 50 mm, DBL = 22 mm.

Suppose, a base in 1Δ effect is desired in final spectacle glasses, then two steps calculations are needed for proper fitting of this minus power lens in the spectacle frame to produce this desired prismatic effect.

First step: Placement of major reference point (MRP) in alignment with pupillary center

Second step: Decentration of lens in the frame to produce prismatic effect.

First step: As discussed before, the frame PD is sum of frame size and DBL, i.e. 50 + 22 = 72 mm (in our example).

Therefore, MRP = Frame PD − IPD, i.e. 72–66 = 6 mm

Hence, in this case the pole of each lens should be moved 6 /2 = 3 mm inward (nasally) to the center of pupil when no prismatic effect is required.

Second step: According to Prentice's rule, the pole of a −5 D lens must be displaced 1Δ/5 D = 0.2 cm or 2 mm to produce 1Δ effect.

Direction of lens displacement must be outward (minus lens) to achieve a base in effect for each eye.

So, in a nutshell in first step we need to move the lens pole 3 mm inward (nasally) from geometrical center and in the second step we need to move the lens pole 2 mm outward (temporally) from pupillary center of the each eye. Hence, the total decentration of this prescription lens is 1 mm inward (nasally) from geometrical center of each lens to produce a prismatic effect of base in 1Δ.

Rule of thumb in determining the direction of decentration to produce a desired prismatic effect is that when a lens or meridian of a lens has
- A plus power then the lens decentration is done in the same direction of the base of prism.
- A minus power then the lens decentration is done in the opposite direction of the base of prism.

In the above example we needed a base in 1Δ effect for a minus 5 D lens, hence we displaced lens 2 mm in outward direction, i.e. opposite to the base of prism.

Decentration of plano-cylindrical lenses: Prismatic effect of a cylindrical lens is always perpendicular to its axis, hence a cylindrical lens can be decentered to produce a desired prismatic effect only in cases where the desired base direction is coinciding with the direction of power meridian.

So a plano-cylinder having a horizontal axis, i.e. 180° can only be decentered to produce vertical prismatic effects like base up or base down. On contrary, plano-cylinder having vertical axis, i.e. 90° can only be decentered to produce prismatic effects like base in or base out.

For example, a spectacle lens prescription has OD +2.5 DC × 90°.

Suppose we need 1Δ base in or 2Δ base out prismatic effects, then decentration of lens to be fitted in spectacle frame can be find as follows

To produce 1Δ base in effect, the spectacle lens must be decentered (using Prentice's rule) as follows

$$d = 1Δ/2.5 D$$
$$= 0.4 \text{ cm inward, because plus power in the meridian.}$$

Similarly, to produce 2Δ base out effect, the spectacle lens must be decentered (using Prentice's rule) as follows

$$d = 2Δ/2.5 D$$
$$= 0.8 \text{ cm outward, because plus power in the meridian.}$$

Decentration of spherocylindrical lenses having principal meridians as horizontal and vertical axis.

For example, a spectacle lens prescription has OD + 2 DS × −4 DC × 90°

Calculate the direction and amount of decentration to produce 1Δ base down and 1Δ base out prismatic effect.

The first step is to determine the power in each of the two principal meridians, so that we may apply Prentice's rule to each meridian, using the rule-of-thumb for the direction of decentration.

As shown in Fig. 7.21, power in the vertical meridian is +2 D and in the horizontal meridian is −2 D.

Hence, on applying Prentice rule

Base down is 1Δ/ 2 D, i.e. 0.5 cm downward displacement

Base out is 1Δ/2 D, i.e. 0.5 cm inward displacement

Hence, the spectacle lens decentration will be 0.5 cm downward and 0.5 cm inward in the above prescription to produce a 1Δ base down and 1Δ base out prismatic effect.

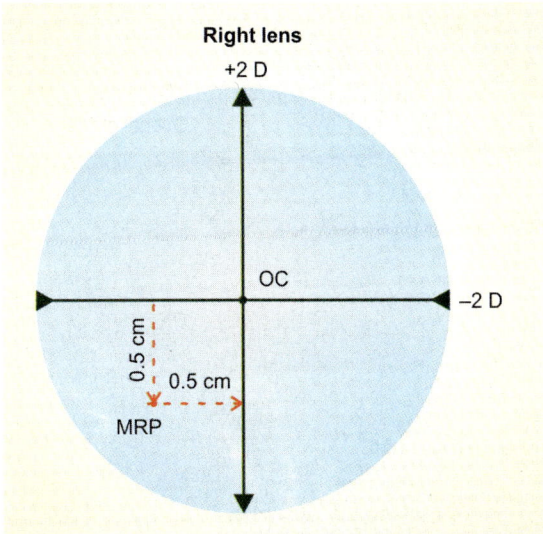

Fig. 7.21: Application of Prentice rule. MRP: Major reference point; OC: Optical center

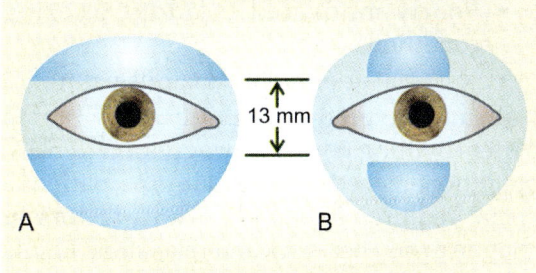

Fig. 7.22: Fitting of various double segment lens designs. A. Double executive design; B. Double straight top design

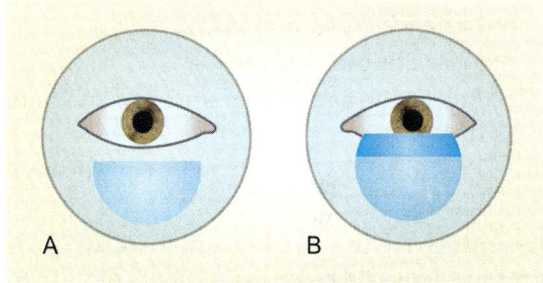

Fig. 7.23: Fitting of trifocal lens and comparing with D bifocal

Fitting of double segment bifocals: In most types of double segment bifocals separation distance between upper and lower segment is 13 mm, whereas normally cornea is vertically 11–12 mm in size. Hence, an ideal way of fitting a double segment bifocal lens is as shown in Fig. 7.22A and B.

Fitting of trifocal lenses: Although, trifocal lenses are not so commonly used nowadays but a proper fitting should be known to every practitioner. Upper edge of the trifocal near segment is kept 2–3 mm below the lower lid margins same as that in a straight top segment bifocal lens as shown in Fig. 7.23A and B.

Fitting of a progressive lens: Various factors are considered in proper fitting of a progressive lens, because it is not as simple as that of regular monofocal or bifocal lenses.

Patient selection: For better results a proper patient selection is an important concern for progressive lens fitting. The main purpose of progressive lenses is to provide a continuous vision for all distances, however, many patients and optician consider it just as an invisible bifocals. Hence, it is not a good choice for those patients who want only in invisibility in lens; however, round fused bifocal lens is a good choice for these patients but intermediate vision remains blur through these bifocal lenses. Hence, if a patient wants no visibility and his requirement is for intermediate vision, then the best choice is progressive lenses.

Normally, progressive lenses should not be prescribed for the patients who are
- Having large interpupillary distance or very wide nasal bridge.
- Satisfied with their existing bifocals or trifocals spectacles.
- Comfortable with their present reading glasses and are satisfied with it.
- Need vertical prism for correction of refractive error, because progressive lenses are not available with vertical prisms.

Note

To avoid the sensation of blurring or swimming of objects in lateral visual fields, progressive lenses wearer must be essentially a head mover, not an eye mover.

- Poorly motivated to adopt wearing conditions.
- Nervous or of highly anxious nature.

In a motivated and emotionally stable patient willing to wear progressive lenses, practitioner needs to evaluate the patient's visual requirements and various factors in relation to his/her work and relaxation. Points to be considered are

- Pupil size
- Habitual eye and head movements
- Distance correction power
- Near addition power
- Relative usage of near and intermediate distance
- Previous experience with progressive lenses

Essential fitting measurements for progressive lenses: The measurements require to fit progressive lenses differ from conventional bifocal lens fittings in the following ways

- Interpupillary distance measurement should be taken monocularly by pupilometer so that each pupil aligns with progressive corridor correctly, however, single measurement is taken by a ruler binocularly for bifocal fittings.
- In progressive lens the reference point in vertical meridian (similar to segment in bifocal lenses) is the center of pupil, not the lower lid margins or ciliary line as in conventional bifocal fittings.

The progressive addition lenses consist of two types of markings

Temporary markings as shown in Fig. 7.24A consist of a fitting cross, which corresponds to center of the pupil. A distance reference point (DRP) and a near reference point (NRP) are used to check the distance and near powers of refractive correction, respectively. The height and PD of fitting cross can be confirmed from manufacturer's centering or verification chart.

Permanent markings as shown in Fig. 7.24B are partially visible; consist of two carved circles which represent the beginning of

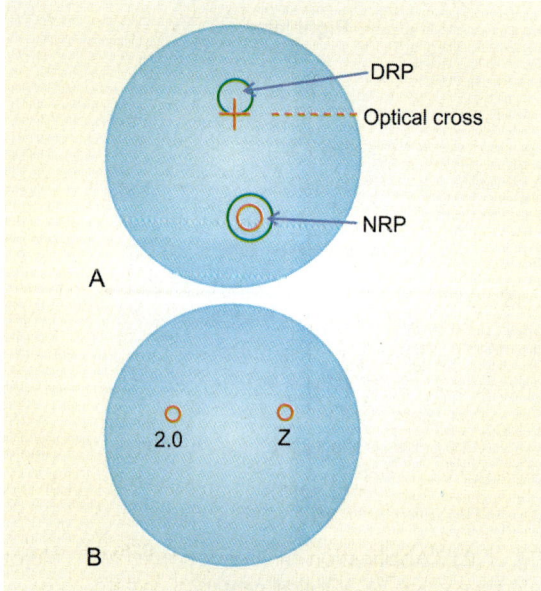

Fig. 7.24: Temporary and permanent markings on progressive lens. A. Temporary markings (DRP—distance reference point, NRP—near reference point); B. Permanent markings

progressive zone or corridor in the form of horizontal line. Some manufacturers also put their identification mark and addition power on temporal side of lens.

A precise fitting of progress lens is mandatory, because width of progressive zone or corridor is limited. Monocular distance PD measurement is essential to ensure that line of sight of each eye always remains in the progressive zone, while eyes are moving downward. Fitting steps of progressive lens are

- The distance PD is marked by corneal reflection pupilometer or by special device provided by lens manufacturer.
- Then measure the vertical distance (D) from the center of pupil to a horizontal line tangent situated at the lowest point on bottom edge of progressive lens as shown in Fig. 7.25A.
- Now place the temporary marking commonly called fitting cross on the finished lens corresponding to the center of pupil as shown in Fig. 7.25B.

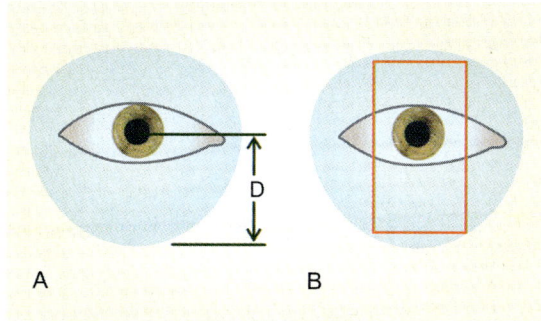

Fig. 7.25: Measurement for fitting of progressive lens. A. Vertical distance (D); B.Optical fitting box

- This center marking should be done on the same frame in which the patient's lenses will be mounted.
- Once the target spots are centered before each pupil, remove the frame and transfer target spot location on plastic lens using fine point pen.

There are two systems which are especially designed for progressive lens measurements are
- Grolman fitting system developed by American Optical: This system gets directly attach with patient's spectacle frame and has horizontal and vertical scales for marking of various measurements.
- Magna/Mark system: This is a magnetic based system consists of translucent targets to mark the various measurements.

In majority types of progressive lenses, the progressive corridor begins about 2 mm below the fitting cross; hence fitting techniques are modified according to the need of patient. Patients who like to use intermediate distance vision too much, fitting cross needs to be placed 1–2 mm above the pupillary center.

Glazing of Lens

Glazing of lens is the fitting process of an uncut ophthalmic lens inside the selected frame. The process of glazing has the following steps
- Lens shaping
- Lens cutting
- Lens edging and fitting

Lens Shaping

First of all the shape of lens is measured optically or mechanically, so that either manually or by a computer controlled lens grinding machine we can get an exact image of the desired lens before cutting begins.

Lens formers as shown in Fig. 7.26 also called patterns are usually supplied by lens manufacturers. These formers have similar shapes as that of desired spectacle lens, and are used to outline the shape of spectacle lens.

Lens former has a central hole which corresponds to the geometrical center and a line representing 0–180° plane. The geometrical center of former should be made coincide with the optical center of lens and by marking the side holes an axis can be marked accordingly on uncut lens.

Manual shaping of desired lens can be drawn by using Indian ink keeping the pattern on a sheet or hard board paper. Cylindrical axis, if present, is marked over the uncut lens by lensometer as three dots using greased pencil or Indian ink.

Once we had marked the uncut lens with axis of cylinder and outlined the shape of lens, the center mark and nasal side of lens is marked by using specially designed protectors in relation to cylindrical axis of lens.

Lens Cutting

After proper marking of uncut lens the extra part of lens is cut, usually a little extra than

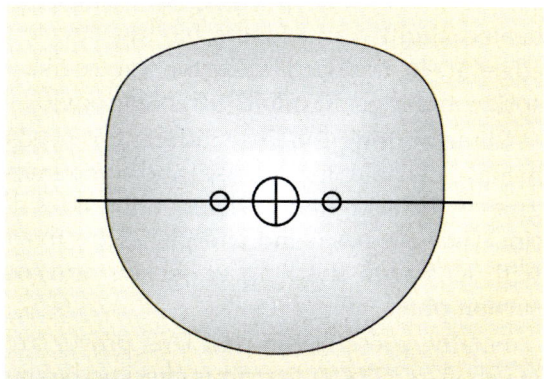

Fig. 7.26: Lens former showing 0 to 180° line for marking.

the shape marked because some margins are needed to form the edge of lens for proper fitting. After cutting the formed rough lens shape should be matched with size and shape of the frame.

The lens cutting can be done manually by using a chipper (before using chipper groove the outline of lens shape with a diamond pencil) or alternately a diamond cutter wheel or fully automated cutting machine can be used.

Lens Edging and Fitting

The partial finished lens formed after cutting also need proper edges so that it can fit properly inside the frame. Therefore, edging of lens is done either manually on a rotating diamond wheel or by fully automatic machines, although edging by manual way is more economically viable than automatic machines. For manual edging various types of grit wheels are available to grind the lens edges and to make it smooth and shiny. Nowadays diamond wheels are also present which produce faster, accurate and smooth edges of lens at an economical price. Various edge shapes which can be produced are flat, bevel, groove and mid-bevel as shown in Fig. 7.27.

After formation of well-edged lens, the next step is to fit this polished finely shaped lens into the spectacle frame. In metallic frames usually a bevel-edged lens is fitted by opening the frame sides and refitting the side screw, whereas in plastic frames the lenses are fitted by a method called springing in. Frames are heated slightly and lenses having beveled edges are just pressed inside the frames like a spring and it get fit into the frame groove.

Rimless fitting is a little different, it needs to make the holes in the lenses and sometimes grooves are also cut near holes on the sides of rim. Then the nasal and end pieces are fixed with lens with the help of screws and/or suction plugs.

Finally, prescription and lens power are matched, quality of lens fit is checked before cleaning and packing for dispensing of

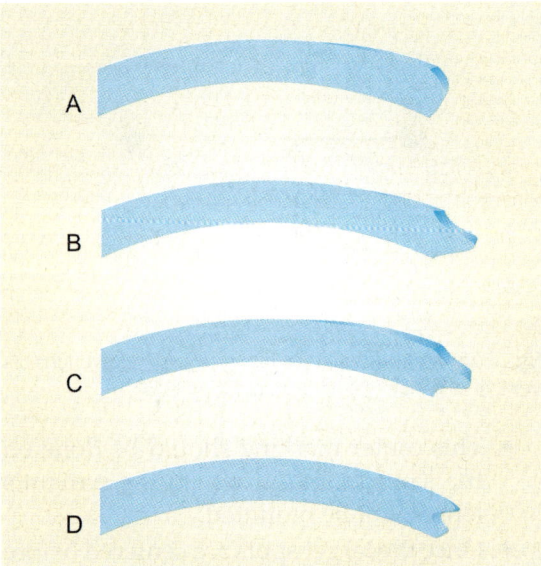

Fig. 7.27: Various types of lens edges. A. Flat; B. Bevel; C. Mid-bevel; D. Groove

spectacle. With an expert fitter whole glazing process may take 10–15 minutes.

Verifications of Spectacles

Sometimes, the patient may complain that the lenses prescribed to him/her are not proper and there was an error in evaluating the degree of refractive error. However, on careful examination, it may be found that the problem was due to an error of either dispensing or fitting of lenses. Hence, it is mandatory to verify the spectacles before dispensing.

Spectacle verification means to verify the lens powers, cylindrical axis, optical center and prismatic effect of spectacle lenses along with any surface defects, if present. It is also essential to check the fitting of lens in the frame along with the frame alignment. Before dispensing the spectacle we should check

* Surface defects
* Lens power measurement
* Frame alignment

Surface Defects

Sometimes there may be defect in the surface which may occur during manufacturing (waves in lens) or during glazing and fitting (aberrations, chipping or dents) and can be missed many a times by dispenser.

Lens Power Measurement

Lens power and cylindrical axis of a spectacle lens can easily be measured by lensometer; however, in the absence of instrument manual neutralization can be done to assess the parameters of spectacle lens.

Hand neutralization techniques for spectacle lenses

For spherical lenses

For neutralization of an unknown spherical spectacle lens the following method is used

- Hold the spectacle lens at about 1 meter distance while keeping its back surface towards examiner and then observe an object at 20 feet distance.

- The object should have both vertical and horizontal shapes. For example, a large cross or square or 6/60 size letter A.

- Focus on the image at central zone of the lens and slowly move the spectacle lens, both in vertical and horizontal meridians.

- Observe whether the transverse movement of object appears to be in the same direction or in the opposite direction in comparison to the movement of the spectacle lens.

- Same direction movement or 'with motion' indicates that it is a minus lens as shown in Fig. 7.28. An opposite direction movement or 'against motion' indicates that it is a plus lens.

- In plus lenses, 'against motion' is seen until the distance between the plus lens and observer's eye is less than focal length of plus lens (Fig. 7.29). If this distance is more than focal length of the lens, then 'with motion' will be seen like minus lenses, but the image will be inverted.

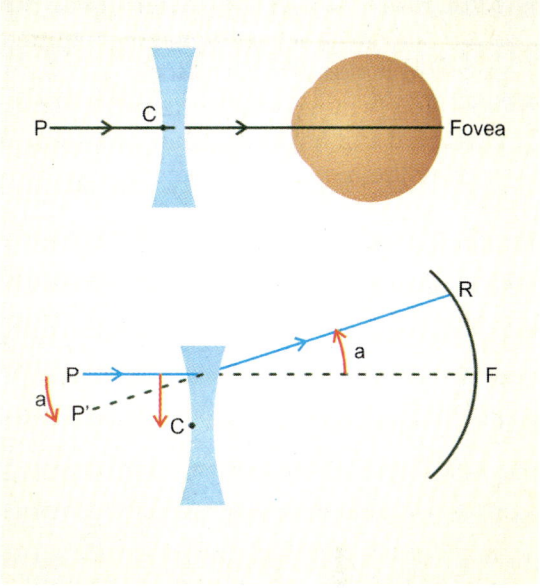

Fig. 7.28: Downward movement of minus lens, showing downward movement (same direction) of object from P to P' position

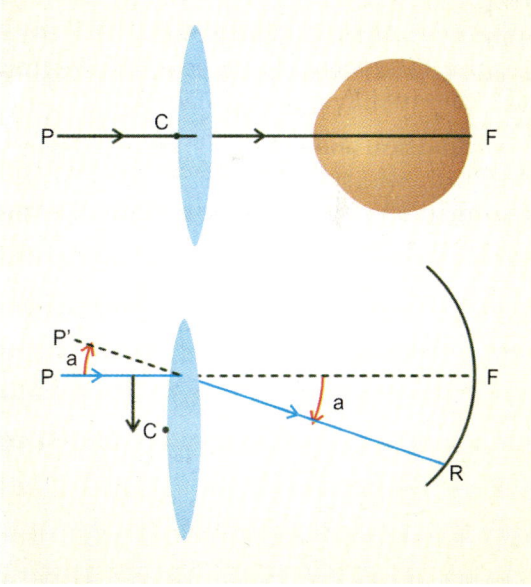

Fig. 7.29: Downward movement of plus lens, showing upward movement (opposite direction) of object from P to P' position

- Now take a lens of opposite power from trial lenses and keep its back surface in contact with the front surface of this unknown power spectacle lens.

- With more and more experience, the examiner can closely estimate the required power of neutralizing trial lens.
- Now slowly move both the lenses together in vertical and horizontal meridians while judging the motion of object simultaneously.
- Suppose the power of neutralizing lens is inadequate, then a movement of object will be seen ('with motion' with low power and 'against motion' with high power) and if power of neutralizing lens is sufficient or equal, then no movement of object image will be noticed. For example, if no motion is observed when a +2.5 DS power trial lens is used as neutralizing lens, then the power of unknown spectacle lens is –2.5 DS.

In case of spherical lenses the examiner observes the motion in the same speed and same direction in both horizontal and vertical meridians. However, the situation will be different with unknown cylindrical or spherocylindrical type spectacle lenses because the speed and direction of motion may vary in different meridians.

For cylindrical and sphero-cylindrical lenses:
Neutralization of cylindrical or spherocylindrical spectacle lens is done by the following method

- Similar to a spherical lens, examiner holds the spectacle lens at one meter distance keeping its back surface towards him/her and observes an object, e.g. a plus (+) mark at 20 feet distance.
- Then examiner rotates the spectacle lens either clockwise or anticlockwise and observes a scissors like motion of the object.
- When a cross target is observed through spectacle lens, the displacement of its vertical and horizontal lines will be seen as compared to their original positions present outside the spectacle lens as shown in Fig. 7.30A.
- During rotation when spectacle lens gets oriented in a way that two limbs of target cross become parallel and continuous with principal meridians of spectacle lens, then the displacement of vertical and horizontal limbs of cross target disappears as shown in Fig. 7.30B.
- Once examiner reaches to an orientation where both limbs of target cross are parallel and continuous both inside and outside the spectacle lens, then a further rotation of spectacle lens will show a scissors motion either with or against the rotation of spectacle lens.

Hand neutralization method to determine the cylindrical power and axis.

- Observer holds the spectacle lens firmly in position where the spectacle lines are parallel and continuous with cross target

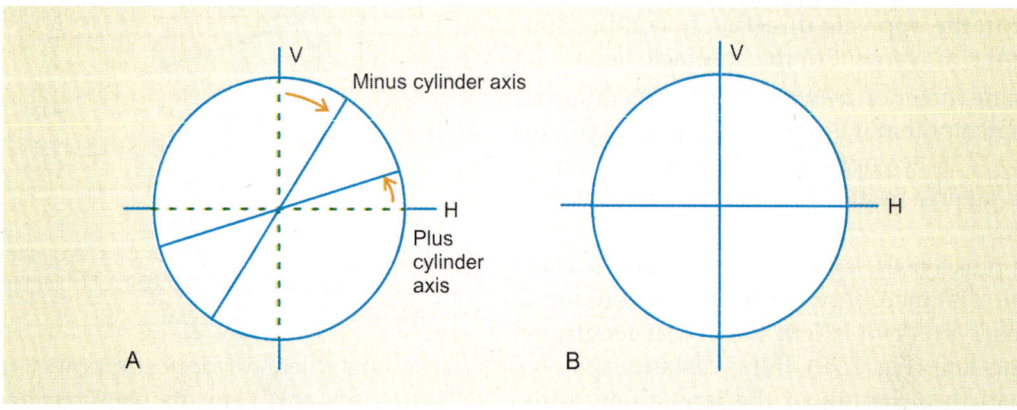

Fig. 7.30: Hand neutralization of spectacle lens containing cylindrical power. A. Off-axis cylinder showing scissor movement; B. On-axis cylinder

limbs both inside and outside the spectacle lens.

- Then examiner draws line ABOCD in vertical axis as shown in Fig. 7.31A over limbs seen inside the spectacle lens using grease pencil on the back surface of the spectacle lens.
- Examiner then rotates the spectacle lens and observes the movement of this vertical line ABOCD.
- Suppose line seen inside the spectacle lens rotates as 'with motion' in the direction of the rotation of spectacle lens, means that line ABOCD of cross target is parallel to the minus cylinder axis as shown in Fig. 7.31B.
- When line inside the spectacle lens rotates against the direction of rotation of spectacle lens, means that line ABOCD of cross target is parallel to plus cylinder as shown in Fig. 7.31C.
- Once two principal meridians of spectacle lens of unknown power are localized, then neutralize each meridian separately using spherical lenses.
- Examiner firmly holds the spectacle lens against the line of cross on trial lens representing the axis of neutralization inside and outside the spectacle lens. Then examiner marks the axis on unknown cylindrical spectacle lens with grease pencil. This axis can be measured with the help of a lens protractor, however, an approximate ±5° will occur in manual assessment of axis.

- After neutralizing each principal meridian, power and axis are noted and a prescription of spectacle lens is written in a minus cylinder form. For example, if spectacle lens gets neutralized in horizontal meridian with –5 DS trial lens and in vertical meridian with –3 DS trial lens, it means power of unknown spectacle lens is +5 DS in the horizontal meridian and +3 DS in the vertical meridian. Prescription for unknown lens would be written as + 5 DS/–2 DC × 180°.

Another difficult task in hand neutralization method is to mark the optical center or pole of spectacle lens.

- To mark the optical center of spectacle lens, examiner identifies the point where the two lines of target cross meet inside and outside the spectacle lens. Then mark a small dot on the lens while holding the spectacle lens in a position where the lines inside and outside are parallel and continuous as described above.

Frame Alignments

As we normally consider that the standard alignment of frame has been already done by the manufacturers, so we prefer to fit the lens

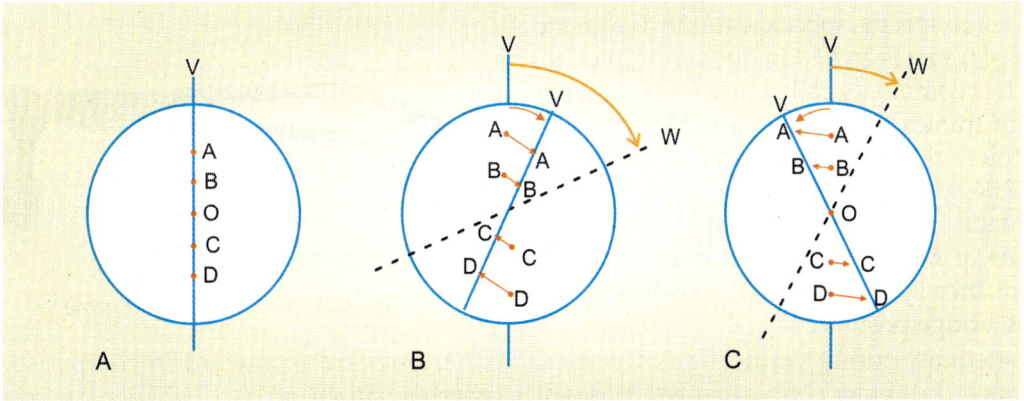

Fig. 7.31: Determination of cylindrical axis. A. Marking of axis line ABOCD over spectacle lens; B. With movement in case of minus cylinder; C. Against movement in case of plus cylinder

directly. However, this is not always true and often it becomes necessary for dispenser to check the frame alignment before dispensing.

A proper frame alignment is done by the following methodology

- Front alignment
- Temple alignment

Front alignment: Front alignment is done in two steps with the help of device having straight border, e.g. a millimeter ruler.

First step: examiner places the millimeter ruler against the back of spectacle frame below the end pieces as shown in Fig. 7.32, while spectacle frame is held horizontally. Then examiner observes whether right and left end pieces are at equal distances above the ruler or not. If they are at equal distance, then no adjustment is needed, however, if they are at unequal distance, then the frame bridge is either raised or lowered so that they become equal.

Second step: Examiner then verifies the vertical alignment of spectacle frame by placing the ruler along the back surface of frame underneath or above the nose pads with temples extending upwards while spectacle frame is held vertically as shown in Fig. 7.33. In proper alignment situation the ruler should touch four points on spectacle frame. Two points are back surfaces of each lens (or eye wire above each lens) and one point each at nasal and temporal edges of spectacle frame.

In some specific spectacle frame design the front of frame is arched in outward direction, which is commonly called face form. In these design frames the nasal edges of frame will not touch the millimeter ruler as shown in Fig. 7.34. Mostly aviation types of sunglasses are made in this design. Suppose preferred degree of face form or four point touch is absent, then it can be rectified by adjusting the frame bridge position.

Sometimes during verification of vertical alignment, examiner notices that two lenses of spectacle frame are in different vertical planes (X-ing of frame), means one side lens is tilted

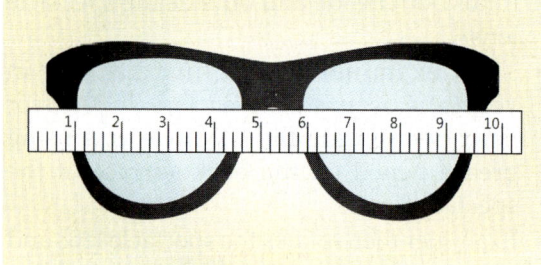

Fig. 7.32: Examination for front alignment of spectacle frame

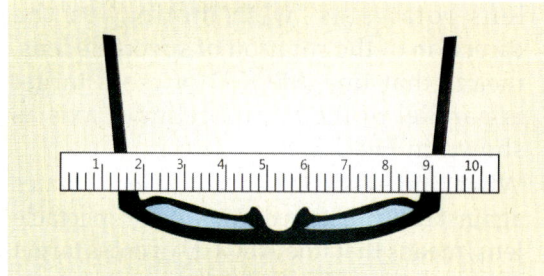

Fig. 7.33: Examination for vertical alignment of spectacle frame front

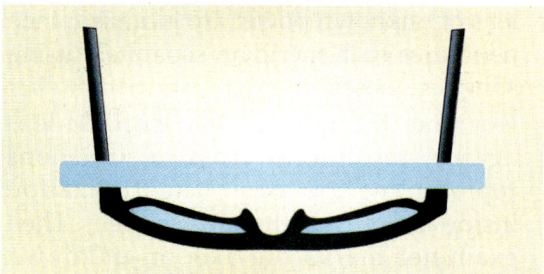

Fig. 7.34: Face form in spectacle frame

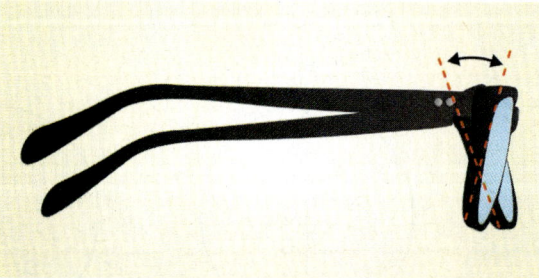

Fig. 7.35: X-ing of spectacle frame

either outward or inward in comparison to other as shown in Fig. 7.35. Similar to face form correction X-ing can also be corrected by adjustment of frame bridge rotation.

Temple alignment: Normally in a properly aligned spectacle frame a pantoscopic tilt (generally 6°–10°) and temple angle of 92°–95° (a little greater than a right angle) is present. This procedure is done for the adjustments of pantoscopic tilt and temple angle in case if they are disturbed. Equality in pantoscopic tilt of the spectacle frame is checked by placing the spectacle frame on a glass top table with temples facing downward. Suppose one of the temples does not touch the glass surface fully as shown in Fig. 7.36, it means that end piece on that side of frame has a larger degree of pantoscopic tilt compared to the end piece of the other

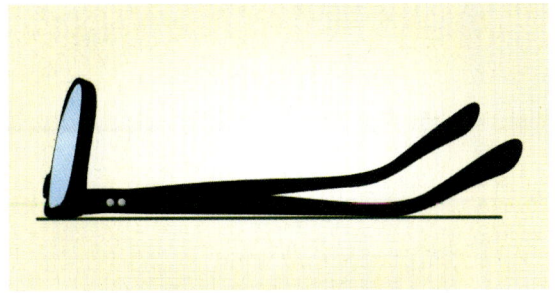

Fig. 7.36: Unequal pantoscopic angles

side. Similarly, both sides of spectacle frame should have the same degree of temple angle. This can be easily assessed by examination of frame.

Contact Lens: An Overview

INTRODUCTION

Contact lens is a small piece of plastic which is designed to rest on the cornea and/or sclera in such a way that they are in direct contact of cornea and correct the refractive errors of eye. Along with optical uses, a contact lens can be used for various other purposes also including therapeutic, cosmetic and diagnostic.

History and Events of Progress

Basis aim of several researchers was to neutralize the front surface of cornea with the help of various devices.

- In the year 1508, Leonardo da Vinci came up with an idea that a vision of a person can be altered by immersing head up to ears with face down in half water filled specially designed bowl.
- In the year 1636, Descartes suggested that corneal surface can be neutralized by placing a tube filled with water on the cornea having a watch glass on the other end.
- In the year 1801, Thomas Young on the basis of principle of Descartes tried to neutralize his refractive power by designing long tube filled with water, having a lens of 20 mm focal length on the other end.
- In the year 1827, John Herschel done experiment with application of animal jelly in the form of glass capsule on the eyes in order to eliminate the astigmatic errors.

- In the year 1886, first proposal of hydrophilic contact appliance came from Galezowsky, who suggested the use of a gelatin disc soaked in cocaine and sublimate of mercury for post-cataract extraction cases.
- In the year 1887, FA Muller used a glass blown lens to cover the eye of a patient whose eyelids had been removed.
- In the year 1888, Fick was the first to coin the term contact lens and used a non-optical corneal contact lens for treatment of keratoconus. He also suggested the use of contact lens for aphakia and cosmetic purposes.
- Nearly for 40 years period (1895–1930) all contact lenses were made up of glass. Basically of two types
  - Blown glass from Muller
  - Ground glass from Carl Zeiss
- For another decade methods were developed to take eye cast by using material like Negocolle, a seaweed extract mainly used for dental purposes.
- In the year 1938, Obrig diagnosed that contact lens intolerance was due to limbal pressure. He also discovered that fluorescein solution with blue light can be used to check the contact lens fit.
- In the year 1937 Feinbloom first time used the plastic material for contact lens. Lenses

made by him had a glass optic with a plastic scleral zone.

– Subsequently, in the year 1943 the true corneal lenses having diameter of 11–12 mm were introduced, popularly called Tuohy lens.

- During 1950–1960 Gyorrfy revolutionalized the contact lens manufacturing world by introduction of Polymethyl methacrylate (PMMA) contact lenses for production of soft contact lenses, which shortly followed by use of hydroxyl methyl methacrylate (HEMA) in the year 1963.

- In the year 1970, rigid contact lenses (made up of PMMA) were introduced. Later on in the year 1978, rigid gas permeable (RGP) lenses were also manufactured by using Cellulose Acetate Butyrate material (CAB).

- Silicon acrylate material was introduced in the year 1975–78. Around the same period, CIBA Vision Company introduced tinted and bifocal contact lenses.

- Later on, in the year 1986, it was Johnson and Johnson Company who manufactured the weekly disposable contact lenses.

Contact lenses differ from spectacle lenses in many aspects. Important difference is that the spectacle lenses are worn about 12–15 mm away from the corneal surface, hence only vergence of incident rays hitting the corneal surface is altered. However, in case of contact lens, as it remains in contact with corneal surface, the vergence of the incident rays not altered, rather vergence of eye itself is altered. Hence in case of spectacle lens the refractive power of eye gets an accessory effort and there is no real change in refractive status of eye, on contrary, in case of a contact lens, the real refractive status of eye is changed. This change in refractive status of eye is contributed by the fact that when contact lens is in place, the anterior surface of cornea becomes optically absent, as it becomes the posterior surface of a liquid or glass lens. Furthermore, there is a chance of independent viewing movement of eyes behind the spectacles which is not seen

with contact lens. The prismatic effects are observed more with the use of spectacle lens than contact lens.

Concept of Contact Lens Forms

To understand the function of a contact lens, it is essential to know the concept of glass lens and liquid lens. As we know that tear film play a significant part in corneal integrity to perform the refractive role, we should know the dynamics of tear film and contact lens together for functioning of a contact lens as corrective device.

Depending upon the curvatures of contact lens and corneal surface various lens forms are seen as

- Afocal segment
- Liquid lens
- Glass lens or focal segment
- Combined lens system

Afocal segment: When curvatures of both the surfaces of contact lens are the same, then they form an afocal contact lens. For example, contact lens having anterior surface of +6 D and posterior surface of –6 D.

As we can see in Fig. 8.1 that when three curvatures (two surfaces of contact lens and one surface of cornea) are same, the contact lens serves as afocal segment, where anterior surface of contact lens becomes anterior surface of refractive system.

Liquid lens: When two curvatures of contact lens surfaces (both anterior and posterior) are

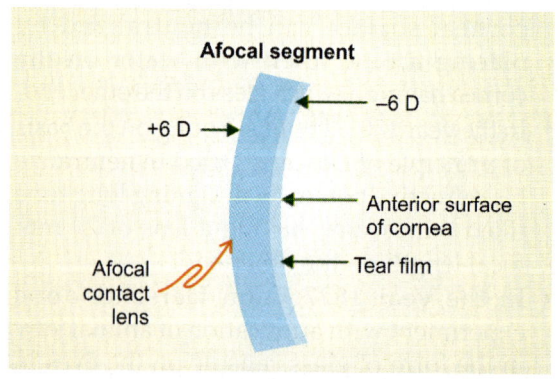

Fig. 8.1: Afocal segment

same like afocal segment but they are different from the anterior surface of cornea, then it forms a liquid lens. The elements of refraction in this kind of system are contact lens, tear film lens (liquid lens) and anterior surface of cornea, which are separated by an invisibly thin air film. Hence in this system the effective refractive power will be exerted by back vertex power of liquid lens in the air.

As we can see in Fig. 8.2, the posterior surface of contact lens and anterior surface of the cornea forms a lens filled with liquid (tear film), called liquid lens or tear lens or fluid lens. The correction of ametropia will be due to the refractive power of this lens, which is equal to a sum of anterior and posterior surfaces of tear lens.

Glass lens: When curvature of posterior surface of contact lens is the same as that of cornea, but curvature of anterior surface of contact lens is different, then they form a glass lens or focal segment or powered lens.

As shown in Fig. 8.3, a focal segment is formed due to difference in curvatures of anterior and posterior surfaces of contact lens. To understand the refractive power of this type of system, if we know the power of posterior surface of contact lens (which is usually kept fixed), then only task remains is to know the power of anterior surface of contact lens (which usually has a relationship with anterior corneal surface and decided empirically).

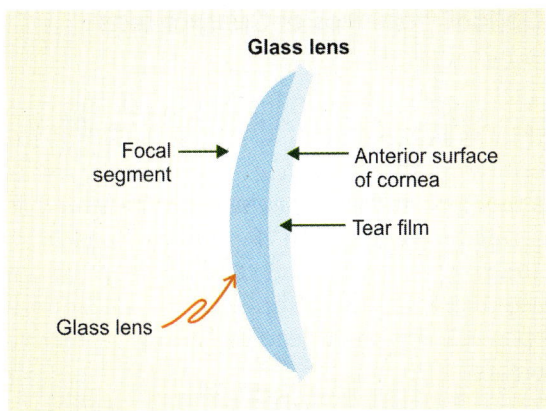

Fig. 8.3: Glass lens

Suppose the posterior contact lens surface is parallel to anterior corneal surface, then back vertex power of contact lens will be equal to ocular refractive status.

Combined lens: When the curvatures of three elements, i.e. anterior and posterior surfaces of contact lens and anterior surface of cornea, are different to each other, then the effective power of system is determined by power of both the liquid lens and glass lens.

As we can see in Fig. 8.4, that two lenses are formed: Anteriorly a glass lens and posteriorly a liquid lens. Refractive status of this system is a combined power of these two lenses. Although ametropia can be corrected by tear lens alone, but in routine practice both the liquid lens and glass lens in combination are used to neutralize the refractive error.

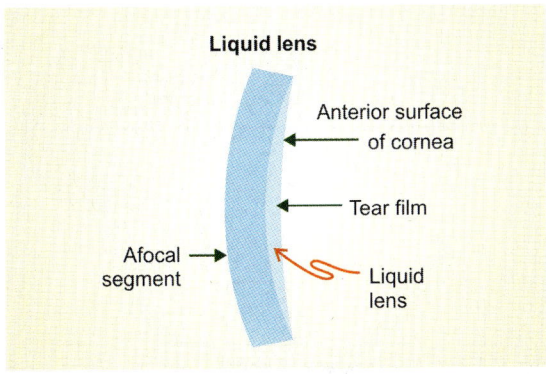

Fig. 8.2: Liquid lens

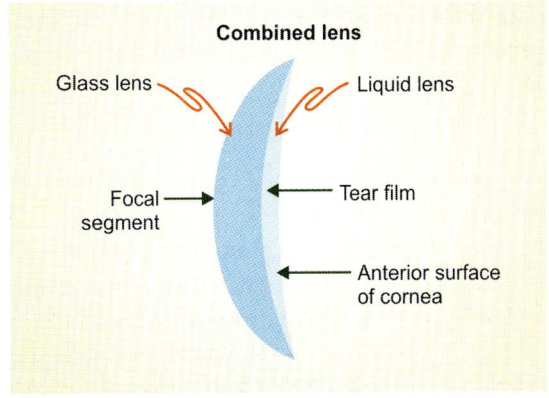

Fig. 8.4: Combined lens

Optical Properties of Contact Lens

Thick Lens

Although a contact lens physically appears thin as compared to spectacle lens but for optical reasons spectacle lens is considered as a thin lens and a contact lens is considered as a thick lens. Because the contact lens is so steeply curved, that application of an approximate power formula, as in case of a spectacle lens, will lead to serious refractive errors.

Effective Power of Contact Lens

The effective power of a correcting lens (contact lens or glasses) changes as we bring it nearer to eye. In case of a contact lens the correcting lens is brought very near to eye, i.e. it touches the eyes. Effective lens power is determined by the relative position of correcting lens with that of vertex plane. While in case of spectacles, the lens is placed at 14–15 mm in front of vertex plane, whereas in case of a contact lens, the lens is placed on vertex plane. For example, a minus lens becomes more effective when moves towards the eye, whereas a plus lens becomes more effective when moves farther away from the eye. This means that for a myope a contact lens must be weaker than a spectacle lens, whereas for a hypermetrope a contact lens power should be stronger than a spectacle lens for correction of the same amount of refractive error.

Effective power of a contact lens can be calculated from spectacle power or lens prescription by this simple formula:

$$P_A = \frac{P_O}{1 - d\,P_O}$$

Here P_O = power at original position of lens

P_A = power at altered position of lens
d = distance the lens has been moved (in meters), is given a plus sign if moved towards the eyes and a minus sign if moved away from the eyes.

To understand this, let us consider a myope of –8 D spectacle lens power at vertex distance of 12 mm (12/1000 meters), calculate the contact lens power (Fig. 8.5).

As per formula

$$P_A = \frac{-8}{1 - 0.012(-8)}$$

$$= \frac{-8}{1 + 0.096}$$

$$= \frac{-8}{1.096}$$

$$= -7.29 \text{ D}$$

Similarly, suppose an aphakic patient needs +12 D spectacle power at vertex distance of 12 mm, then the contact lens power will be calculated as shown in Fig. 8.6.

As per formula

$$P_A = \frac{+12}{1 - 0.012\,(+12)}$$

$$= \frac{+12}{1 - 0.144}$$

$$= \frac{+12}{0.856}$$

$$= +14.01 \text{ D}$$

The abovementioned examples clearly indicate that for myopia the power of contact lens will be less than power of a spectacle lens, whereas for hypermetropic eyes it will be more than a spectacle lens.

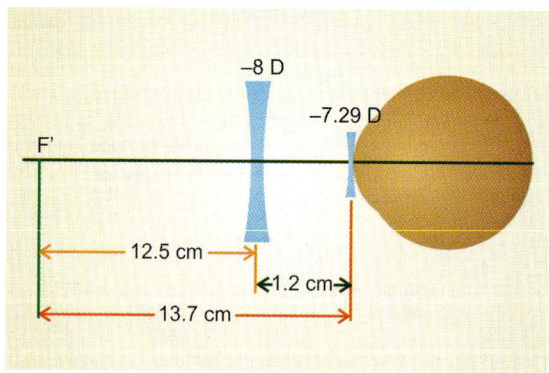

Fig. 8.5: Effective power of a contact lens for a 8 D myope; when refracted at vertex distance of 12 mm

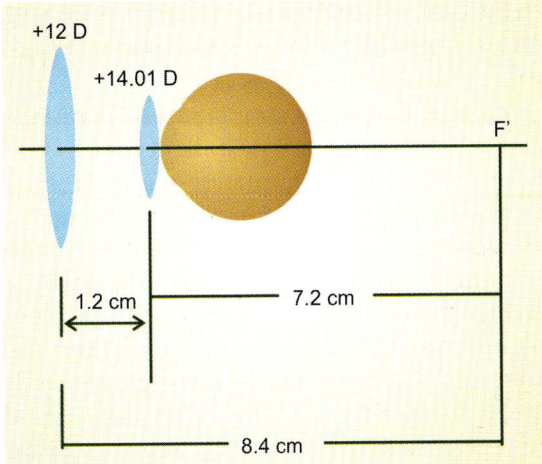

Fig. 8.6: Effective power of a contact lens for an aphakic having +12 D power; when refracted at vertex distance of 12 mm

> **Note**
>
> When refractive errors in eyes are of less than ±3 D, then the power difference between contact lens and a spectacle lens will be about 0.12 D, which can be considered as negligible for all practical purposes.

Change in Retinal Image Magnification

The change in magnification of retinal image is another optical effect of contact lens which is due to more closeness of contact lens to eyes. So, when a person shifts from spectacles to contact lens, he/she will observe change in size of the image of objects.

It is due to the fact that during calculation of magnification by spectacles, the distance between back of lens and entrance to pupil of eye is also included. It means if a correcting lens is brought near to eyes, the retinal image magnification will change which is seen with contact lens. Therefore, in a myopic person, the contact lens will produce a retinal image bigger in size than a spectacle lens, hence a myopic patient who starts wearing a contact lenses will usually feel happy by the fact that everything looks larger than before. On contrary, in hypermetropic patient the contact lens will produce retinal image smaller in size than spectacle lens, hence a hypermetrope

> **Note**
>
> Usually, aphakics wearing spectacles lens have an image magnification of about 22% which is difficult to adjust binocularly, however, with contact lens the same person will have an image magnification of only 7% which is easier to adjust binocularly.

especially an aphakic will be pleased by the fact that now the objects are looking nearly to their normal sizes.

Effect on Refractive Status

As contact lenses are in direct contact of eyes, the refractive status of eye may change especially with the use of hard contact lens. On contrary, eyes are also capable to change the refractive power of contact lens especially of a soft contact lens. These changes in refractive power are of important in cases of astigmatism. A spherical hard contact lens usually hide or eliminate the corneal astigmatism, whereas a spherical soft contact lens remain confine with the toricity of cornea and produce very little or no effect on corneal astigmatism. Hence, to correct astigmatism by means of soft contact lenses, toric contact lenses should be used.

Effect on Accommodative Demand

Shift of spectacle glasses to contact lens in both myopes and hypermetropes also cause change in accommodative demand. Myopes using minus glasses has an advantage over an emmetropic person in terms of accommodative demand because the use of minus spectacle glasses decreases the accommodative demand in myopes. Suppose a myope switch over to contact lens from spectacles, then he/she has to exert more accommodative power. On contrary, in hypermetropes use of plus spectacle glasses causes increase in the accommodative demand and when they switch over to contact lens the need of accommodative demand is decreased.

The change in demand of accommodation in contact lens wearer myopes and hypermetropes as compared to spectacles lens wearer has important role at presbyopic age. In contact lens wearer myopics, the addition power for near work will be required at earlier age, whereas contact lens wearer hypermetrope will need additional power for near work at a later age as compared to spectacle worn counterpart.

An average amount of accommodation needed while wearing contact lenses is about 2.5 D irrespective to the amount or type of refractive error. Consider this fact in example, a +10 D hypermetrope wearing spectacles require 3.29 D of accommodation for a 40 cm reading distance, whereas a −10 D myope counterpart needs only 1.8 D for the same reading distance. So in this example hypermetrope has to accommodate about 0.75 D less (i.e. 2.5 – 3.29), while myope needs to accommodate 0.75 D more (i.e. 2.5 – 1.8), when these hypermetrope and myope patients wear contact lenses instead of spectacles.

> **Note** _____
> Persons having very high degree myopia ([3]14 D) will face problems in wearing contact lenses, due to a significant increase in demand of accommodation.

Effect on Accommodative Convergence

An increase demand of accommodation in myopes due to wearing of contact lenses will lead to use of more accommodative convergence. On the other hand, hypermetrope wearing contact lens will use less accommodative convergence. As a result, contact lens wearer myope having esophoria will have to apply more negative fusional vergence than glasses wearer myope, resulting in increased eye strain. While in an exophoric contact wearer myope, increase in the accommodative convergence will decrease the use of positive fusional vergence, and thus results in reduced exophoria. Similarly, an exophoric hypermetrope contact lens wearer will require more positive fusional vergence than glasses.

The change in accommodative demand and fusional vergence due to contact lens are practically insignificant for refractive errors of small degree, however, the changes may have significant effects in cases of large refractive errors, especially if there is an associated high AC/A ratio.

As in the above example, a −10 D myope and + 10 D hypermetrope both needs more or less 0.75 D of accommodation respectively, if they wear a contact lens in place of spectacles. However, a change in accommodative demand of almost 0.75 D will be accompanied by a change in accommodative convergence. Now if they have an AC/A ratio of 6, then the change in accommodative convergence at 40 cm distance will be of 6 × 0.75 which is equal to 4.5 prism dioptres (Δ). Hence, in an exophoric myope, exophoria will be reduced by 4.5 Δ, while in esophoric myope esophoria will be increased by 4.5 Δ at 40 cm distance. It means an exophoric myope having a refractive error of −10 D will use 4.5 Δ less positive fusional vergence, when uses contact lens in place of spectacles. On the other hand, an esophoric myope in the same situation will use more negative fusional vergence of 4.5 Δ.

Similarly, a +10 D hypermetrope when switch from spectacles to contact lenses, then an exophoria at 40 cm will be increased by 4.5 Δ and an esophoria will be decreased by 4.5 Δ at the same distance.

Routinely, majority of contact lens wearers has a refractive error in the range of ±1 D to ±5 D, hence the change in accommodative convergence, needed with use of contact lenses instead of spectacles; do not present a significant clinical problem.

> **Note** _____
> In an aphakic patient due to absence of crystalline lens, the accommodative convergence does not exist because of lack of accommodation, hence when they switch from spectacle to contact lenses, there is no change in the demand of fusional convergence for near vision.

Prismatic Effects as Compared to Spectacles

Spectacles lens induces prismatic effect which occurs because line of sight moves away from major reference point of lenses as spectacle lens remain fixed and do not move with movement of eyes, while contact lens moves with the movement of eyes, hence no significant prismatic effects are produced with contact lenses.

For example, in case of myopes "base in" effect is produced by minus lenses, while "base out" prismatic effect is produced by plus lenses for near vision. Hence, when an exophoric myope switches from spectacles to contact lenses, he/she will be at disadvantage due to lack of base in prismatic effect for near work, whereas an esophoric hypermetrope when switches from spectacle to contact lenses, similarly will have disadvantage because of lack of base out prismatic effect for near work. A vertical prismatic effect during up and down gaze and change in demand of vergence during right and left gaze in anisometropia is seen with spectacles lenses, but wearing of contact lenses eliminate this prismatic effect.

> **Note** _____
>
> Although use of contact lens eliminates many unwanted prismatic effects of spectacles lens but due to contact lens some beneficial prismatic effects are also eliminated. For example, spectacle lens can correct a lateral prismatic deviation which is lost with contact lens.

Aberrations and Field of View

Most important types of aberrations which can be experienced with spectacle lens are oblique astigmatism, curvature of image, and distortion. All of these aberrations are minimized by the use of contact lenses which move with the movement of eyes.

Oblique astigmatism and curvature of image aberration happens when spectacle wearer rotates his/her eyes to look through the periphery of spectacle lenses, however, contact lens wearers has no such issue to look through the periphery.

Distortion of image occurs due to distance between aperture of spectacle lens and aperture (pupil) of eye. However, in case of contact lens, this distance is negligible, hence very minimum distortion of image.

Field of view is larger in majority of the contact lens wearers as compared to spectacle glasses. In a moving eye, contact lens wearer has an additional advantage of unlimited macular field of view which is absent in a spectacle worn person because due to presence of rim of spectacle's frame the macular field gets restricted as a field of fixation.

CONTACT LENS MATERIALS

Introduction

History about contact lenses tells us that initially for manufacturing of contact lens the glass material were used, mainly blown glass of Muller and ground glass of Carl Zeiss. However, a constant hunt for an ideal contact lens material was on, because contact lens of glass material were brittle, heavy and were difficult to manufacture in mass.

A revolution in contact lens material took place in the year 1943 when Kevin Tuohy introduced plastic material for manufacturing of contact lens. Although a few years back Obrig had already started the use of methyl methacrylate to produce contact lenses.

Subsequently, Gyorrfy introduced PMMA for lens, and then Wichterle changed the picture of contact lens world by introducing the hydroxyl methyl methacrylate in the year 1963. Gradually, acrylic, silicon and cellulose acetate butyrate were also introduced as contact lens materials for mass manufacturing.

Properties required in an ideal contact lens material are

- *Optical property:* Lens material should have a good percentage, i.e. 95–98% of light transmission and have a refractive index compatible with tears and cornea.
- *Ocular compatibility:* Material should be safe to wear and has no harmful effects on ocular surface especially cornea.

- *Gas permeability:* In absence of contact lens the cornea receives oxygen through tears, thus lens material should have good oxygen transmission through it so that cornea does not suffocate. Hence gas permeability through material is a major factor to decide tolerance and duration of wearing of lens.
- *Physical properties:* Specific gravity and density of the material are important properties to keep the contact lens in position because a high density material will not stay for a long period on the corneal surface.
- *Chemical properties:* Lens material should be easily wettable and water should not spread over its surface (hydrophilic), so that tear film can serve better when contact lens is in position.
- *Material strength:* This property decides that whether lens will maintain its shape and curvatures after fitting. This is important to maintain the optical property of contact lens.
- *Resistant nature:* Contact lens material should be highly resistant to chemical agents and microbial contamination, so that it will remain sterile during wearing. It should have a property to easily get sterilized by chemicals or radiations.
- *Moulding:* An easy mouldability of lens material is a prerequisite to give proper shape and curvatures to manufacture lens in large scale.

Terminologies in Contact Lens Material

For better understanding of properties of contact lens material, we should be well versed with the following related terminologies.

Water Properties Related to Lens

A hydrated contact lens has the following water elements
- Water content
- Water absorption
- Wettability

Water content: Water content means the quantity of water present in a lens. We can measure it in terms of volume or weight. It can be expressed as:

Water content = wet weight – dry weight/wet weight × 100

Water content of a contact lens is usually equilibrated in presence of 0.9% saline and change in conditions like pH and tonicity of solution and temperature can alter the water properties of lens.

Water absorption: It means the quantity of water that a contact lens can absorb, means it measures the water uptake capacity of lens and can be expressed as

Water absorption = wet weight – dry weight/dry weight × 100

Wettability: This is important to maintain the corneal tear film. Wettability indicates the adherent property of a liquid to a solid surface, despite that the liquid is held by cohesive forces. This can be assessed by contact angle which is inversely proportional to wettability. Thus a lower value of contact angle indicates better wettability than a higher contact angle. On the basis of contact angle various contact lens materials can be grouped as
- Hydrophilic = 0° contact angle
- Hydrogel = 20° contact angle
- Hydrophobic = > 150° contact angle

Oxygen Related Contact Lens Properties

Oxygen related properties of contact lenses play an important role in its usage for longer duration and to keep the cornea healthy. This includes various elements such as
- Oxygen permeability
- Oxygen transmissibility
- Equivalent oxygen percentage
- Oxygen tension

Oxygen permeability (*Dk*): It is the property of a contact lens material, which indicates the ability of oxygen to pass through contact lens material without any effort. This is called as

Clinical Importance

- Increased in water content of lens improves the wearing comfort by increasing the transfer of oxygen through lens. Oxygen permeability of a contact lens doubles with an approximate increase in 20% water content, which is more significant with high absorption property of lens.
- Increased in water content also enhances the mechanical strength of contact lens by increasing its thickness.
- Low wettability increase the wearing duration and comfort of contact lens by maintaining tear film stability.

 Note

Oxygen permeability (Dk) is a feature of contact lens material, not of contact lens.

Dk value of that material, where D means the diffusion co-efficient of oxygen and k indicates the solubility of oxygen in that contact lens material. The value of Dk of a lens material can be calculated by using oxygen electrodes in a gas chamber device. Units of Dk are expressed as Fatt units or Barrer

$$Dk = \frac{10^{-11}(cm^2 \times ml\ O_2)}{sec \times ml \times mmHg}$$

Oxygen transmissibility: It is the property of a contact lens which indicates the ability of oxygen to pass through contact lens of known thickness. It means it tells about the rate of oxygen transfer across the different contact lenses of varying thickness. This is represented as Dk/L, where Dk is oxygen permeability and L is the central thickness of contact lens in centimeters (cm).

The oxygen transmissibility across a contact lens can be known by formula:

$$J = \frac{Dk\ (P_l - P_o)}{L}$$

Here P_l = oxygen pressure in front of contact lens

P_o = oxygen pressure behind the contact lens

Oxygen transmissibility is a characteristic of contact lens, not of its material and is inversely proportional to thickness of lens. It means thinner is the lens, greater will be its oxygen transmissibility.

L = thickness of center of contact lens (cm)

Units of oxygen transmissibility is 10^{-9} (cm $\times$ ml O_2)/(sec $\times$ ml $\times$ mmHg).

Equivalent oxygen percentage (EOP): Cornea being avascular in nature, receive oxygen mainly from the atmosphere. Presence of contact lens on the cornea will hamper the supply of atmospheric oxygen to cornea. Thus EOP indicate the amount (%) of atmospheric oxygen (in volume) reaching at cornea in presence of contact lens, for a known thickness of contact lens. For example, as we all know that normally about 21% oxygen is present in the atmosphere, however, if it is stated that EOP is 4%; means that cornea is receiving 4% atmospheric oxygen, instead of 21%.

Oxygen tension: It is expressed as partial pressure applied by oxygen in a specified atmospheric condition. This is an interchangeable term with EOP and helps in deciding the health status of cornea during usage of contact lens for a long period.

Broadly, contact lens materials are divided as

- Focons
- Filcons

Focons: These are hydrophobic material, primarily used to manufacture rigid contact lenses.

Filcons: These are hydrophilic material, primarily used to manufacture non rigid contact lenses. However, elastomers of silicon rubber are highly hydrophobic, but due to its other properties these are also grouped as Filcons. On the basis of different types of substances focons and filcons are grouped as summarized in Table 8.1.

Table 8.1: Lens materials and their characteristic properties

Focons	Substances	Filcons	Substances
1a (Dk = 0)	Pure PMMA	1a (hydration = 38)	Pure HEMA with <0.2% ionisable chemical (e.g. methacrylic acid)
1b (Dk = 0)	Copolymer of PMMA with 10% other monomer	1b	Pure HEMA with > 0.2% ionisable chemical
2a (Dk = 2–8) (hydration = 38)	Pure cellulose acetate butyrate (CAB)	2a	Copolymer of HEMA + hydroxyalkyl MA + dihydroxyalkyl MA with < 0.2% ionisable chemical
3 (Dk = 12)	Copolymer of Allyl methacrylate (MA) + Siloxanyl MA	2b	Same as 2a with > 0.2% ionisable chemical.
4	Polysiloxones	3a (hydration = 71)	Copolymer of HEMA + N vinyl lactum with < 0.2% ionisable chemical
5 (Dk = 71)	Copolymer of Allyl MA + Siloxanyl MA + 0.5% fluroalkyl MA	3b	Same as 3a with > 0.2% ionisable chemical
		4a (hydration = 79)	Copolymer of alkyl MA + N vinyl lactum + alkylacrylamide with < 0.2% ionisable chemical
		4b	Same as 4a with > 0.2% ionisable chemical
		5 (Dk = 200)	Polysiloxanes

Rigid Contact Lens Materials

Initially all contact lenses were manufactured using rigid materials such as glass and thermosetting plastics like PMMA. Because of several clinical drawbacks associated with these materials subsequently better rigid lens materials such as cellulose acetate butyrate (CAB), silicon and polymers of silicon, etc. for manufacturing of contact lens were developed.

Broadly, these rigid contact lens materials can be grouped as
- Rigid non-gas permeable materials
- Rigid gas permeable materials

Rigid non-gas permeable material: Mostly the hard contact lenses were made up of thermosetting plastic like spectacle lenses. PMMA was the first commercially available plastic in this category for mass manufacturing of contact lenses. PMMA material is not permeable for water or oxygen, hence wearers have to depend on a tear pump action of eye for hydration and oxygen supply to cornea.

Advantages
- It is inert and free of toxic chemicals, because PMMA is prepared by a process of annealing (successive heating and cooling), so does not cause hypersensitivity reactions.
- Can be moulded or lathed with high degree of precision.
- Excellent visual properties and safe to wear.
- Requires minimum use of cleaning, soaking or wetting solutions.
- Can be tinted easily to reduce excessive light sensitivity.

- Durable and can be repolished to remove minor scratches, hence lasts for nearly 5–6 years.
- Economical as compared to any other type of contact lens.

Disadvantages

- Oxygen permeability of PMMA lens is negligible, hence cannot be worn for long duration, otherwise person will develop dryness, swelling and ocular discomfort.
- PMMA material is very hard in nature so can cause corneal abrasions.
- Because of hydrophobic nature of PMMA, it has poor wettability. In PMMA lens the oxygen transmissibility is very poor so oxygenation of tears depends on renewal of tears due to blinking. As the contact lens wearer blink, there is slight movement of contact lens over the cornea so that interchange of tears occurs underneath the lens and as a result oxygen is exchanged and provides necessary oxygen to cornea.

In subsequent years many researchers tried to improve the permeability of contact lens by drilling small holes or fenestration in the lens. Hydrogel (polymers that imbibe water and swell) were also added with PMMA to improve its permeability, but still gas impermeability of material remained a major issue in its wide usage. Because of impermeability property these lenses are kept light, thin and of small size so that they do not cover a large portion of cornea. In addition, these lenses cannot be used for correction of high degree of corneal astigmatism because of their light and thin nature.

Rigid gas permeable lens material: Materials which are used for production of RGP lenses maintain the property of PMMA in terms of rigidity, but unlike PMMA these materials have good oxygen permeability, hence became popular for a long-term usage. Primarily, cellulose acetate butyrate (CAB) and silicon were used to manufacture these rigid gas permeable lenses, however, several polymers of silicon and allyl methacrylate later introduced in the market for manufacturing of better tolerable contact lens.

Contact lenses formed from these materials are also called semisoft contact lenses because of their good oxygen permeability and better Dk value.

Cellulose acetate butyrate (CAB): It was first widely used material to manufacture rigid gas permeable contact lenses. This biodegradable thermoplastic polymer was derived from yellow poplar wood fiber (YPWF) having good wettability. Advantages of this material over PMMA were good oxygen permeability, relative wettability and reduced hardness; however disadvantages as compared to PMMA were poor scratch resistance and tensile strength. Due to these reasons a constant search for better material was on, which leads to development of silicon acrylate material.

Styrene: A highly gas permeable, surface wettable, and relatively hard contact lens material used for manufacturing of RGP contact lenses is styrene (T-butyl dimethyl siloxy). This contact lens material is a copolymerization product of a reaction mixture consisting styrene, esters of vinyl alcohol and polyethylene glycol, polysiloxane along with a cross-linking agent like divinyl benzene. Initially this material looks promising, however, due to brittle nature of this material mass manufacturing became a problem.

Silicon: Silicon is highly permeable oxygen than water. Contact lenses with more silicon will be more permeable than less silicon lens. However, silicon has its own problem like hydrophobic nature (less wettability) and relative stiffness and because of these properties it is a less friendly material for large production of contact lenses.

Silicon acrylate: In the year 1974, Norman Gaylord produced first siloxane (oxygen and silicon are combined together) based rigid lens material by cross-linking silicon acrylate with MMA, resulted in formation of trimethylsiloxy

(Tris) silane. The presence of silicon provides good oxygen permeability to material while MMA provides good wetting and physical property to material. Many rigid materials now are used for production of contact lens are on the basis of these properties.

Silicon can be added in various proportions with varying *Dk* value in the range of 15–60 and oxygen permeability. As silicon increased, the oxygen permeability of lens increases but it also alters the surface characteristic of lens.

Fluoropolymers: Fluoropolymers were discovered during 1930 and are considered as most desirable material for mass manufacturing of RGP contact lenses because of their high oxygen permeability, wettability and resistibility to surface deposits. Fluoropolymers can also withstand high temperature and chemical attack. Free radical polymerization is basic industrial synthesis method for fluoropolymers. The polymerization process is mainly water-based method, which uses either aqueous suspension or aqueous emulsion polymerization in presence of fluorinated emulsifiers. For manufacturing of contact lenses fluoropolymers can be used either in pure form or in co-polymer forms. Flurofocon A is a polymer having high fluorine content which is commercially developed by 3M Company for mass production of extended wear contact lenses. As compared to earlier available fluoropolymers, an excellent wettability and flexibility is present in Flurofocon A. This material has very high levels of oxygen transmissibility and remarkable resistance against deposit formation. Hence, combination of physical properties and optical stability of Flurofocon A makes it the most desirable new lens material for manufacturing of contact lenses.

Soft Contact Lens Materials

First monomer material for soft lens, i.e. hydroxyethyl methacrylate (HEMA) was introduced by Otto Wichterle in the year 1950. As the name suggests that this material has a hydroxyl group, in contrast to PMMA where only methyl group was present. These soft lens materials are also termed hydrogel because they are cross-linked polymer and being hydrophilic absorbs water, get swell and make lens soft and elastic. The cross-linking provides physical stability to lens material.

During production of soft gel materials, monomers such as HEMA with the aid of a catalyst undergo polymerization which results in formation of sequence of repeating units termed Poly hydroxyethyl methacrylate or P-HEMA. This polymer is made by polymerizing two molecules of hydroxyethyl methacrylate (HEMA) monomer and using a cross-linking agent like ethylene glycol dimethacrylate (EGDMA) or polyvinylpyrrolidone (PVP). The hydrophilic nature of P-HEMA is due to the presence of hydroxyl group (OH) which creates small pores in the polymers through which fluid can enter.

When more than one type of monomer is used in production of the material, then this type of material is termed copolymers. A polymerized HEMA EGDMA lens has water content of about 38–50% and used as daily wear lens while HEMA-PVP has high water content (>50%) and used as extended wear lens. However, by using various different types of monomers different materials can be produced varying in terms of water contents, refractive indices, hardness, and strength and oxygen permeability.

Advantages

- Good hydration equilibrium of material provides better comfort of wearing. These soft lenses can be either low hydration lenses having water content of 38–50% or of high hydration lenses having water content of >50%.
- Refractive indices of these lenses is comparable with cornea, hence quality of vision is better.

- High oxygen permeability is a major advantage and permeability increases proportionally with an increase in the water content, whereas decreases with an increase in the thickness of lens.
- Soft in nature and hence a larger portion of cornea can be covered for better field of vision and correction of refractive error.

Disadvantages

- Due to high water content and soft material nature these lenses are very fragile and get damaged easily.
- Swells up due to high water content, hence clarity of vision is less as compared to rigid contact lenses.
- Higher incidence of microbial keratitis as compared to RGP lenses.

Soft contact lenses can be produced by using several materials either as monomers, polymers or co-polymers. Broadly, we can group these soft hydrogel materials into
- Conventional hydrophilic hydrogel materials
- Silicon hydrogel materials

Conventional Hydrophilic Hydrogel Material

Conventionally, hydroxyethyl methacrylate (HEMA) is most commonly used hydrophilic monomer material for manufacturing of hydrogel lens. Although nowadays, cross-linking polymers are more used because of their better stability.

HEMA: HEMA is most widely used, original, water insoluble soft contact lens material which is used as monomer for mass manufacturing of soft contact lenses in our country. Pure HEMA lens has water content of about 38–40%. It is mostly copolymerised to form various hydrogel which are used for manufacturing of soft hydrogel contact lenses. For example, materials such as dimethyl acrylamide (DMA), glycerol methacrylate (GMA), methacrylic acid (MA), methyl methacrylate (MMA) and vinylpyrrolidone (VP) are used for polymerization in currently available contact lens materials.

HEMA has important properties like it is not easily damaged by biodegradation, chemical or thermal sterilization and by enzymes present in tears, hence makes this material most suitable for making contact lenses used for a long period.

HEMA-NVP: Subsequently, HEMA copolymers were developed to improve water content or hydration of lens material. Copolymerization of HEMA with N-vinyl-pyrrolidone (NVP) was first commercially successful contact lens material having equivalent water content of up to 90%. These types of copolymers have rubbery feel as compared to slippery feel of P-HEMA. In addition, the amide group present in these material bind weakly with water molecule as compared to hydroxyl group, therefore, evaporation rates of water through these lens is relatively high leading to chances of instability of lens and discomfort.

Disadvantages

- Sensitive to change in temperature: Parameters of copolymers of HEMA-NVP can change with change in the temperature, hence caution is required during lens fitting because lens parameters may change after its contact with eye.
- Corneal staining: Use of NVP containing lenses with solutions which contain polyhexanide in high amount may cause staining of cornea and increase level of discomfort. Hence, it is essential to keep in mind that if staining occurs, then solution must be changed which contains negligible amount of polyhexanide.

MMA-VP: MMA (methyl methacrylate) and VP (vinylpyrrolidone) monomers were combined to produce MMA/VP copolymer. MMA/VP copolymer showed different characteristics than HEMA/VP copolymer. MMA/VP copolymers based contact lenses may have water content from 60–85% depending upon the composition.

MAA-HEMA: To increase the equivalent water content (EWC) of material, a different hydrophilic monomer methacrylic acid (MAA) was used to manufacture hydrogels. Addition of MAA during formation of soft lens material results in formation of ionized groups within the matrix of polymer which increases water absorption property of lens. Addition of MAA with HEMA usually increases the water content up to range of 50–60%, which in turn results in significant increases in the oxygen permeability through lens.

The use of MAA in lens material is also associated with some disadvantages such as

- The lens containing MAA are very sensitive for changes in the tonicity. For example, in solutions having less tonicity (hypotonic like water) the effective water content (EWC) of lens increased, while opposite occurs in hypertonic solutions.
- EWC of this type of lens material also change with change in the pH of solution. The EWC of lens decreases in low pH conditions.
- Significant amount of protein depositions can occur on surface of lens and within its matrix. However, recently it has been found that these proteins are in non-denatured form.
- During heat-disinfection process the lens may loss its dimensional stability.

MMA-PVD: These are copolymer of polyvinyl pyrrolidone (hydrophilic), monomer VP and methyl methacrylate (hydrophobic).

Glyceryl methacrylate: Glyceryl methacrylate (GMA) monomer consists of two hydroxyl groups as compared to HEMA and thus more water soluble than HEMA. GMA in combination with other monomers or hydrogels is used for manufacturing of contact lens materials. Combination of GMA with MMA (Crofilcon A) produces a material which is more stiff and strong than P-HEMA as well as contains water contents in range of 30–42%. In addition, it can be combined with HEMA, which results in formation of non-ionic material having high water content (up to 70%). Moreover, the water balance ratio of these types of lens material is excellent because their rate of rehydration is fast, while dehydration occurs at slow rate. The chances of deposition are very less and the property of material remains unaltered with the change in pH in the range of 6–10.

Silicon hydrogel material: In the year 1999, silicon hydrogel material was successfully introduced in manufacturing of contact lens which within a decade became main type soft contact lens material representing almost 70% of total lens materials. Similar to conventional hydrogels, in silicon hydrogel materials the main chain consists of siloxane derivates like polydimethylsiloxane (PDMS), Bis (trimethylsiloxy) methylsilane, tris-propyl vinyl carbamate (TPVC) and polydimethylsiloxy bisvinyl carbamate (PBVC).

Initially two silicon hydrogel materials, Lotrafilcon A and Balafilcon A were available which were having high oxygen permeability but having low water content (25 and 38%, respectively). Hence these materials were stiffer and hydrophobic than poly-HEMA based (water soluble) materials. However, silicon containing materials are highly oxygen permeable. Later on better silicon hydrogel materials were produced and currently more than 12 different types of materials are available having desired relationship between water content and oxygen permeability. The increase in the silicon content increases permeability of material. The silicon hydrogen materials developed later on have high Dk values as well as maintain medium to high water content (>45%).

Following surface properties of silicon hydrogels material are desirable for manufacturing of contact lenses.

- Topography and roughness
- Friction (less)
- Wettability (improved by surface treatment)
- Surface charge/ionicity (mostly non-ionic)

Several following bulk properties of this material are also contributing for manufacturing of extended wear contact lens.

- Equilibrium water content and water activity; has high percentage of free water, bound water and intermediate water.
- Oxygen permeability and transmissibility.
- Hydraulic and ionic permeability

Advantages of silicon hydrogels are

- Less chances of microbial contamination.
- Less mechanical interactions to corneal surface.

> **Note**
>
> Silicon hydrogels are most desirable material for manufacturing of extended wear contact lenses throughout world.

- Less protein depositions over lenses.
- Release of moisture agents like polyvinyl alcohol.
- Can also be used as drug delivery system.

A few disadvantages like sensitivity to lipid deposition, hydrophobic surface and non-ionic nature are also present in silicon hydrogel materials.

Manufacturing and Design of Contact Lenses

MANUFACTURING AND TYPES OF CONTACT LENS

Various processes used to manufacture contact lenses are
- Lathe cutting
- Melt pressing
- Spin casting
- Cast moulding

Lathe Cutting

Earlier this process was used for manufacturing of corneal PMMA and rigid lenses. Later on, it was also used in the manufacturing of soft hydrogel lenses. This process is used for production of both soft and rigid types contact lenses by using various types of lens materials.

Various steps in the process of lathe cutting are
- Manufacturing of buttons from material
- Back surface cutting of a lens blank
- Front surface cutting of a lens
- Wet processing of the lenses

Manufacturing of buttons from material: Firstly, the monomer material is polymerized to prepare button-shaped moulds or alternatively can be cast in the form of rods from which button can be cut later on. These buttons act as lens blanks. Polymerization process takes time, hence these button or rods are kept in a water bath at a definite temperature (depending on the type of material used) for several hours. It is followed by annealing process of buttons where the material or buttons are heated at high temperature followed by cooling at room temperature. Annealing makes the material soft so that stress is relieved inside buttons. In addition, it also prevents grooving of edges or rolling up (like cigarette) of finished lens when in hydrated state.

A soft contact lens is lathed in dry state means a smaller, steeper lens of greater power is prepared by lathe so that when it absorbs water it swells and attains required dimensions and powers.

Cutting of back surface of lens blanks: The buttons are processed on lathe to cut the back surface of lens from the buttons. Nowadays, computer-based lathe are available which can be programmed accordingly to cut buttons into numerous design and of variable parameters. Diamond cutting tools are used to cut back surface from buttons which is a two-step process. Firstly, a rough cut is given on buttons to remove excess material. Then a final cut is given to slice secondary curves and slanted edges of lens. Following the cutting, the polishing of back surfaces is done on a polishing machine. Polished materials usually contain a lanolin base and coarse diamond dust. During lathing and polishing the excessive heating of lens material must be avoided to prevent warpage and errors of curvature. Prepared semi-finished lenses are then kept in a solvent to get rid of excessive polish.

Cutting of front surface lens: The semi-finished lens blank (buttons with cut back surface) is fixed on to a mount or chuck, this process is called blocking. The mount is a cylindrical-shaped tool made of metal or plastic, having one end dome-shaped which match with the curve of posterior surface of lens blank. At this dome end, hot melted wax is applied and the posterior or back surface of lens blank is mounted with the help of this wax at dome end and centered carefully. This assembly is now loaded on the lathe machine for front surface cutting and then centration of lens blank is confirmed followed by cutting of surface by diamond tool. The front lens surface is then polished and deblocked by immersing into a deblocking solvent.

Wet processing of the lenses: The processed dry lenses go through hydration and wet processing steps which will vary according to the type of lens material. For example, non-ionic lenses are usually first washed with deionized water and then with saline. Ultrasonic baths are also used to increase the speed of hydration process. For lenses containing MAA, washing is done in tanks containing sodium bicarbonate to facilitate ionization of the lenses.

Advantages
- Can be used to manufacture both rigid and soft type contact lenses.
- Lenses usually have high quality surface finishing due to diamond cutting edges on an automated lathe machine.
- Variety of lens design, surface curvature to fit for an individual requirement and different size diameter lenses can be produced.
- High quality polishing reduces surface defects and improves the optical property

of lens having a stable visual acuity which does not fluctuate.
- Lathing in dry state of soft lens gives a high dimensional accuracy so even toric lens can be designed.
- Also necessary for production of low volume and high prescription custom lenses.

Disadvantages
- Require intense labor, hence it is both expensive and susceptible to significant human errors.
- It is a slow process.

Manufacturing errors may occur during lathe process like
- Hydrogel or soft lenses are lathed in dry state, hence they undergo final step of hydration which can be a potential manufacturing error.
- Core fractures
- Inclusions, e.g. rust
- Watermarks, bubbles or holes on lens
- Debris, e.g. fibres
- Lathe rings
- Distortion, discoloration and edge defects of lens

Melt Pressing

This method was used to manufacture PMMA and silicon contact lenses, however, now this is not widely used and is an obsolete procedure. Various steps involved in the process of melt pressing are summarized as
- The monomer is polymerized to produce a polymer (polymerization).
- This polymer is then converted into sheets, beads, granules or power.
- Moulds of desired size shape and types are taken from this polymer material.
- Compression or injection moulding is done.
- Semi-finished lens is then removed from mould.
- Lens is edged and polished for packing purposes.

Spin Casting

In the year 1961, Wichterle described a new method for manufacturing of soft lens and patented it, which is known as spin casting. Subsequently, in the year 1971 this method was further refined by Bausch & Lomb (B&L). Nowadays, manufacturing of contact lens by spin casting process is based on the same principle as developed by B&L.

Principle: The cast or mould containing mixture of desired monomers (monomer solution + cross-linking agent + initiator) is spinned at a controlled speed. During spinning the generated centrifugal forces cause ascending of the monomer mixture to the walls of cast and take the required lens shape, while simultaneously polymerization also occurs.

This process has the following steps of manufacturing the contact lens as shown in Fig. 9.1.

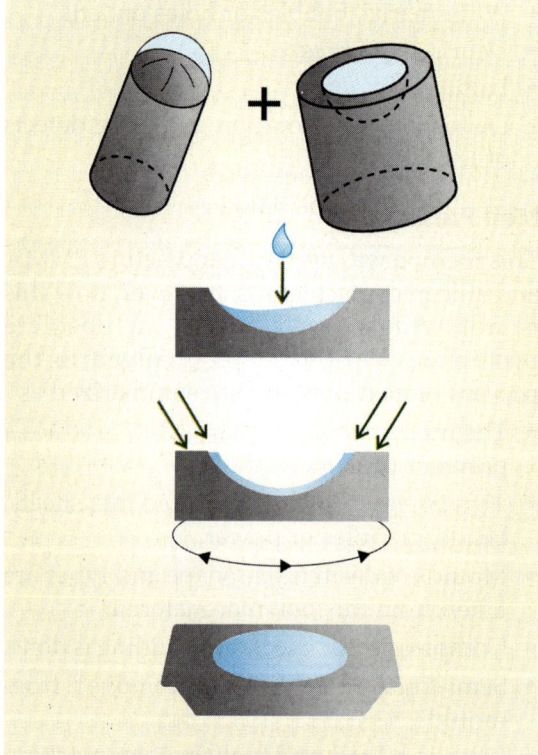

Fig. 9.1: Contact lens manufacturing by spin casting method

Manufacturing of inserts: First step is to produce inserts of excellent quality which are then used as mould to produce the casts because the quality of anterior surface and edges of each lens depend on quality of the inserts prepared.

Manufacturing of cast: Casts are usually prepared by using materials like poly propylene or polyvinyl chloride. Occasionally, the surface treatment of resulting casts is done to ensure the wetting of cast material, but this treatment also increases the cost of production of lens.

Spinning process: Most important step of entire process is spinning of the cast which determines the final power and shape of the produced contact lens. Various other factors, such as combined effect of gravity, surface tension, centrifugal force during spinning, quantity of liquid monomer and the rate of spin determine the final outcome. If the radius of the produced cast is predetermined, then a contact lens of desired central thickness and back vertex power can be made by controlling the speed and dose of monomers. The rate of spin speed will decide the back vertex power while dose will decide the central thickness of lens.

- The anterior surface of lens is spheric and curvature of front or anterior surface of desired lens is provided by the inner surface of cast or mould.

- Back or posterior surface of contact lens is aspheric and the curvature of this surface depends on factors like shape and amount of speed of mould, physical properties and amount of liquid monomers in the cast.

- It is considered an ideal method for production of minus power contact lenses because the manufactured lens by this process has power of approximately equal to −3 D lens.

- However, for manufacturing of positive powered contact lens, casts with more complicated designs are required. Another method which has been adopted by manufacturers to produce the lens of desired power and curvatures is that after the spinning, lathe is also done on spin cast lens.

- The final lenses are demoulded, either manually or by an automated production line.
- These finished lenses are wet processed in a similar way to lathed lenses as explained above.

Advantages

- Generates a homogenous, consistent and properly cross-linked polymer, because a thin film of monomer is polymerized.
- Produces best quality optical surfaces.
- Accurate spin speed and precise dosing produces perfect parameters contact lenses.
- Minimum surface defects and edging errors, because surfaces formed are free and independent to cutting.
- Less expensive and easily reproducible.

Disadvantages

- Unpredictable fitting.
- Fitting of lens is not dependent on kerato-meter reading of patient.

Cast Moulding

Primarily this process was used as cost effective method to manufacture plastic goods but later on it was also used for production of contact lenses.

Principle: During the cast moulding procedure to prepare a contact lens the liquid monomer undergo polymerization process between two casts. The formed semi-finished lens before packaging again processed to produce desired lens.

Cast moulding: Cast moulding and its modified methods are now commonly used for production of high volume soft lenses because the unit production cost is potentially low by this method. Various steps of this process as shown in Fig. 9.2 are as follows

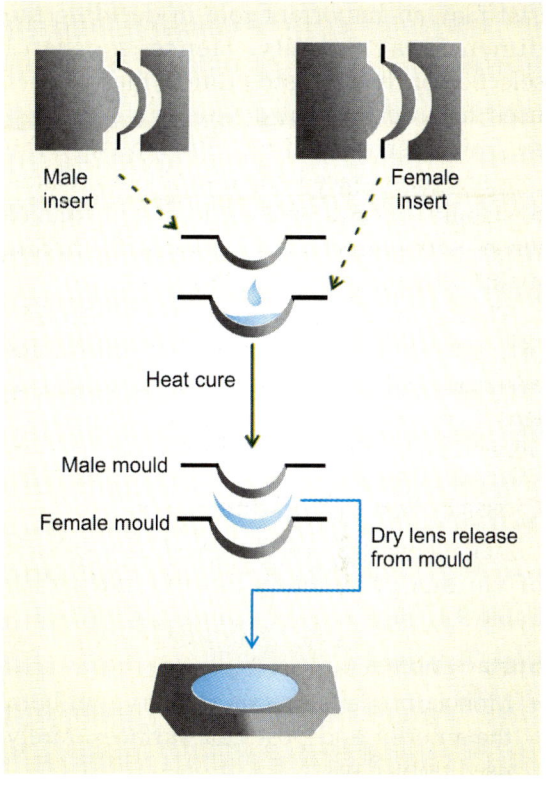

Fig. 9.2: Contact lens manufacturing by cast moulding method

Manufacturing of inserts: During cast moulding process both male and female type inserts along with auxiliary insert housings are manufactured. Front or anterior surface of final contact lens is formed by using female cast which is created by the female insert, whereas back or posterior surface of the final contact lens was created by male cast which is formed by the male insert.

During this process the male inserts are manufactured in less number than female inserts, because contact lens of different powers can be produced by altering the female insert, as the radii of anterior surface and altogether thickness profile of lens get change by changing the female cast.

Manufacturing of cast: During manufacturing by cast moulding both the material used for cast and design of the casts play a vital role. The material that is used for development of cast play an important role in deciding the dimensional stability. Hence, a careful selection of chemical structure of the polymer used to produce contact lens is a vital step during cast moulding. Previously, the manufacturers faced some problems related to stability of casts which lead to low yield of lenses with correct specification for a specific manufactured batch.

The design of the cast during manufacturing of lens will decide the optical property, curvatures of surface, pattern of edge and diameter of final lens, hence resultant lens is also significantly dependent on the design of the casts.

Classification of Contact Lenses

Contact lenses can be classified on the basis of various parameters as summarized in Table 9.1.

Surface curves

- Monocurve lens has single curve on both the anterior and posterior surfaces, rarely used nowadays.
- Bicurve lens has single anterior curve, but two back curves (a central curve and flatter peripheral curve), most commonly used.
- Tricurve lenses are similar to bicurve except that an intermediate curve is present on back surface.
- Multicurve lenses are also similar to bicurve lenses but have more than one intermediate curve.
- Toric lens has a toric back surface, mainly used for highly toric cornea (astigmatic) cases.
- Bitoric lens has a cylindrical power on anterior surface of lens along with the toric posterior surface, mainly used in high degree of astigmatism with low corneal toricity like in cases of lenticular astigmatism.

Anatomical position in the eye

- Scleral lenses are also known as haptic or corneo-scleral contact lenses. These lenses cover the cornea, conjunctiva and sclera and are mainly used for therapeutic purposes, rarely used for optical, cosmetic or diagnostic purposes.
- Corneo-limbal contact lenses cover the entire cornea and limbus to lay over conjunctiva. Mainly used for optical and cosmetic purposes.
- Corneal contact lenses are entirely confined to cornea and are mainly used as optical and diagnostic contact lenses.

Physical properties

- Soft contact lens
- Semisoft contact lens
- Hard contact lens

Table 9.1: Classification of contact lens (CL) on basis of various parameters						
Surface curves	Anatomical position	Physical properties	Chemical nature of lens material	Hydration status	Duration of lens wear	Clinical uses
Monocurve CL	Scleral lens	Soft CL	Rigid non-gas permeable CL	Low hydration CL	Long-term or yearly wear	Optical CL
Bicurve CL	Corneo-limbal lens	Semisoft CL	Rigid gas permeable CL	Medium hydration CL	Monthly wear	Therapeutic CL
Tricurve CL	Corneal CL	Hard CL	Soft CL	High hydration CL	Weekly wear	Cosmetic CL
Multicurve CL					Daily wear	Diagnostic CL
Toric lens					Extended wear	Occupational CL
Bitoric lens						

Chemical nature of lens material

- Rigid non-gas permeable lenses, usually hydrophobic in nature made up of PMMA. These lenses are also called Focons.
- Rigid gas permeable lenses, made up of cellulose acetate butyrate and silicon, most commonly used as long-term wear contact lenses.
- Soft contact lenses, usually hydrophilic in nature made up of acrylic and HEMA. These lenses are also called Filcons.

Hydration status of lens material

- Low hydration lenses: Having water content in a range of 0–38%.
- Medium hydration lenses: Having water content in a range of 40–60%.
- High hydration lenses: Having water content more than 60%.

Duration of lens wear

- Long-term or yearly wear
- Monthly wear
- Weekly wear
- Daily wear
- Extended wear

Clinical uses

- Optical contact lens
- Therapeutic contact lens
- Cosmetic contact lens
- Diagnostic contact lens
- Occupational contact lens

CONTACT LENS DESIGN

Contact lens can be designed in various ways to achieve the requirement of an optimized contact lens so that it is fit for different clinical conditions.

- Regular lens designs
- Special lens designs

Regular Lens Design

These types of lens are used most commonly and usually designed for correction of simple refractive errors, because refractive status of eye in simple errors is not affected due to

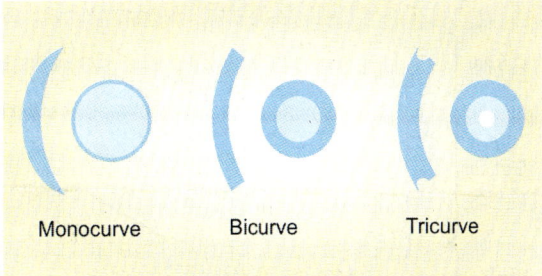

Monocurve   Bicurve   Tricurve

Fig. 9.3: Single cut contact lens designs

rotation of contact lens on the cornea. These lenses are designed as

- Single cut design
- Lenticular cut design

Single cut designed lenses may be monocurve, bicurve or tricurve containing a single continuously curved front surface as shown in Fig. 9.3. Desired base curve and peripheral curves are cut from the back surface of contact lens.

Special Lens Design

Several special types of design features are done in lens to optimize the fitting of contact lens and to prevent rotation of lens in the eye. These modifications are

- Lenticular edge modification
- Prism ballast lenses
- Truncated design lenses
- Fenestrations design
- Blending design

Lenticular edge modification: These lenses have a central optical portion which is surrounded in periphery by a carrier edge (either minus or plus powers) as shown in Fig. 9.4. This carrier edge is supported by eyelids and prevents the decentring of lens. These types of modified contact lens are designed for those persons where the optical power of gas permeable contact lens becomes more than –6.00 D or + 4.00 D. The lenticular edge modification of anterior surface of contact lens helps to improve the edge profile as well as also decreases weight and thickness

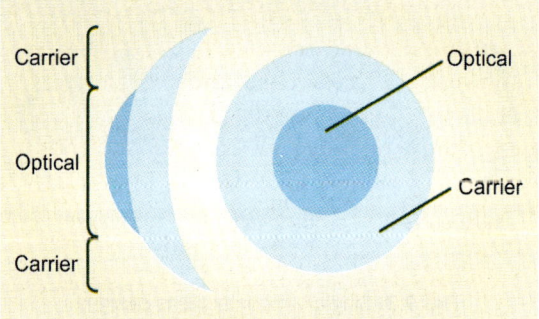

Fig. 9.4: Lenticular contact lens design

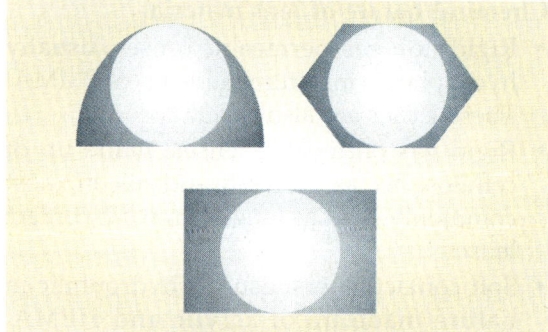

Fig. 9.6: Truncated contact lens designs

of contact lens which further improve the tolerance and centration of lens. The curve of posterior surface of lens is kept same.

Prism ballast lenses: These lenses are heavier at bottom and are indicated for correction of problems related to binocular vision related problems as in vertical phoria. As the name indicates, a prism is given in contact lens for proper orientation and to prevent rotation as shown in Fig. 9.5. The vertical base-down type of prism is prescribed in contact lens. Usually prisms are prescribed in toric (front surface) and bifocal contact lens, in both gas permeable and hydrogel material to maintain orientation.

Truncated design lenses: In these design lenses a circumferential zone in contact lens is present, which is made flat by removing lens material from a circular contact lens as shown in Fig. 9.6, the process is called truncation of lens. Like prism ballast lens, the truncation of a lens also helps in decreasing the rotation of

contact lens especially with bifocal or toric (front surface) contact lens.

Fenestrations: In these design contact lenses small holes are present, which are drilled through the surface of a contact lens as shown in Fig. 9.7. This design is mainly used in contact lenses of rigid type, either PMMA or gas permeable types. The insufficient oxygen permeability through these lens material may cause corneal edema. The holes help to facilitate the oxygenation of cornea, either directly or by enhancing tear exchange.

Blending: Chances of corneal abrasion or trauma can be decreased by smoothing or blending the junctions between multiple curvatures present on posterior surface of

> **Note**
>
> Heavy blending helps in multicurve contact lenses, to improve the quality of vision.

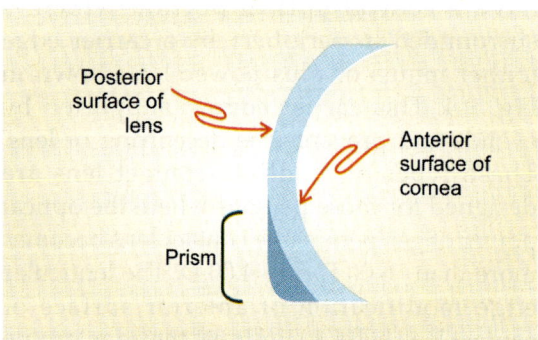

Fig. 9.5: Prism ballast contact lens design

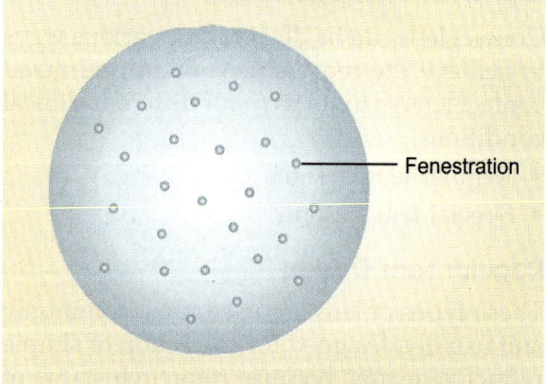

Fig. 9.7: Fenestrated rigid contact lens design

contact lenses. Thus, blending increases the tolerance and comfort of wearing. Blending is generally conducted on gas permeable contact lenses. This can be classified as

- Light blending: When transformation or blending is clearly visible between two posterior curves of a contact lens.
- Medium blending: When transformation is minimally visible between two posterior curves of a contact lens.
- Heavy blending: When transformation is invisible between two posterior curves of a contact lens.

Terminologies in Contact Lens

Most important purpose of knowing the details of contact lens design is that the posterior surface of lens must fit optimally on surface of the cornea because any discrepancy in fitting will lead to positional instability of contact lens on the cornea.

Contact Lens Dimensions

To know specifications of contact lens and to improve the fitting of lens on the cornea, it is important to know some basic information about lens dimensions which are as follows (Fig. 9.8).

Total diameter (TD): It is the linearly measured longest distance between the two boundaries of contact lens and is measured in millimeter. This is also called overall size, chord diameter or overall diameter and should not be confused with a double of radius of curvature of lens. Lenses of various types have different total diameters as follows

- Rigid non-gas permeable lenses or PMMA lenses have a TD of 7.5–8.5 mm.
- Rigid gas permeable lenses have a TD in the range of 9–9.6 mm.
- Soft contact lenses have a large TD in the range of 13–14 mm.

Back optic zone diameter (BOZD): It is a linear distance of central optical zone of contact lens which focuses rays on the retina. It is the distance between the two junctions or blend of lens and measured in millimeter. This is also called posterior optical zone diameter, back central optic diameter or optic zone diameter. Normally it should be more than 7 mm for good vision.

Peripheral curve width: It is the width of peripheral curve of lens which is flatter than the base curve and it decides the fitting of lens on the cornea. This is also called peripheral

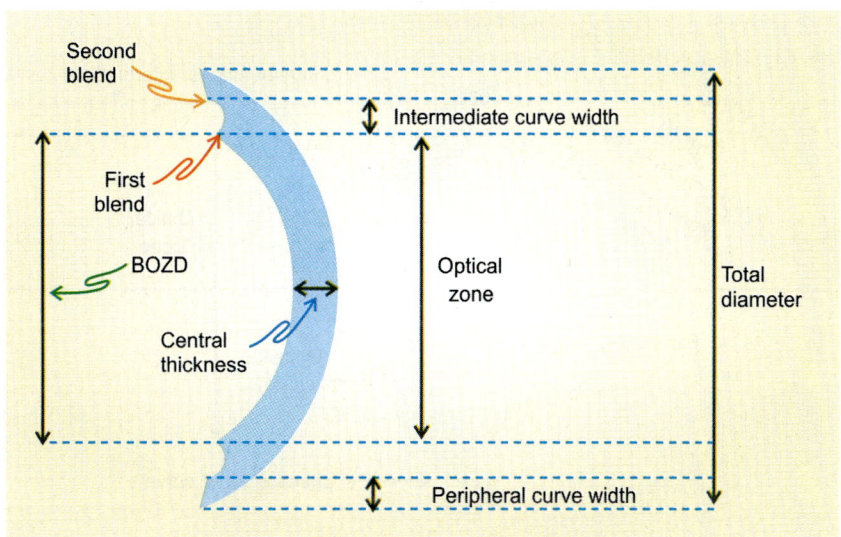

Fig. 9.8: Dimensions of contact lens

curve diameter. There may be an intermediate curve width, if an intermediate curve is present as in cases of trifocal or multifocal contact lenses.

Central thickness: It is the thickness of lens measured at optical or geometrical center of a contact lens. This is also called as geometrical central thickness (GCT). It is an important factor to decide the hydration and oxygenation of lens and is measured in millimeter. The value of central thickness of a lens depends on its posterior vertex power.

Contact Lens Curves and Radius

Various contact lens curves and their related radius as shown in Figs 9.9 and 9.10 are as follows

Base curve: It is the curve of back surface of contact lens which rests on the cornea and is responsible for good fit. This is also called

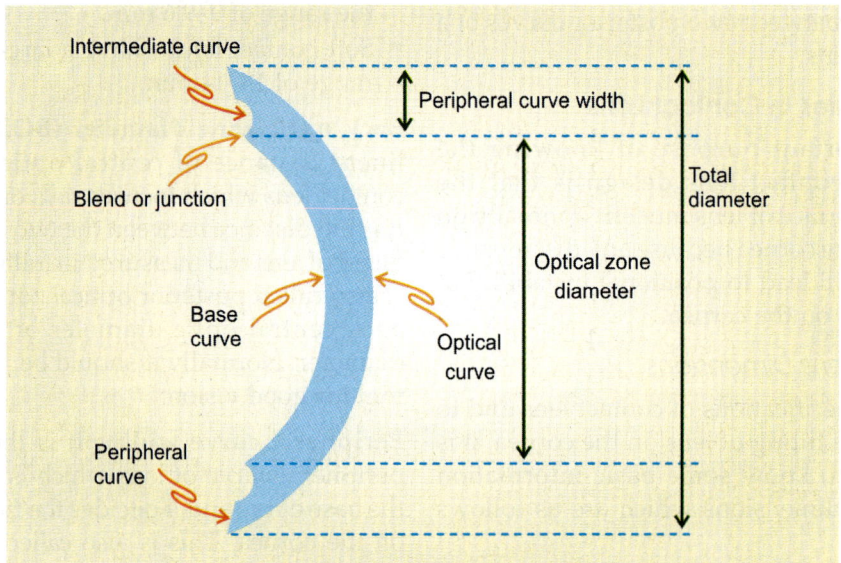

Fig. 9.9: Various terms and structures of contact lens

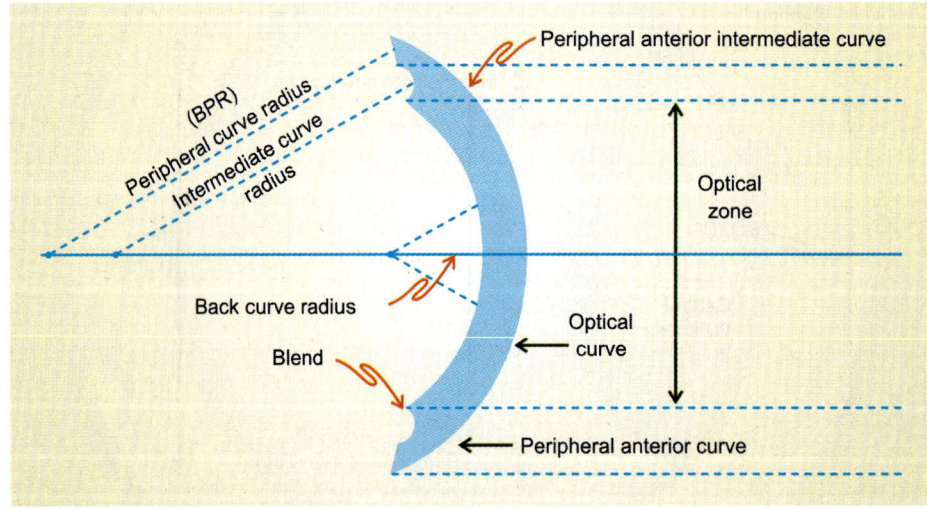

Fig. 9.10: Curves in contact lens

central posterior curve or back central optic portion. In a given lens design, back curve radii may be present in a range from 7.5 to 9.0 mm, at 0.5 mm intervals.

Optical curve: It is the curve of anterior surface of contact lens, in optical zone. Optical power of a contact lens is determined by the amount of curvature of optical curve. This is also called front curve.

Peripheral curves: These curves are present on the posterior surface of lens and include intermediate curve and peripheral curve. These curves are concentric to base curve and act as reservoir of tears to facilitate a smooth lens movement over the cornea. This is also called back peripheral optic portion. Simple bicurve lens has a single peripheral curve which is larger than optical zone in radius, although two or more peripheral curves are present in tricurve or multicurve contact lenses.

Back peripheral radius (BPR): This is also known as back peripheral optic radius or peripheral curve radius. Similarly, in specific cases of high refractive errors, a contact lens with an intermediate curve and its radius are used.

Peripheral anterior curves: The slope on the anterior surface of contact lens which starts from boundary of optical curve and goes up to the edge of lens is called peripheral anterior curve, however, in specific cases there may be a peripheral anterior intermediate curve in between the optical curve and peripheral anterior curve. In high hypermetropes or high myopes the intermediate anterior peripheral curve is designed in lens for better visual quality.

Indications and Fitting of Contact Lenses

INTRODUCTION

Contact lens wear can be prescribed for various indications which can be grouped as

Optical indications: Contact lenses are used as an alternative to spectacles for correction of various refractive errors like myopia, hypermetropia and astigmatism. Several other ophthalmic conditions like aphakia, anisometropia, aniseikonia, presbyopia, keratoconus, field restrictions as seen in retinitis pigmentosa are other important indications where contact lens are advised as a better optical correction device than spectacles.

Contact lens versus spectacles: Comparison of various characteristics of contact lenses with spectacles summarized in Table 10.1.

Therapeutic indications: Contact lenses can be used as curative, supportive, palliative or preventive devices in various ocular conditions.

a. **As curative device:** As curative therapy can be used in pathology of cornea, conjunctiva, etc.
   • *Corneal pathologies:* Contact lens can be used in various disease of cornea including non-healing corneal ulcers, corneal abrasions, recurrent epithelial defects, bullous keratopathy, traumatic epithelial defects, filamentary keratitis, small corneal perforations, corneal trauma, exposure keratitis and descemetocele. The extended wear type contact lenses are mainly prescribed which are also called bandage contact lens (BCL), because they serve like a bandage over a

Table 10.1: Comparison of characteristics of contact lenses with spectacles		
Characteristics	*Contact lenses*	*Spectacles*
Irregular astigmatism	Corrected (hard CL)	Not corrected
High anisometropic	Binocular vision possible	Not possible
Field of vision	Larger field obtained	Smaller field
Peripheral aberrations	Eliminated	Not eliminated
Prismatic distortion	Eliminated	Not eliminated
Wearer skill	Reasonable skill	No skill
Precautionary wearing measures	More	Less
Cosmetic acceptability	Higher	Lower
Cost	Expensive	Economical

Long duration wearing of contact lens may cause damage of ocular surface

wound. Use of these lenses in corneal pathologies help in decreasing the ocular pain and discomfort by preventing mechanical trauma due to lids, also improves hydration and drug penetration which help in enhancement of the epithelial healing.

- *Conjunctival melanosis:* Lenses are used to deliver high doses of continuous radiation to conjunctiva.
- *In glaucoma:* Contact lenses are used as drug delivery device.

b. **As palliative device**
  - *Iris pathologies:* Coloboma, aniridia and albinism to avoid excessive entry of light rays.
  - In amblyopia for occlusion therapy (opaque contact lenses used).
  - Post-surgical procedures: Pterygium excision, lamellar keratoplasty, photorefractive keratotomy, laser sub-epithelial keratomileusis, C3R for keratoconus.
  - X-chrome lenses for red green color deficiency.
  - In lagophthalmos to support the globe.
  - Leaking conjunctival filtration bleb.

c. **As preventive device**
  - Lid conditions like trichiasis, entropion and ptosis to prevent corneal abrasions.
  - Giant papillary conjunctivitis to protect cornea.
  - In chemical injuries to prevent symblepharon and to restore anatomy of fornix.
  - Neuroparalytic keratitis to prevent corneal ulcerations.
  - Glare producing iridectomies.

> **Note**
> Orthokeratology in high myopia and/or astigmatism rigid contact lens with progressive flat fit, believed to mould cornea (technique is now obsolete).

Cosmetic indications
- Corneal scars
- Microcornea

- Microphthalmos
- Heterochromia
- Deformed eyes

Occupational indications
- Actors/Actresses to change looks. Sports person involved in archery, football, etc.
- People using telescope.
- Defense people, in pilots, in shooters.

Diagnostic and operative indications
- Goldman's three mirror contact lens
- Fundus photography
- Electroretinography
- Fundus examination in irregular astigmatism
- A-scan biometry
- Gonioscopy
- For intraocular foreign body localization.
- High minus lenses for fundus examination during vitrectomy and endolaser photocoagulation.
- Goniotomy lenses during surgical goniotomy.

Research indications
- Corneal temperature measurement
- Intraocular pressure measurement

Contraindications of Contact Lens Use

a. **Diseases of Eyelids**
  - Stye
  - Chalazion
  - Blepharitis
  - Meibomitis

b. **Diseases of conjunctiva**
  - Conjunctivitis (bacterial, viral, fungal)
  - Chronic hyperemia
  - Bulbar conjunctival papillae

c. **Diseases of lacrimal apparatus**
  - Acute or chronic dacryocystitis

d. **Diseases of cornea**
  - Corneal dystrophies
  - Dry eyes
  - Tear film abnormalities

- Corneal anesthesia as in fifth nerve palsy
- Pannus

e. **Other ocular pathologies**
  - Episcleritis
  - Scleritis
  - Iritis
  - Choroiditis

f. **Systemic conditions**
  - *Diabetes mellitus:* There are frequent fluctuations in refractive status and corneal erosions heal very slowly.
  - Perimenopausal period.
  - Oral contraceptive usage: Lens poorly tolerated.
  - Pregnancy: Corneal shape can change due to oedamatous swelling.

g. **Allergies**
  - Contact dermatitis
  - Asthma
  - Atrophic rhinitis

h. **Occupational hazards**
  - Smoky, dusty and hot job environment
  - High altitude flyers
  - Construction workers
  - Automobile mechanics

i. **Poor general and mental health**
j. **Low hygienic patients**
k. **Old age patient with poor motivation**
l. **Arthritis or parkinsonism patient unable to use hands properly**

CONTACT LENS FITTING

Contact lens fitting require a protocol to achieve the desired results. We need to do a good work up in desired patients. Patient work up and examination remains constant in all types of contact lenses fitting whether it is soft hydrogel contact lens, rigid contact lens, cosmetic or therapeutic contact lenses.

Patient Work up for Contact Lens Fitting

Patient requiring either soft or RGP, and /or any other types of contact lenses, thorough examination is required to produce a satisfactory result which can be achieved by following examination

History: Proper history plays a major role in the outcome of a contact lens wearing results, whether a patient is new or an old patient already wearing a contact lens. Patient should be evaluated considering these facts

- Whether patient is enough motivated to wear a contact lens or not, and is mentally prepared to take all necessary precautions regarding contact lens wear.
- Understanding of patient about the advantages and disadvantages about contact lens and with this knowledge emotionally he/she is prepared to wear a contact lens.
- History of any chronic systemic illness or systemic allergy is present or not, i.e. to rule out presence of any contraindication of contact lens wear.
- Previous experience with wearing of contact lens, if present. Details of types and methods of wearing schedule of previous contact lenses.
- Occupational history (dust exposure, chemical exposure, etc.) of patient is also important.

Ocular examination: Cycloplegic refraction with a detailed anterior segment examination using slit lamp biomicroscopy should be done to rule any ocular pathology. Detailed examination includes

- General examination
- Refraction
- Keratometry
- Corneal topography

General examination

- Eyelids should be examined to check force of lid closure, and also for any infective pathology like blepharitis, meibomitis, etc.
- Conjunctiva is examined using slit lamp to rule out any infiltrates, concretions, surface defects, limbal injection, papillae, follicles and any other infective pathology.

- Cornea transparency is noticed and detail examination is done to rule out any opacity, infiltrate and vascularization abnormality of surface.
- Tear film status is checked by Schirmer's' test and tear break up time by using fluorescein dye.
- Blink rate is calculated by a time clock. Blink rate <15 and/or >30 blinks per minute are considered as defective blink mechanism and cause should be established. Blink characteristics like partial or full blink should be noticed because a partial blink is unable to wet the contact lens and chances of improper tear exchange underneath the contact lens increases.
- Corneal diameter, pupil diameter and interpalpebral width are recorded by using a plane transparent ruler. Horizontal visible iris diameter (HVID) is an important parameter to assess the best contact lens fit. It is measured from temporal end of limbus to nasal end of limbus by PD ruler. This diameter will guide clinicians to select total diameter of desired lens.

Refraction

- Refraction under cycloplegia should be done to know the exact amount of refractive error. The recorded refraction value is expressed in minus cylinder form for those cases where we desire to prescribe only spherical contact lens.
- Vertex distance should be measured for accurate calculation of power of desired contact lens. Refractive errors with more than ± 5 D require a zero vertex distance correction at cornea because with this much refractive error effective power of contact lens will be significantly different. However, an error of ±2 D or less seldom needed any vertex distance correction at cornea.
- Spherocylindrical power should be converted to spherical equivalent power in cases of rigid lenses and in case of soft lenses where either toric lenses are contraindicated or practitioner decides to give only spherical powers. Simply half of the cylindrical power becomes spherical equivalent power, which is added with spherical power mathematically.

Keratometry

- Corneal curvatures are measured at least in its two principal meridians (vertical or 90° and horizontal or 180°) by using keratometer either manual or automated.
- Keratometry reading is important data which is required to select the base curve radius in both rigid and soft type contact lenses.
- Any major difference in keratometry values indicates high degree of corneal astigmatism and contact lens wearing should be avoided in these cases.

Corneal topography

- Corneal topography is performed to locate the apex of cornea because centration of lens is done according to the central corneal apex not according to geometric center of cornea which is the central point of pupil. Displacement of corneal apex will lead to the decentration of contact lens. Hence, locating of the apex will help in determining the best optical outcome with contact lens.
- Orbscan can be used to study the curvatures and surface characteristics of cornea which helps in a proper fit and avoid a flat or steep fitting of contact lens.

Various types of contact lenses will be considered as follows in detail to understand their uses and fitting methods in a better way

- Soft contact lenses
- Rigid contact lenses
- Extended wear contact lenses
- Disposable contact lenses
- Scleral RGP contact lenses
- Therapeutic contact lenses
- Colored contact lenses
- Contact lenses in special conditions such as high myopia, aphakia, presbyopia, and high astigmatism

Soft Contact Lens Fitting

- Soft contact lenses can be manufactured by using different types of polymers but mostly hydroxyethyl methacrylate (HEMA) is used because of its properties like more stability, transparent, non-hazardous and non-allergic nature.
- Soft lenses are usually bigger in size than cornea which provides a fit, where the lens edges fall under the upper and lower eye-lids.
- These lenses are much more comfortable as compared to the rigid contact lens, due to its softness and an ability to bend with blinking of eyes.
- Most commonly used lenses in routine practice are soft contact lenses because of their comfort, flexibility, oxygen permeability, less glare and minimal over wear reaction.

Fitting procedures: Recommendations for fitting of soft contact lenses are provided by many lens manufactures in their brochures supplied with contact lenses. These brochures give the details of that particular lens series along with desired data and fitting parameters, however, a practitioner should be well-versed with various parameters and related nomenclature in the brochure provided with soft contact lenses.

Usually majority of lens manufactures give three choices for selection of the base curve and the overall diameter (TD) of contact lens. Practitioners need to decide the parameters for selection of contact lens on the following grounds to get the best fit of lenses.

Fitting steps include
- Trial lens selection
- Trial lens fit evaluation
- Trial lens ideal fit
- Ocular factor influencing lens fitting
- Contact lens factors affecting lens fit

Trial lens selection: Trial lens selection is done on the basis of these following criteria

- *Total diameter or overall diameter:* It must be larger (by approximately 2.5 mm) than the HVID of cornea to permit full coverage of cornea. However, this value may be more depending upon the limbal sulcus in particular eyes.
- *Lens power:* To decide the power of contact lens to be prescribed, the refraction for spectacle should be corrected for vertex distance which is distance between the posterior surface of spectacle glass/contact lens and cornea. Suppose on refraction the cylindrical power of spectacles is more than ±1.5 D, then toric contact lenses can be used or otherwise a spherical equivalent power can be used as described above.
- *Back vertex power:* To get the benefits from contact lens, the back vertex power of contact lens should be kept as close as possible to the patients' spectacle prescription. It also helps to facilitate adaptation. If it is not possible to get same power, then it is preferred to choose a contact lens of less power to avoid accommodative spasms. For monovision, trial lens should be chosen of power as close to correct power.
- *Back optic zone radius:* Suppose choice of base curve is available with lens, then manufacturer's guidelines must be followed regarding the selection of trial lens to be tried first. This trial is done without taking the Keratometry readings in consideration. When no choice is available, then a lens with base curve flatter than keratometry reading is chosen. Amount of flattening is decided by the TD and water content of that contact lens which is taken for trial.

Following guidelines can be used to decide about selection of the trial lens parameters
- *Depending on TD:* Principle is that if larger the TD of lens, then prefer the flatter lens. For example, in a lens with TD of 13.0 mm, a lens having base curve 0.3 mm flatter than the flattest keratometry reading should be selected. Similarly for a further increase in 0.5 mm diameter, increase the flattening of base curve by 0.3 mm, means for a 13.5 mm diameter lens a flattening of 0.6 mm is

needed from the flattest keratometry reading.

- *Depending on water content:* Principle is that lens of high water content usually require more steep fitting as compared to low water content lens. For example, if a high water content lens with TD of 14.5 mm needs a flattening of base curve by 1 mm than the flattest keratometry reading, then a low water content contact lens of the same diameter will require flattening by 1.2 mm.

Trial lens fit evaluation: Once the trial lens with correct parameters for fitting is selected, a sterile selected trial lens is inserted into the patient's eye. A proper fit of trial contact lens is evaluated by these parameters

- **Adaptation and patient's response**
  - *Adaptation period:* After placing the soft contact lens in the eye of patient, it is always necessary to wait for some time before (settling or adaption time) assessment of the fitting of lens because soft lenses have tendency to lose water once they are inserted in the eye. This loss of water may alter the parameters as well as fitting characteristics of a soft lens. Hence, it is recommended that the lens fit should be assessed only when the contact lens becomes in equilibrium with the tear film and established in the environment of eye. Traditionally, it is advised that about 25–30 minutes should be given for settling of a lens, however, some recent studies suggest that initial evaluation of fitting can be carry out after 5–10 minutes of insertion.
  - Although it is difficult to judge the physiological response as well as patients comfort for lens in five minutes period but its assessment should be based on lens sensation and eye movements.
  - Patients comfort is evaluated by the fact that lens should feel imperceptible on the eye by patient, especially on insertion. Lens sensation should be steady, having

no appreciable difference in lateral eye movements or blinking.

- **Over refraction**
  - Normally to check the correct fitting of contact lenses, examiner should perform an "over refraction", means refraction is done while patient is wearing a pair of trial contact lenses. Advantage of an over refraction is that, rather than depending on the predictions, whether the given contact lenses are able to correct ametropia or not, examiner can determine the actual refractive status.
  - An over refraction is done with binocular balancing. There must be a clear endpoint and stable visual acuity. Any disparity in these factors show poor fit of lens and repeat retinoscopy should be carry out to confirm it.
- **Biomicroscopy examination:** Subsequent to over refraction, examination by slit lamp using a diffuse, direct illumination under medium to high magnification (which enable us to visualize the contact lens on eye) should be done to check lens fit.

Trial lens ideal fit: *"Fluorescein dye is not used to assess the lens fit in case of a soft contact lens".* The fitting is assessed by observing following parameters

- **Coverage of cornea:** Contact lens should cover full cornea before, after and during the blink in the primary position of eye. Minimum 1–1.5 mm conjunctival overlap should be seen in all movements of eyes.
- **Centration:** Lens should remain in center of cornea in primary position of gaze and should retain full coverage of cornea even during extreme lateral gaze (lens lag) and up gaze (lens sag) as shown in 10.1A and B respectively.
- **Post-blink movement:** Amount of post-blink lens movement should be judged in primary gaze, ideally recorded using a reticule marking on slit lamp. Lens movements are observed at the bottom part

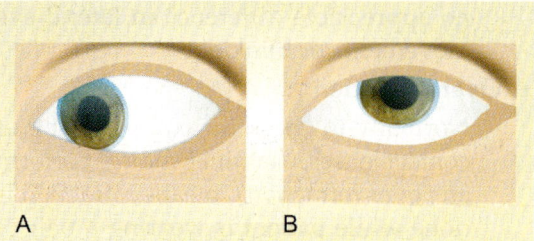

Fig. 10.1: Centration of contact lens. A. Lens lag; B. Lens sag

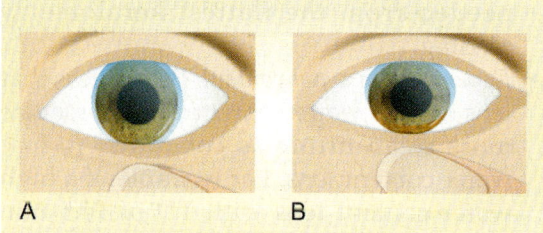

Fig. 10.2: Push test. A. Finger in position; B. Lens moved up

(inferior edge) of contact lens during the blink. Alternatively, if lower eyelid is obstructing inferior edge of lens, then we can observe lens at 4 or 8 o'clock position for movement. Sometimes, we can displace the lower eyelid using index finger, before assessing the movement. An ideal post-blink lens movement should be of 0.5–0.7 mm. If with each blink movement of lens is more than 1 mm, then it indicates too flat fitting of lens, if it is less than 0.5 mm, then lens fitting is steeper.

> **Note**
>
> Recent available contact lenses has more water content and are thin with less elasticity as compared to older lenses, which were usually thicker and lower in water content; hence they show less post-blink movement.

- **Push up test:** Many a times it is difficult to assess lens movement by blink alone, hence a better assessment of lens movement can be done by Push up test. It is considered most useful way to judge dynamic fit of a contact lens in relation to eye.

  Test procedure: To do this test, the examiner applies pressure on the lower eyelid by finger to move the contact lens vertically upwards and then remove the finger to release pressure on the eye so that lens returns to its original position as shown in Fig. 10.2A and B. During this test aim is to observe how easily the lens displacement occurs on pressure and then how rapidly it returns to its original position on releasing pressure.

Results: These are represented in a percentage grading system where 100% means that lens movement is not possible and 0% means that lens will fall away from the cornea without support of eyelids. A correct and optimum fit is considered when lens movement recorded is 50%. In addition, tightness of lens as measured by the push-up test shows a linear relationship with squeeze pressure (it is the force which exist between posterior surface of lens and front surface of the eye) and so it can also be considered in judging lens fit.

Effect of blinking is noticed not only on lens movement but also on visual acuity, retinoscopy reflex and keratometer mires.

- **Post-blink visual acuity:** Change in clarity of vision due to blinking should be checked. In case of an ideal lens fit, no change in visual acuity will be noticed by the patient. However, in a flat fit the patient complaints of blur vision while in steep fit, the vision improves immediately after blinking.
- **Post-blink retinoscopy reflex:** The changes in retinal reflex are in correlation with clarity of vision means in an ideal lens fit the reflexes are sharp, whereas in flat fit reflex becomes blur and in steep fit, it becomes clear instantly after blinking.
- **Post-blink keratometer mires:** Even the distortion of keratometer mires are in correlation with vision clarity, means in an ideal lens fit the mires appear crisp and sharp, whereas in flat fit they are blur and in steep fit they become clear immediately after blinking.

- **Conjunctival congestion:** On slit lamp the status of conjunctival vessels and scleral indentation should be observed. In case of a steep fit limbal vessel nipping, conjunctival congestion and scleral indentation (on long duration usage) is present.

To summarize these observations and evaluations of a trial lens fit following points to be remembered as shown in Table 10.2.

Ocular factors influencing lens fitting

- *Ocular sag:* This is determined by corneal diameter, radius and shape factor and also by scleral shape and radius and any factor among these if altered will affect the lens sag, which can only be assessed by a trial lens fit.
- *Corneal apex:* Position of corneal apex will affect the centration of lens. Displacement of corneal apex will cause the lens decentration, which can be corrected by increasing the total diameter (TD). An increase in TD will increase the corneal coverage, if exposed, while changes in base curve will not affect centration.
- *Pressure of lids:* Too much pressure caused by tensed lids may lead to high riding of lens and also an excessive movement of lens. To overcome it a thin lens design and/or lens with more diameter can be used. Loose lids usually have less effect on lens fits than tight lids.
- *Tear characteristics:* The change in pH and osmotic pressure of tear has important part

to alter the parameters of lens, finally affecting the lens fit. Decrease in the pH of tear film causes steepening of ionic contact lens. Change in osmotic pressure like decrease in tonicity of tear will cause tight fit of both ionic and non-ionic lenses. Hence it is important to remember that if an acceptable fit is not obtained with contact lens material, then it is necessary to change the ionicity or water content of another lens material.

Contact lens factors affecting lens fit

- *Total diameter (TD):* Variation in the total diameter of lens will affect the fitting of lens. For example, increase in the TD of lens will enhance sag of lens, resulting in tight fit, while reduction in TD of lens will produce opposite effect. In case of lens with displaced apex, the TD can be increased to improve the corneal coverage by this lens. Lens fit is usually more affected by change in lens diameter as compared to change in BOZR.
- *Back optic zone radius (BOZR):* Change in the base curve of lens cause change in the movement of lens. However, studies indicate that change in the BOZR does not cause much effect on lens fit.
- *Peripheral design of lens:* The peripheral lens design may also influence the lens fit. The peripheral design indicates correlation between front and back peripheral curves of lens. It should be kept in mind that it is

Table 10.2: Various indicators of loose fit and tight fit of contact lens	
Indicators of loose fit of contact lens	*Indicators of tight fit of contact lens*
Too much movement of contact lens	No movement of contact lens
Poor centration in primary gaze, usually in inferior lag	Constriction of limbal vessel or 'nipping'
Buckling of lens edge after wearing	Indentation of conjunctiva at lens margins
Presence of lens awareness sensation	Conjunctival congestion with redness
Change in vision, especially immediately after blinking	Ocular inflammation of low degree
Blurring of retinoscope reflex and keratometer mires, immediately after blinking	Visual improvement, immediately after blinking

not necessary that lenses with different peripheral design having same TD and BOZR will show fitting characteristic in similar fashion.

Soft Contact Lens Ordering

After a detailed evaluation of the lens parameters and checking a proper trial lens fit with these parameters, soft contact lenses are ordered from a known manufacturers' series, by specifying the desired power. Usually we can specify the total diameter and power of lens, to get a proper fit soft contact lens from various manufacturers' guide.

Examination of delivered contact lens: Contact lens delivery received from the lens manufacture should be examined thoroughly before inserting it into the eye of patient as shown in Fig. 10.3. Following parameters are checked for received contact lens:

- Lens total diameter: This is checked by using a diameter gauge.
- Contact lens power: Power of the lens is determined by using lensometer, specially designed to measure the contact lens power.
- Lens edges and curves are inspected by keeping the lens on the tip of finger and observing it in bright light for any defect or abnormality.
- Lens quality and clarity is also observed while checking for its edges.

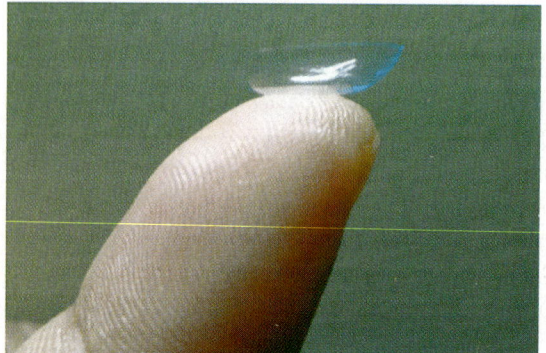

Fig. 10.3: Examination of soft contact lens before insertion

Evaluation of ordered lens fit: Once all the parameters of delivered lens are checked thoroughly, this lens is ready to use in the patient's eye. Following instructions related to lens fit along with explanation of methods of lens insertion and removal are taught to the patient.

Contact lens handling instruction to the patient: Although most of the patients are enthusiastic about wearing of a contact lens, but many of them are first time wearers. Hence, a detailed instruction about handling and caring of contact lens along with the insertion and removal techniques should be taught to majority of patients.

General instructions: Patients should be instructed that contacts should not be considered as fashion accessories or cosmetics; rather it is a type of medical devices that need proper cleanliness as explained and is vital to prevent infections of eyes. These infections are potentially hazardous for eyes; hence patients are advised to take care of lenses as per direction. Cleaning is done both before insertion and after removal of contact lens from the eye before putting the lens back in lens case.

Following instructions are important to be remembered by patients

- Strictly follow the schedule for insertion and removal of lens.
- Daily wear lenses should not be worn at time of sleeping.
- To protect from water contact lenses should be removed before bath, swimming, or doing anything, where water can go inside the eyes.
- Never touch contact lens with dirty hands. Hands should be washed with soap and water before touching lens.
- Never use tap or sterile water and saline solution prepared at home for rinsing or storage of contact lens. Use sterile contact lens solution (not tap water) for washing of case of lens followed by its drying in air.

- For disinfection of lens proper disinfectant solution should be used. Saline solution or artificial tear drops should not be used for disinfection.

- Always use a "rub and rinse" cleaning method, before insertion, after removal or before placing lens in the lens case. The contact lenses should be rubbed with clean fingers followed by rinsing with solution and then soaking. This process must be done every time for cleaning and disinfection of contact lens.

- Soft contact lenses are always stored in normal saline solution because if exposed to air, may get dehydrated and breaks due to brittleness. Rehydrate the lenses by placing them in saline solution, and wait until they become soft and regain their original shape.

- Old contact lens care solution should not be reused for cleaning and rinsing purpose and also contact lens solution should not be transferred into different container as solution may loss its sterility and infection may occur.

- Tip of lens solution container should not contact any surface. The solution bottle should be kept tightly closed after use.

- Contact lens case must be clean and ideally it should be replaced at least once in 3 months. Damaged and cracked cases should be replaced immediately.

- Over a period of time, contact lenses get damage and also its shape can alter due to cornea. Hence, check at intervals that that lenses fit is proper and the visual acuity is perfect, if not report immediately to practitioner.

Insertion and Removal of Soft Contact Lens

Before insertion of contact lenses in the eyes, we should ensure that the lens have not turned inside out, while removing from their blister packs or lens case. There are two methods to check this

- Keep the contact lens on the tip of index finger and examine its shape and edges as shown in Fig. 10.4A. In correct lens an even cup shape is seen, whereas if lens is not correct, then lens appears shallower with more pointed at its edges as shown in Fig. 10.4B.

- *Taco test:* It is another method to check whether lens is proper or in an inside out position. To do this gently folds the soft contact lens in between the index finger and thumb. Suppose the lens is in correct position, lens edges should fold inward like a Mexican Taco and touches each other edges as shown in Fig. 10.5A, whereas if lens is inside out, then the lens edges will curls outward and flips out onto fingertip as shown in Fig. 10.5B.

> **Note** _____
>
> Important point to be remembered while testing the position of lens is that the lens should be held from its center not from its edges.

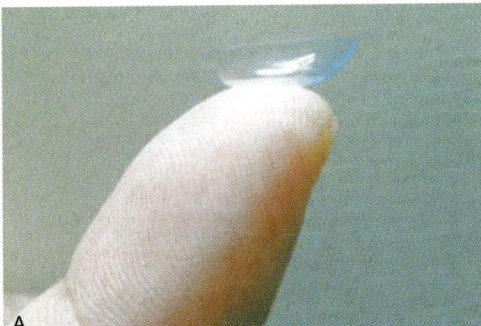 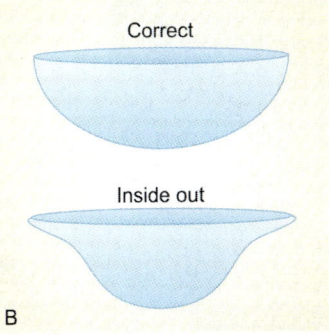

Fig. 10.4: Contact lens checking. A. CL position on fingertip; B. Check position

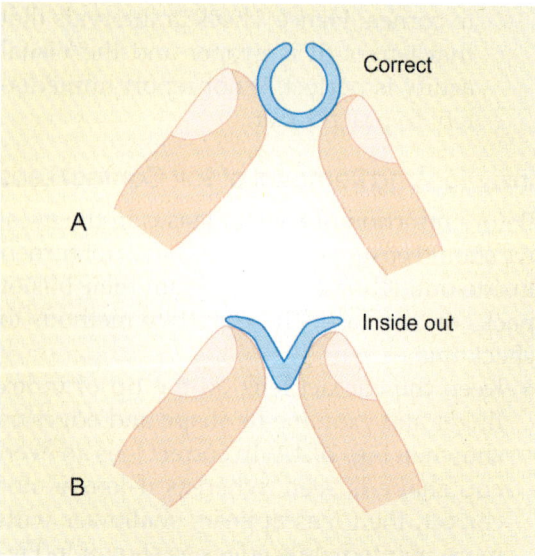

Fig. 10.5: Taco test for checking correct position of contact lens. A. Inward rolling of lens margins; B. Outward rolling of lens margins

Lens insertion technique: Insertion of a soft contact lens is done as follows

- Wash the hands thoroughly using soap, for a few minutes and then air dry.
- Remove the lens from its case and clean as we already discussed above.
- Rinse the contact lens with cleaning solution.
- Place the lens on the tip of the index finger of hand as shown.
- Look up while the lower lid is retracted with the middle finger of same hand as shown in Fig. 10.6A. This is called as one hand technique.
- Alternately, the eye can be spread wide open with the index and middle finger of left hand and contact lens is placed on the tip of index finger of right hand, while the middle finger of right hand is placed over cheek bone to avoid any jerky movement of right hand. This is called as two hand technique as shown in Fig. 10.6B.
- While looking upward, gently touch the contact lens to the lower part of eye. Then slowly remove the finger, when contact lens is placed on the eye.
- Then very gently and slowly first release the lower and then upper lids.
- Close the eye and give a gentle massage over lids, to remove any air bubble in case if present underneath of contact lens.
- Open the eye and move it gently in all gazes, to center the lens. Then observe the correct centration of lens while the other eye is covered with hand.
- Similar instructions are repeated in other eye for lens insertion.

Lens removal technique

- Wash the hands thoroughly using soap, for a few minutes and then air dry.
- First turn the eyes upwards and with middle finger retract the lower lid while keeping the tip of index finger on the lower edge of the lens.

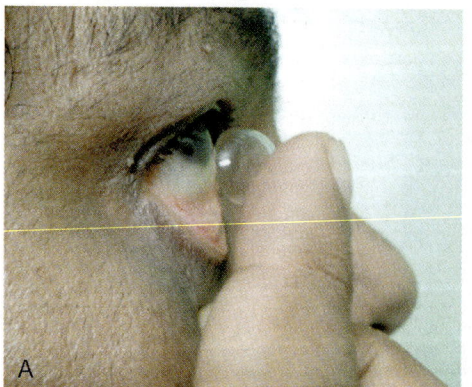
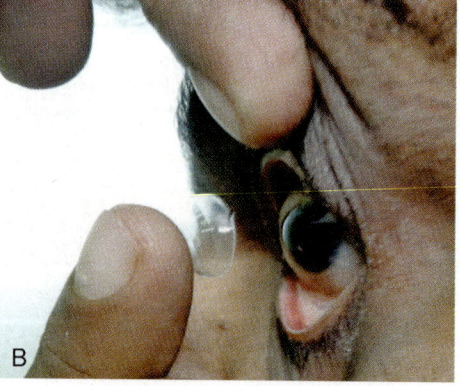

Fig. 10.6: Insertion technique of soft contact lens. A. One hand method; B. Two hands method

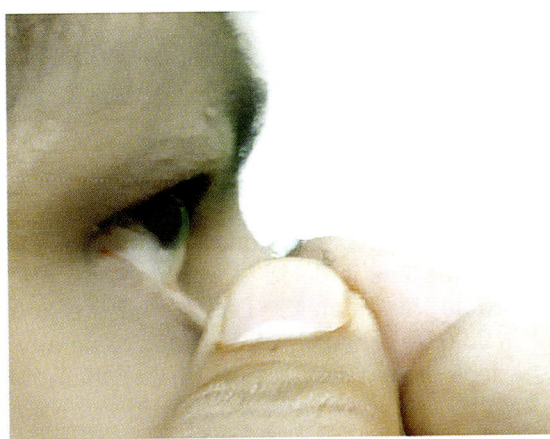

Fig. 10.7: Removal technique of soft contact lens

- Disengage the lens slowly by sliding the lens downwards, over to the white portion of the eye.
- Once lens slides downwards, pinch out the lens between thumb and the index finger, so that suction created under lens is broken by air as shown in Fig. 10.7.
- Slowly remove the lens from eye and do the cleaning with lens solution and place it in the lens case containing solution.

Wearing schedule for soft contact lenses: Normally soft contact lenses are well accepted and comfortable to wear from day one; hence there is tendency in patients that they may over wear it from day one. Patients should be informed about the disastrous results of over wearing of contact lenses and should be advised to follow a strict wearing schedule for best visual outcomes.

Generally the wearing schedule is totally dependent on the individual patient's profile, however, on an average patients' are instructed to wear a soft contact lens for continuous 2–3 hours and then remove the lens for a minimum period of one hour. They are advised to follow this schedule for initial 10–15 days, or till they become comfortable for longer duration wear.

Follow up: Regular follow up is must to achieve a comfortable contact lens wearing period without any complications. Patients'

are instructed to report immediately if develop any discomfort, redness or pain, otherwise can come on a regular follow-up schedule as below

- Day one
- Day seven
- After a month
- Every six months

On every follow-up visits following evaluations are performed

- *History:* Questions are asked in terms of visual and non-visual symptoms like change in vision, intermittent blurring, foreign body sensations, heavy lids or ocular movements, excessive watering, discharge or decreased visual fields, etc. Examiner should be able to differentiate between physiological/psychological symptoms arising due to adaptation and actual clinical abnormalities. Usually adaptation symptoms are not present with soft lenses, however, even if present will subside on its own within 10–12 days, however, symptoms due to clinical abnormalities will start after 2–3 days and persist constantly even after 15 days.
- *Vision:* Check the visual acuity with lens in position, if visual acuity is less, then do an over refraction and recheck vision with a pin hole.
- *Ocular examination:* Detailed ocular examination is done to record head posture, lid position, periorbital edema, blinking rate and conjunctival congestion.
- *Slit lamp examination:* It is done with contact lens in the eye, and then after removal of contact lens. Position of contact lens, cornea and conjunctiva are examined in detail.

Rigid Contact Lens Fitting

Rigid contact lenses are broadly classified as **Rigid non-gas permeable lenses:** Mainly manufactured from PMMA (Plexiglas) and are rarely used nowadays due to their disadvantages overweighing the advantages.

Rigid gas permeable contact lenses: These are most widely used contact lenses and are also called semisoft contact lenses. These lenses are made up of a unique plastic material which has an ability to permit oxygen to diffuse inside and carbon dioxide to diffuse outside the lens. Various polymers materials are used to make these lenses such as CAB (cellulose acetyl butyrate), silicon acrylate, butyl styrene, polystyrene, fluorine copolymers and polysulfone copolymers.

Fitting procedures: Since PMMA lenses are obsolete nowadays, hence we will discuss fitting of rigid gas permeable (RGP) contact lenses in detail.

Fitting of rigid contact lens is usually considered as more difficult than fitting of soft contact lens, but actually many fitting steps are essentially the same when practitioner needs to judge the fitting of either lens. Modern RGP lens designs are available in a wide range of lenses; which can be fitted easily in majority of normal ametropic population.

Nowadays to receive a rigid contact lens, practitioners just need to specify the total diameter (TD), back vertex power (BVP) and back optic zone radius (BOZR) of a particular lens design to manufacturer.

Fitting steps include
- Trial lens selection
- Trial lens fit evaluation
- Trial lens fit interpretation
- Corneal factor influencing lens fitting
- Contact lens factors affecting lens fit

Trial lens selection: The initial trial lens should be selected using the following parameters:

- *Total diameter:* Selection of total diameter (TD) of lens is decided by the horizontal visible iris diameter (HVID) and position of lid (size of palpebral aperture). Generally, a lens having TD 1.4 mm smaller than the HVID should be chosen. In addition, on the basis of size of palpebral aperture, the lens with smaller TD should be selected if aperture is small and vice versa.

  – Choice of TD according to HVID can be made as shown in Fig. 10.8. For small palpebral aperture, rigid lens of approximately 9.2 mm size, for an average size aperture lens of 9.6 mm diameter can be chosen, however, for very large apertures 10 mm TD size rigid lens may be required.

  – Choice of lens is also in inverse relationship with corneal curvature as summarized in Table 10.3. It means flatter the cornea, larger diameter of RGP lens will be required for a proper fit.

- *Center thickness of lens:* To enhance the oxygen transmissibility contact lenses are made as thin as possible. In majority of rigid

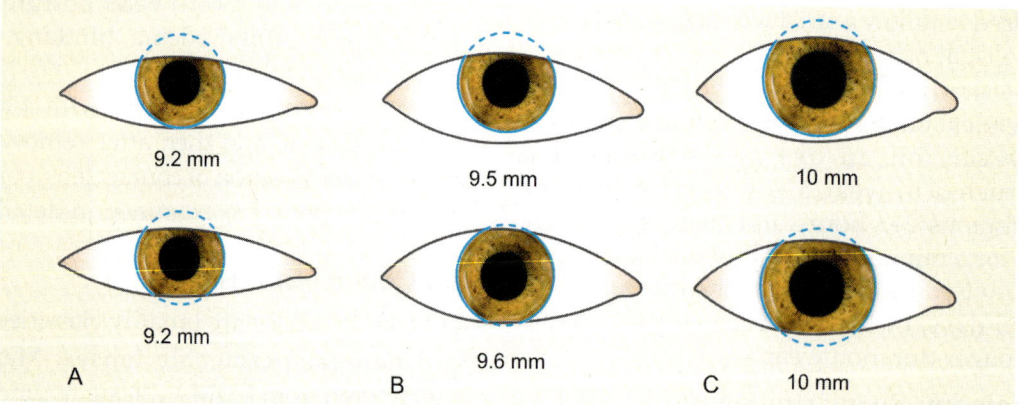

Fig. 10.8: Total diameter selection according to HVID and lid positions. A. Small palpebral aperture; B. Average size palpebral aperture; C. Very large palpebral aperture

Table 10.3: Relationship between corneal curve and contact lens diameter	
Corneal curve	Diameter of contact lens
40–43 D	9.5 mm
43.25–45 D	9.2 mm
> 45.25 D	9.0 mm

lens materials (available nowadays), the center thickness is kept about 0.14 mm.

- *Calculation of power of trial lens:* Refraction should be done to determine spectacle power and then power of trial rigid contact lens is calculated. First convert the spectacle lens power into a minus cylinder form, if present. Now correct this spectacle power for a zero vertex distance by applying appropriate formula or from a ready reference chart provided by the contact lens manufacturer.

  For example, suppose spectacle power is: 8.5 × + 1.5 × 90°, at 15 mm vertex distance.

  First convert it in minus cylinder form as: –7 × –1.5 × 180°

  Then correct it to a zero vertex distance as: –5.75 × –1.0 × 180°.

Note _____

Spherical powers can similarly be corrected to a zero vertex distance and contact lens of corrected power is used directly.

_____

- *Back vertex power:* To provide normal vision and to decrease probable changes in lens fit due to difference in lens power, the back vertex power must be approximate to patient's final prescription. The fit may vary with minus powered lens and plus power lens due to difference in their edge design and center of gravity. Hence, myopes should be assessed with negatively powered lenses and vice versa with hypermetropes.
- *Back optic zone diameter (BOZD):* BOZD is usually kept larger (≥ 1.0 mm) than average pupil size to avoid flare due to lens. To maintain corneal alignment also it is necessary to adjust BOZD because as the flattening of cornea increases, lens of larger BOZD will be required to maintain proper alignment over the cornea.

- *Back optic zone radius (BOZR):* Design of back surface of rigid lenses could be aspherical, spherical or their combination. Spherical RGP lenses can be bicurve, tri-curve or multi-curve in nature where every lens has different BOZR with different peripheral curve design. In case of spherical RGP contact lenses, initial trial lens is selected on the basis of keratometer readings using recommendations provided by the manufacturer or using the values as shown in Table 10.4. In case of an elliptical type of aspherical contact lenses usually more flat fitting is required than spherical lenses so that an alignment across the corneal surface is adequately achieved.

BOZR is chosen on the basis of keratometer readings; usually on flattest K- reading (called as fit 'On-K'), especially for spherical RGP lenses or an astigmatism <0.5 D. But for astigmatism of > 0.5 D, guidelines as shown in Table 10.4 are used to decide about the BOZR of RGP lenses.

For understanding Table 10.3 values, we can take an example, suppose keratometer readings are 45 D/46 D, means having astigmatism of 1 D; then the base curve selected will be 45.25 D. Similarly if readings are 46 D/47.5 D, then a base curve of 46.5 D

Table 10.4: Guidelines for selection of BOZR of RGP lenses in astigmatism > 0.5 D	
Astigmatism	BOZR
Spherical to 0.5 D	Fit 'On-K', means flattest keratometer reading
0.5–1.0 D	Fit on 0.05 steeper than the flattest keratometer reading
1.0–2.5 D	Fit on 0.05–0.10 steeper than the flattest keratometer reading
Over 2.5 D	A toric back optic zone is suggested

will be selected, however in case where readings are 46 D/50 D, then it is better to choose a toric back optic zone contact lens.

Trial lens fit evaluation: Once the trial lens is chosen, then a sterile trial lens is inserted in the eye under all aseptic precautions. Just before lens insertion, patient is instructed that there may be feeling of foreign body sensation after insertion of lens. To reduce feeling of foreign body sensation patient is advised to look downwards after insertion of lens. *"Fluorescein dye is used to assess the lens fit in case of a rigid contact lens".*

- **Adaptation and patients' response**
  - *Adaptation period:* After insertion of lens, as reflex tearing get stop (usually within 5 minutes), lens fit by bare eye and under white light should be examined to check the stability and centration of lens during trial period. Once an adequate lens fit is achieved, patients are advised for a longer trial period (minimum 30 minutes) which allows them to judge the comfort and problems of rigid contact lens. After trial period the subjective response of the patient is assessed. Patient must be comfortable and there must be no reflex tearing. Vision must be stable in all positions of gaze with the used power of trial lens.
- **Over refraction and visual acuity**
  - Initially to check the spherical power of contact lens, an over refraction with binocular balancing is done. The purpose of binocular balancing is to relax the accommodation, which might have been induced due to foreign body sensation of contact lens.
  - Visual acuity achieved with contact lenses should be crisp and stable in all gazes. An unstable or improper acuity indicates that a cylindrical refraction is also needed to correct the refractive status.
  - Both by subjective and objective response should be evaluated during refraction by retinoscope. The results are used to

calculate the tear lens power and to adjust the central fit of contact lens, if needed.

- **Biomicroscopy examination**
  - Dynamic fit of a rigid contact lens can be evaluated and measured by using either a slit lamp or Burton lamp in the same way as for the soft contact lenses.
  - Lens-corneal alignment is assessed by help of either white light or a cobalt blue light as follows

  White light
  - Using diffuse white light and with an optic section examiner should make a judgment about centration of contact lens in the primary gaze as well as during lateral movements of eyes.
  - Along with centration, the movement of lens with blink is also judged. Ideally, RGP lens should move downward with each blink, under the influence of upper eyelid, however, it returns to cover the pupil immediately.

  Cobalt-blue light
  - Alignment of posterior surface of lens with front surface of the eye can be assessed by means of fluorescein because it causes staining of the tear film, which creates a tear lens. On illuminating by appropriate wavelength of blue light (cobalt-blue filter) the fluorescein emits a fluorescent green color. The intensity of this green color is related to the thickness of the fluorescein tear film; means thicker the tear lens, more yellow will be the appearance.
  - As fluorescein dye occupies the tear space present between posterior surface of lens and front surface of the cornea. The distance between these two surfaces (known as fluorescein pattern) can be assessed by looking change in the intensity of fluorescent light which occurs due to excitation by cobalt blue filter. More

is the intensity (brighter) of color; more will be the distance between two surfaces.

Burton lamp

- Burton lamp is used to visualize various fluorescein patterns. It acts as a source of UV light which is used to excite the fluorescein dye. However, as compared to slit lamp the magnification achieved with Burton's lamp is less. In addition, it cannot assess pattern when polymer materials used in manufacturing of contact lens also contain a UV inhibitor where cobalt blue light with slit lamp is the choice.

- **Fluorescein assessment**
  - In RGP lenses, a fluorescein assessment of the contact lens fit is done. Fluorescein dye in small amount is introduced into the conjunctival sac while patient is instructed to blink gently 2–3 times, which spreads the dye all over the eye.
  - Lens fit should be evaluated using slit lamp or Burton lamp with a diffuse, direct illumination under medium to high magnification.
  - The brightness of fluorescein dye is assessed systematically mainly in three regions of contact lens, i.e. peripheral, mid peripheral and central. Guillon proposed a simple grading scale for the assessment of contact lens fit. According to grading if fluorescein dye is seen under the contact lens during assessment of fit, then it can range from
    - Little amount (0), means in alignment or minimal apical clearance
    - Moderate amount (+1)
    - Too much or excessive amount (+2)

Trial lens fit interpretation: Now it is important to interpret the lens fit to know whether it is correct or not, which can be done by

- **Patient's subjective response**
  - RGP lenses usually cause more discomfort after insertion as compared to soft contact lenses, however, after adaptation period of 30 minutes, patient should not feel discomfort. If after adaptation period also the patient complaints of pain and excessive reflex tearing, then it indicates that the contact lens is not correct and require modification in parameters.

  - By means of correct spherical correction the patient must have stable and crisp visual acuity. However, if vision is not stable with use of spherical lenses then a cylindrical overcorrection might be needed.

  - If residual astigmatism is suspected for the poor vision, then before prescribing a toric correction, it is essential to confirm the site of residual astigmatism because bending or curving of lens may be also one of the causes of poor vision. If no site of residual astigmatism detected on examination, then it is most probably the lens bending causing poor vision and lens-eye fitting relationship require modification to correct the vision.

- **Over refraction**
  - Over refraction is done to calculate the tear lens values, i.e. difference in refractive power between the ocular refraction and final contact lens power required to correct ametropia.

  - In case of steeper fitting of lens than cornea, a positive tear lens will form as shown in Fig. 10.9C and final contact lens power will be either less plus or more minus as compared to the ocular refraction.

  - In opposite situation, i.e. flatter fitting of contact lens, a negative tear lens will form as shown in Fig. 10.9A and final power of the contact lens required will be either more plus or less minus than the ocular refraction.

  - In case of an ideal fit as shown in Fig. 10.9B, a slight central touch is seen.

- **Lens centration and movement:** During lateral gaze and in between blinking, the

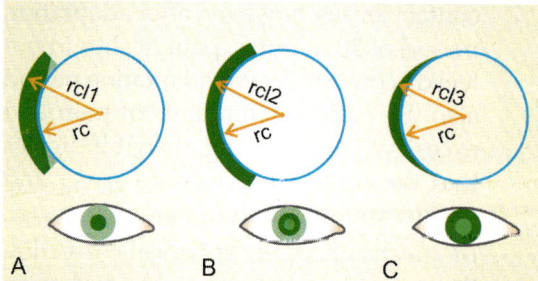

Fig. 10.9: Various tear lenses and over refraction. A. Flatter fit; B. Ideal fit; C. Steep fit

> **Note**
>
> Simple guidelines in calculating tear lens powers are that if there is 0.5 DS difference in over refraction, it means a 0.1 mm difference is present between corneal radius and contact lens radius.

position of lens must be centered over the visual axis. Various positions of lens may be seen due to these factors.

– Corneal opacities, against the rule astigmatism and oblique astigmatism may

decenter the contact lens either temporally or nasally. Smaller lens with a steeper fit will correct this horizontal decentring.

– Vertically lens movement is about 1–1.5 mm, but sometimes lens may ride high, means the upper edge of lens crosses the upper limbal margin or lens hook on to upper lid.

– Similarly, lens may ride too low or rapidly drop after blink, means lower edges of contact lens crosses the lower limbal margin.

– Some degree of decentration is acceptable in case of rigid contact lens fitting.

Various contributing factors and the management of lens decentration are summarized in Table 10.5, along with the available options to improve the centration of contact lens.

- **Fluorescein patterns**
  – Analysis of fluorescein patterns helps to find out the tear lens shapes in relation

Table 10.5: Various possible causes and management of lens decentration		
Lens location	*Possible causes*	*Management*
Lens riding high or not dropping after blink (superior decentration)	Flat and wide peripheral zone High minus lens Large diameter lens and tight lid Too thick edge lens With the rule astigmatism Displacement of optic cap in upward direction	Steepen the base curve Use plus carrier lenticular design Reduce diameter and use prism ballast lens Reduce Tc and Te of lens Use toric peripheral design
Lens riding low or dropping rapidly after blink (inferior decentration)	Lens too small in diameter Lens too thick No lid attachment Displacement of optic cap in downward direction	Use large lens (increase TD) Reduce Tc Add peripheral negative carrier
Continue to be on one side (lateral decentration)	Corneal apex decentered Too small lens Flat contact lens Against the rule corneal astigmatism	Increase the diameter of lens and use soft lens Steepen the base curve of lens Use back surface with toric design or toric periphery design
Stationary Lens	Too steep lens	Flatten the fit
Excessive decentration of lens (beyond limbus)	Excess lacrimation Lens too flat Excess corneal astigmatism	Correct symptoms Steepen the design Use back surface in toric design

to lens fit. Thus help to confirm the relationship of contact lens and the eye. For example, steep looking fit will show positive tear lens pattern while a flat looking fit will show a minus tear lens pattern.

– Sometimes, even when using the contact lens with BOZR which was matched with keratometer readings of cornea, then also a steep or flat fit looking fluorescein patterns may occur. It may be due to either BOZR of trial lens is inaccurate or due to difference in the eccentricity of cornea.

Corneal factors influencing lens fit: Eccentricity (e) of cornea decides rate of flattening of the cornea toward the periphery. Normal cornea has average eccentricity value of 0.2 to 0.5. If cornea has e value lower (i.e. e <0.5) than average, means it indicates that cornea has steepen central cornea (more flat peripheral cornea), while high e value (i.e. e >0.5) indicates flatter central cornea than peripheral cornea. Relationship of corneal eccentricity with contact lens fit is shown in Fig. 10.10.

• *Cornea with average eccentricity:* Spherical contact lens will show an ideal lens fit, as apical appearance, mid-peripheral touch and peripheral clearance pattern as indicated by a bright green periphery with faintly appearing central portion as shown in Fig. 10.10A.

• *Cornea with lower eccentricity than an average eccentricity:* Means cornea steepens out faster towards periphery at faster rate, hence spherical contact lens of the same central radius prescribed for this type of cornea will show peripheral pooling as shown in Fig. 10.10B. This lens fit will need a modification, as if dealing with a flat fitting lens.

• *Cornea with more eccentricity than an average eccentricity:* Means cornea flattens out faster towards periphery at faster rate, hence spherical contact lens of the same central radius will show central pooling as shown in

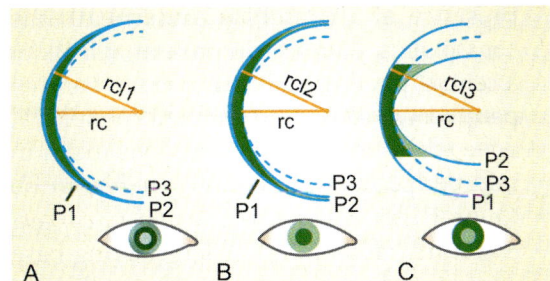

Fig. 10.10: Corneal eccentricity and respective contact lens fit. A. Average eccentricity, ideal fit; B. Lower eccentricity, flat lens fit with peripheral pooling; C. Higher eccentricity steep lens fit with central pooling

Fig. 10.10C. This lens fit needs a modification, as if dealing with a steep fitting lens.

Contact Lens factors affecting lens fit

• *Contact lens base curve is flatter than corneal curvature (flat fitting):* Chances of excessive movement of lens and fluorescein pattern will show a central black area with peripheral pooling. Fluorescein pattern in this case will show a central black area indicating a direct lens corneal touch (means there is no tear layer between lens and cornea) and diffuse green portion in mid-peripheral and peripheral zone due to pooling of dye in these areas as shown in Fig. 10.11.

• *Contact lens base curve is steeper than corneal curvature (steep fitting):* A lens having base curve steeper than corneal curvature will show very little or no movement with

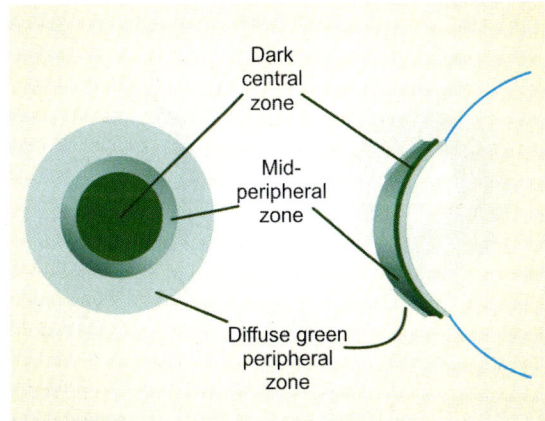

Fig. 10.11: Flat lens fit showing central dark area

presence of air bubbles underneath the contact lens. Fluorescein pattern will show a central pooling and bright green band at periphery, with a broad dark mid-peripheral zone which indicates intense lens touch in mid-peripheral zone as shown in Fig. 10.12.

- *Contact lens base curve is equal to corneal curvature (ideal fitting):* A lens having base curve equal to corneal curvature will show desired movement of lens with rotation of eyeball. Fluorescein pattern will show an apical appearance and light green clearance at periphery, with a dark mid-peripheral zone which indicates that an adequate amount of tear lens is formed with an ideal lens fit as shown in Fig. 10.13.

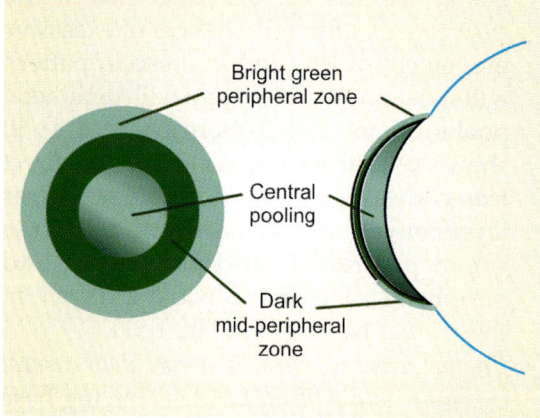

Fig. 10.12: Steep lens fit showing central pooling

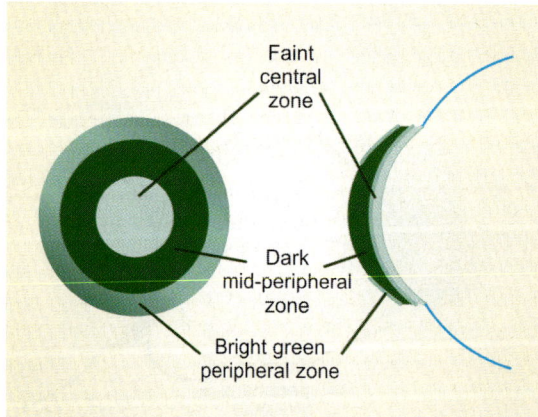

Fig. 10.13: Ideal lens fit showing apical appearance and peripheral clearance

- Base curve in RGP lenses is an important parameter to decide about the lens to be ordered. Sometimes, a selected lens of particular diameter may need change in diameter due to change in the base curve as both are directly correlated to each other. Usually, a large diameter lens should have a small base curve to produce the same effect as that of a small diameter lens with steeper base curve. On an average, a change of 1 mm in the diameter requires a change of 0.01 mm in the radius of curvature of lens.

- Various parameters used for selection of a rigid lens are dependent on each other, so to get an ideal lens fit, if one parameter is changed, then simultaneously it is also required to change other parameter. The fundamental rules which should be remembered to make alterations in lens parameters are as follows.
  - Modification of 0.05 mm in BOZR of lens will cause change in power equal to 0.25 D considering radius of lens is about 7.8 mm.
  - Similarly, 0.5 mm change in BOZD will need change of 0.05 mm in BOZR to retain equal fluorescein pattern.

Rigid Contact Lens Ordering

After doing a detailed evaluation about the lens parameters and checking of a proper trial lens fit with these parameters, the rigid contact lenses are ordered from a known manufacturer's series by specifying the desired power. Following parameters are specified in a contact lens prescription

- Base curve radius (such as 7.8 mm)
- Optic zone diameter (such as 7.0 mm)
- First peripheral curve radius (such as 8.0 mm)
- Second peripheral curve radius (such as 8.6 mm)
- Back peripheral zone (such as up to 8.2 mm)
- Total diameter (such as 9.0 mm)
- Contact Lens power (such as –5 DS)

Above parameters will typically be written in a perception form as

7.8: 7.0/8.2: 8.0/8.6: 9.0, power –5 DS

Examination of the received lens: Contact lens delivery received from the lens manufacture should be thoroughly examined, before inserting it into the eye of patient. Following parameters are checked for received contact lens

- Lens total diameter is checked by using a diameter gauge.
- Contact lens power is determined by using lensometer, specifically designed to measure the contact lens power.
- Base curve is measured by using a specially designed instrument called Radiuscope.
- Contact lens central thickness should be measured by a thickness gauge.
- Lens edges and curves are inspected by keeping the lens on the tip of finger and observing it in bright light for any defect or abnormality.
- Lens quality and clarity is also observed while checking for its edges.

Evaluation of ordered lens fit: Once we had examined the received lens as per specification, this sterile rigid contact lens is inserted in patient's eye under all aseptic precautions. After an extended adaptation period of about 25–30 minutes, evaluation of ordered lens is done to check the lens fit on the same guidelines as described for trial lens fit evaluations. However, some important points of lens fit for evaluation are as follows

- *Position of the lens:* Well-centered lens indicates an ideal fit. High ride or low ride lens indicates an abnormal fit.
- *Movements of lens:* 1–1.5 mm vertical movement or lateral excursion in horizontal gaze indicates an ideal fit. Excessive lens movement in all gazes shows a flat fit and less or no movement indicates a steep fit.
- *Fluorescein pattern:* As described above the distinctive fluorescein patterns will be seen in an ideal, flat and steep fit lenses.

- *Visual acuity:* Should be crisp and clear which remain stable before, during and after the blinks. Over refraction can be done to rule out any under or over correction of power.
- *Psychological and physiological responses:* Patient should feel comfortable and no foreign body sensation should be present. In case of an ideal fit corneal metabolism remain healthy, hence no corneal erosions or edema is noticed after adaptation period.

Patient education: Once we get a satisfactory rigid lens fit, patient is educated about the handling and caring of contact lens. Techniques for insertion, removal and recentration of contact lens are also explained to patient.

Handling and caring of contact lens: To prevent infection, it is essential to educate the patient about proper handling and caring of the contact lens. Following instructions are given to the patient at the time of dispensing of a rigid contact lens

- Thoroughly clean the hands with soap and water and air dry them before inserting, rinsing, cleaning or removing the contact lens.
- Never apply excessive pressure while cleaning the lens, because they are very thin and can easily get fractured.
- Clean the lenses after removal and before placing them in lens case, keeping the concave side upwards.
- Always use antiseptic solution or a commercially available multipurpose contact lens cleaning solution, to rinse, clean, soak or disinfect a RGP lens, never heat or use running tap water.
- These lenses should be disinfected by chemical treatment at regular intervals for maintaining the sterility.
- Patients are advised not to sleep or do underwater swimming, while wearing these lenses.

Insertion and Removal of Rigid Contact Lens

Patient is taught to insert the contact lens in his/her eyes very comfortably.

Insertion Technique

- Insertion steps of a rigid contact lens are similar to that of a soft contact lens as instructed above.
- Lens is kept on the tip of index finger as shown in Fig. 10.14A and is inserted in eye as described for soft contact lens (Fig. 10.14B). Important point in rigid lenses is identification of right and left eye lens, especially in cases where there is a vast difference in refractive powers of two eyes.

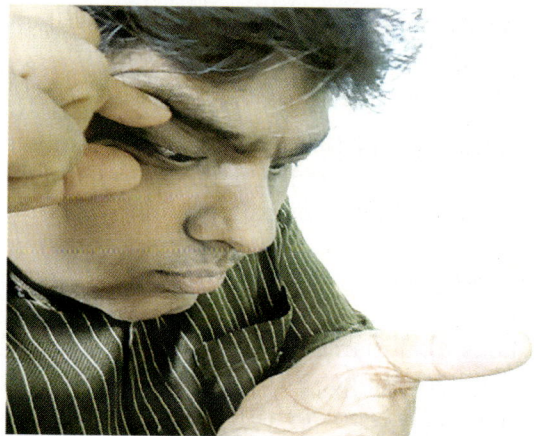

Fig. 10.14: Method 1 for RGP lens removal

Note _____

Letter 'R' is engraved on the lens periphery for right eye lens, hence when patient keeps the lens on the tip of finger, he/ she should search for this mark for right eye.

Removal Technique

Removal procedure for a rigid lens is different from soft contact lens removal technique. Here lens can be removed by two methods as per convenience.

Method 1 (Fig. 10.15)
- Head is bended down to make it parallel to the floor, then patient places the thumb/ middle finger of right hand on right lower lid margin and index finger of the same hand over right upper lid margin.
- Cup the left hand under the right eye to grasp the falling RGP lens.
- Then patient draw both the eyelids away from the lens, while pressing them tightly together and keeping the straight gaze.
- Suppose lens did not fall by this manoeuvre, then alternatively both the hands can be used to pull the upper and lower eyelids using right and left hands.

Method 2 (Fig. 10.16)
- Similarly bend the head down, now place index finger of right hand over the upper lid margin.
- Cup the left hand under the right eye to grab the falling lens.

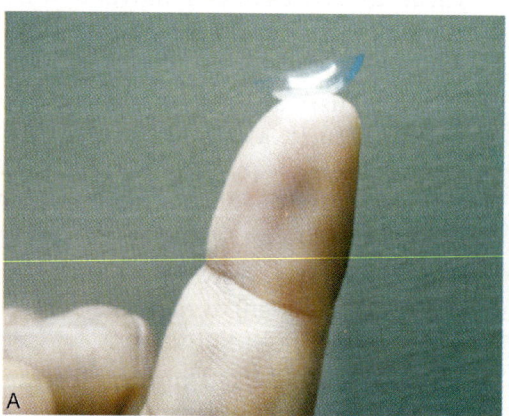
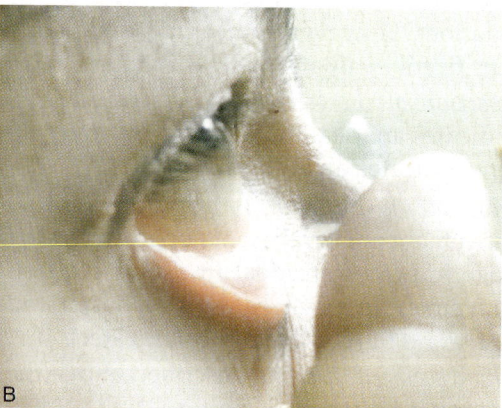

Fig. 10.15: Technique of RGP lens insertion. A. Lens placed on index finger; B. Lens insertion

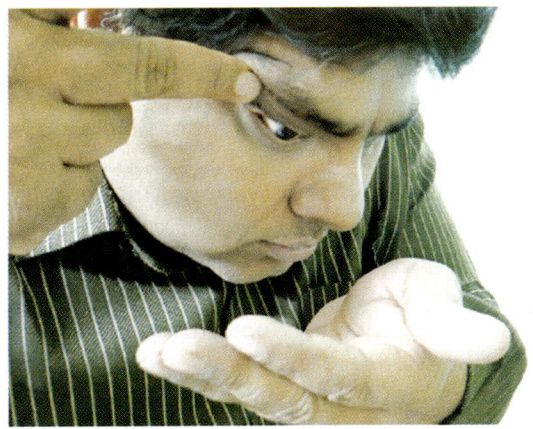

Fig. 10.16: Method 2 for RGP lens removal

- Look downwards keeping both the eyes wide open, now pull the index finger upward and outward.
- Suppose lens did not come out, then patient is instructed to blink simultaneously while pulling the upper eyelid.
- Left hand is used to remove the lens from the left eye.

Recentration Technique

- *Suppose if lens is beneath the upper lid:* Pull the upper eyelid in upward direction and look downwards, while firmly holding the upper lid upwards. Now make rapid horizontal eye movements, slowly look straight, and then downwards, now gently leave the eyelid.
- *Suppose if lens in beneath the lower lid:* First widely open both the eyelids by right hand fingers and locate the contact lens. Slowly slide the lens upwards by placing the upper eyelid margin at lower edge of lens. Once centered, look straight and then downwards, while slowly leaving the eyelids, first leave lower lid then upper lid.
- *Suppose if lens is in the corners of eye:* Wide open the eyelids as above, now locate the lens by lateral eye movements. Once lens gets centered, look straight and then downwards. Now slowly leave the eyelids one by one, first lower followed by upper lid.

Wearing schedule

- Patients are advised to practice the insertion and removal of RGP lenses for initial 2–3 days, once they feel confident and comfortable, regular wearing of lenses should be started.
- Gradually the wearing time is increased, in case of RGP lenses. First wear the lens for 1–2 hours and see the response in terms of visual acuity, comfort and ocular symptoms. If comfortable, then wear the lenses regularly for 2 hours everyday, for 3–4 days.
- When there is no symptom then gradually the wearing time is increased on daily one hour basis, at 3–4 days interval.
- Once a constant wearing of 6–8 hours is reached, say roughly in 30–45 days, then patient can wear these lenses regularly during their duty hours.
- Always remember to remove the lenses after a constant wear for 8 hours and before sleeping time.

Follow-up: Regular follow-up is must to avoid the complication of contact lens wear. Following follow-up visits are mandatory for a comfortable and successful RGP lens wearing

- Day one
- Day three
- Day seven
- After a month
- Every three months
- Every six months
- After one year

Follow-up visit evaluations are essentially similar as in case of a soft contact lens, by taking history, vision and slit lamp examination.

Rigid Contact Lens Related Complications and Management

- **Pain:** Intolerable pain can be experienced after using rigid lenses at various time intervals, which gives a clue about the cause of pain as follows

- Immediately after wearing rigid lenses the pain may be due to improper insertion technique, foreign body behind the lens, torn lens edges or due to dry lenses.
- Severe pain a few hours after wearing rigid lenses may be due to corneal edema or abrasions caused by steep fitting lens. Replace the lens after evaluating the lens fitting with fluorescein dye.
- Sometimes pain may be felt 2–3 hours after removal, which indicates occurrence of over wear syndrome due to micro corneal abrasions and edema caused by tight lens fitting. Give rest period for 2–3 weeks and then advice a flatter lens, once cornea is healed.

- **Watering:** Continuous excessive watering may occur due to unfinished lens edges which cause mechanical irritation, inadequate blinking and corneal edema. Change the lens and advice to clean the lens surface properly before insertion.
- **Burning or scratchy eyes:** Irritation in eye if occurs immediately after insertion of lens, then it is most likely due to contamination of multipurpose cleaning solution or dirty lens. However, if burning or scratchy sensation is felt after 1–2 hours of insertion of lens, then it indicates lens has a steep fit. Sometimes dry eyes, poor blinking and polluted environment may also give this kind of sensation. Change the cleaning solution and sterile the lens. Use a flatter lens if steep fit is found as the cause of irritation.
- **Excessive blinking:** During adaptation period frequent blinking is common however; if it persists even after a few days of wear, then it is essential to find the cause. Small size lens or presence of small foreign body over lens are the common causes of excessive blinking, however, a mucus strand or fogging of lens because of scratches will also induce excessive blinking.

- **Excessive dryness sensation:** Patient may experience continuous dryness feeling due to poor lacrimal secretions, inadequate blinking or tight fit lenses. Treat the cause for better tolerance of lenses and prescribe artificial tears eye drops.
- **Foreign body sensation:** During adaptation period a little foreign body sensations are acceptable, however if they present for a long duration, then search for the causes of it. Mostly the torn edges or too flat lens causes these kinds of sensations, although too thick, large or scratchy lens with conjunctivitis may also give continuous foreign body sensation. Treat the causes and change the lens of appropriate fit.
- **Lens coating in morning:** Sometimes in early morning a milky fluid coating may be seen over the lens. This may be due to collection of Meibomian gland secretions, mucus, proteins or epithelial cells debris over the lens. Rarely, in low grade infections abnormal secretions will deposit over lens. Treat with antibiotics and clean the lens with anti-infective solutions.
- **Lid swelling in evening:** During adaptation period very mild swelling of lids may be seen which subsides on its own once patient is accustomed to lens. If lid swelling is present even after adaptation period, then probably edges of lens or steep fit lens is the cause. Remove the lens and change as per proper fitting guidelines.
- **Visual disturbances:** Several visual disturbances may occur while person is wearing a rigid contact lens. These symptoms can be grouped as
  - *Fluctuation in vision:* Initial fluctuation in vision may be present during adaptation period, which improves on its own. However, if it appears later then excessive watering or small size lens are the causes. Treat the cause of watering

and change the lens size to achieve a stable clear vision.

– *Visual changes with head posture:* Flatter lenses move excessively over the cornea, so patients have tendency to tilt their head upwards to keep the lens in the center position for better vision. Change the lens with smaller diameter for central fit and thus decreases the lens movement. Sometimes the visual acuity may improve by head shaking or head bending, this is due to poorly centered lens. Change the base curve and TD of lens to achieve better centration and stable vision.

– *Blurring in distance vision:* Blurring for distance vision may be seen in early phase of lens wear. Common reasons are excessive watering, improper lens power or uncorrected astigmatism, poor quality lenses or scratched lens surfaces. Do an over refraction and examine the lens in white light, check the power of lens with lensometer. In late phase blurring of distance vision may be caused by corneal edema or warpage of contact lens. In both conditions simply change the lens with appropriate fit.

– *Blurring in near vision:* In a pre presbyopic age group, if distance vision is clear and blurring of near vision is present with contact lens, then the probable causes are improper lens power, decentred lens, and poor fluid exchange underneath lens or severe convergence insufficiency. Change the contact lens if incorrect power or decentration is present. Advice patient to blink frequently for proper tear exchange and do convergence exercises in convergence insufficiency cases.

– *Blurring in vision after contact lens removal:* Many patients experience blurring of vision, when they remove contact lenses and start wearing spectacles commonly called 'spectacle blur'. Reasons for this spectacle blurring are corneal edema or lens-induced corneal curvatural changes.

Specific Type Contact Lenses

INTRODUCTION

Extended Wear Contact Lenses

Since invention of contact lenses, some patients either desired, or were selected by their clinicians to wear contact lenses during sleep also. Hence the need for type of contact lenses arose which could act for extended period. In attempt to this, extended wear and continuous wear contact lenses have been developed. Extended wear (EW) lenses are the one, which the patient can wear for six nights continuously followed by a night of no lens wear. Similarly, continuous wear (CW) lenses can be worn up to 30 nights continuously followed by a night of no lens wear.

Indications of extended wear contact lenses
Ideally every person should be prescribed daily wear contact lenses. However, in following situations extended wear contact lens can be used

- In certain persons who are engaged in night duties or irregular working shifts like in case of doctors and nurses, armed force personnels, security persons and emergency staff members, etc. the use of extended wear contact lens is more convenient.
- Young infant or elderly aphakics may also benefit from these lenses because they are incapable or frightened for contact lens insertion, thus to overcome complications

related to lens handling and vision limitations, extended wear can be used.

- When patient is not keen to use daily wear contact lenses, because of convenience of extended wear lenses.
- Persons habitual of over wearing or sleeping with contact lenses, require extended wear lenses to avoid complications.

Broadly on the basis of material used and properties, we can group these EW lenses into

- Rigid extended wear contact lenses
- Silicon hydrogel extended wear contact lenses
- Soft hydrogel extended wear contact lenses

Rigid Extended Wear Contact Lenses

Almost all types of rigid contact lenses manufactured for extended wear are gas permeable lenses with medium and / or high Dk values. It is well known that insufficient oxygen supply to eye may cause edema of cornea. Extended wear contact lenses either RGP or silicon hydrogel allow sufficient supply of oxygen to the cornea and meet criteria of zero additional swelling.

Indications: RGP extended wear lenses are indicated in the following conditions in addition to abovementioned indications.

- Patients facing visual problems with toric extended wear soft contact lenses.

- Severe metabolic problems such as edema and hypoxia with soft hydrogel extended wear lenses.
- Medical problems like allergies, giant papillary conjunctivitis, or superior limbic keratoconjunctivitis associated with use of soft extended wear contact lenses.
- Patients having high refractive errors (hypermetropia or myopia) requiring thick lenses or toric bifocals lenses.

Several studies showed that rigid contact lens wear is usually associated with greater degree of hypoxia leading to decrease in corneal epithelial barrier function. Hence, recommended RGP contact lenses for extended wear purpose should have the highest oxygen transmissibility and fastest rate of tear exchange so that an adequate barrier function of corneal epithelium remains maintained.

Lens fitting and wearing schedule are essentially similar to basic RGP lenses of daily wear type. Although in some specific cases, such as papillary conjunctivitis, corneal decompensation, etc. extended wear RGP lenses are not recommended.

Initially, patient is advised to wear RGP contact lens on daily basis for a week, and then gradually extend their wear duration, preferably up to 5–6 nights continuously. For a successful, uncomplicated extended lens wear, lens should be removed for one night, then after cleaning and rinsing lens can be worn again for 6 nights.

Follow-up: Regular follow-up is must to prevent complications related to extended wear; a usual follow up schedule is after

- 24–48 hours of initial lens wear
- One week of lens insertion
- One month or at time of removal, cleaning, disinfecting and reinsertion of lens

On every follow-up visit a thorough examination for proper lens fit and clinical signs are done. Generally during slit lamp examination a special attention is given for:

- Contact lens depositions

- Lens adhesion
- 3–9 o'clock staining
- Persistent corneal striae
- Epithelial microcysts
- Contact lens bending or indentation

Complications of rigid extended wear contact lenses: Complications and lens related problems in extended wear lenses are more common and more pronounced as compared to daily wear RGP lenses.

Chances of infections are less but caution is required in case of lens adhesion because of increased risk of corneal ulceration. Low riding lenses should be avoided because there is increase risk of adhesion to cornea. Risk of adhesion further increased with use of lens material having high Dk value, thin lens and inadequate edge lift of lens. To avoid adhesion it is advised to use thick, flatter fitting rigid lens with medium Dk/t value (~100) with adequate edge lift.

3 and 9 o' clock staining usually does not cause discomfort but with continuous use of lens severe injection of conjunctiva can occur. It is more common with use of low riding, thick edge lens as well as in person who blink incompletely. Prolonged 3 and 9 o' clock staining may lead to vascularization in horizontal meridian. Sometimes, there may be contact lens induced papillary conjunctivitis due to hypersensitivity reaction or irritation.

Silicon Hydrogel Extended Wear Contact Lenses

The silicon hydrogel (Si-Hy) lenses were introduced in 1999 with the aim to increase the oxygen transmission through lens which was main limitation factor with the use of soft hydrogel lenses. As a result the wearing of lens for extended period became safer and comfortable with availability of these types of lens. The Si-Hy lenses contain both properties, i.e. increase oxygen permeability due to presence of silicon and hydrophilic nature of hydrogel lens. However, these lens material demonstrated less wettability and more chances of lipid depositions than hydrogel lens materials. As a result to improve the wettability the lenses were surface treated or added with other materials.

A wide range of Si-Hy material extended wear lenses are available, for up to 30 nights of continuous wear and/or for six nights of extended wear. These lens materials show a significant advancement in lens design, so that complications usually associated with lens induced corneal hypoxia, such as limbal redness, epithelial and stromal edema, vascularization of cornea, endothelial polymegathism and myopic shifts are rare.

Although several advantages are present with Si-Hy lenses, but a few disadvantages are

- Si-Hy materials are more stiff in nature as compared to soft hydrogel material (HEMA or Etafilcon A), hence during blinking can create more negative pressure beneath the contact lens. As a result, chances of development of mechanical arcuate lesions and local papillary conjunctivitis are more.
- Increased frequency of formation of mucin balls with overnight wearing for a long period, especially more common in eyes having steeper corneal curvature.

Various hydrogel contact lens materials and their respective properties are summarized in Table 11.1.

Soft Hydrogel Extended Wear Contact Lenses

Soft hydrogel extended wear lenses were familiarized by John de Carle with Permalens and in the year 1981 soft hydrogel extended wear contact lenses got an approval from FDA for cosmetic purpose. Soft hydrogel extended wear contact lenses can be used continuously for 30 nights. After 30 days lens should be removed, cleaned, disinfected and then reinserted. However, these lenses as compared to rigid gas permeable and silicon hydrogel (Si-Hy) do not allow sufficient oxygen to the cornea, thus incapable to accomplish the criteria of zero additional swelling with overnight wear.

Lens fitting: Instrumentation required for fitting of extended wear soft contact lenses is essentially same as for all other basic contact lens fitting. History and symptoms are elicited from patient before fitting extended wear contact lenses, specifically to fully understand and to find out the reasons of patient's desire for overnight lens wear. Although, the fundamental principles of extended wear soft

Material	Water content (%)	Max Dk/t	Min Dk/t	Surface modification	Other technology
Asmofilcon A	40	161	70	Nanoglass plasma coating	Menisilk
Balafilcon A	33	84	38	Plasma oxidation	None
Comfilcon A	48	145	64	None	Aquaform technology
Enfilcon A	46	125	55	None	Aquaform technology
Filcon II 3	58	86	–	None	Aquagen process
Galyfilcon A	47	107	37	None	Hydraclear technology
lotrafilcon B	36	101	45	Plasma polymerization	Aqua moisture system
Etafilcon A	58	26	8	None	None
Narafilcon A	46	118	47	None	Hydraclear technology
lotrafilcon A	24	203	68 to 140	Plasma polymerization	Aqua moisture system

Table 11.1: Various hydrogel contact lens material and their respective properties

contact lens fitting are similar to fitting for daily wear, however, most important concern is to provide maximum oxygen supply to the eye along with enough tear exchange so that debris formed behind lens can be removed effectively.

Wearing schedule: Initially it is recommended to wear soft lenses for 24 hours and observe the symptoms and clinical condition of eyes. If patient is asymptomatic and comfortable, then these lenses wear can be extended for week period. Gradually, these lenses can be worn for longer durations, usually 25–30 days.

Follow-up: Regular follow-up is the key to avoid complications such as microbial keratitis and lens depositions. Normal follow-up visits are planned after:

- Day one
- One month
- Two–four months or during removal and reinsertion of lens

On every visit a detailed slit lamp examination for lens fit and corneal condition is done. In case of any complication lenses are removed and reinserted after resolution of problem.

Complication with soft EW lens: The EW soft lenses can cause all those complications related to daily wear soft lenses. However, use of EW soft lenses carry more risk for development of

- Ulcerative keratitis: Wearing of lens for extended period may alter morphology of corneal epithelium and predispose to infections.
- Corneal vascularization
- Deposition of protein and mucus on contact lens
- Tight lens syndrome: There is sudden development of painful red eye. On examination, lens is immobile and moderately dehydrated. Corneal edema develops due to poor oxygenation, also flare and cells are seen in anterior chamber. To treat this condition, lens should be

removed for 1–2 weeks for healing and to prevent infections. Once the eye is normal, lens with looser fitting should be prescribed.

Rigid versus soft extended wear contact lenses: High Dk/t RGP extended wear contact lenses have several advantages and disadvantages over soft hydrogel lenses as summarized in Table 11.2.

Extended wear versus daily wear contact lenses: Extended wear contact lenses have several advantages over daily wear lenses such as

- Simple and convenient for patients to wear.
- Needs lesser handling and maintenance as compared to daily wear.
- Cost effective.

However, extended wear lenses has a few disadvantages such as

- Greater incidence of overall complications as compared to daily wear lenses.
- Increased risk of microbial keratitis, because of overnight use.

Patients should be given full information regarding associated risks and benefits with an overnight or extended wear and then asked to make the choice of contact lens type. Hence,

Table 11.2: Various advantages and disadvantages of rigid EW lens over soft extended wear contact lenses

Advantages	Disadvantages
Enhanced oxygen transmissibility	Adhesion phenomenon
Active tear pump mechanism	Poor initial wearing comfort
Lesser lens deposits	Difficult fitting procedure
Better reproducibility	3 and 9 o'clock staining
Superior optical quality	
Maintenance of lens parameters for a long period	
Zero additional swelling with overnight wear	

it is important that a discussion should include risk comparison with other lens types and wearing modalities even a comparison to refractive surgery. Once patient accepts this increased risk with extended wear, then clinician decide on best course of action.

Disposable Contact Lenses

These may be grouped as

- Daily wear disposable contact lenses
- Extended wear disposable contact lenses

Daily wear disposable contact lenses: These daily wear disposable lenses are sometimes confused with simple daily wear contact lenses. The daily wear disposable lenses are the one, which are worn during awakening time, only for one day. Once removed from the eye, these lenses are thrown away and not used again, whereas daily wear lenses after removal from the eye can be worn again in the next morning after overnight treatment in cleaning solution.

Over past decade, a significant increase in the demand of daily disposable contact lenses has been noticed all over the world because these lenses provide more convenience of wearing and are associated with decreased risk of complications. Various types of 'comfort enhanced' daily disposable lenses have been developed to decrease the chances of dryness and discomfort among the wearers. Selection of daily disposable contact lens for a patient will depend on the total of convenience offered by lens to the wearer as well as on the health and compliance of patient for wearing the lens. As compliance is better and risk of complications is less in the teenage group, these lenses are more preferred in this age group.

Comfort enhancing daily wear disposable contact lenses is mainly classified into three groups depending on their mechanism of action

- *Lens made up of poly HEMA materials and co-polymers:* The copolymers have property to retain water. For example, Acuvue Moist contact lens (Etafilcon A)

has an embedded copolymer called polyvinyl pyrrolidone (PVP), which works as a water holding agent, hence rate of dehydration of lens is reduced during lens wear.

- *Lens made up of poly HEMA materials with lubricating additives:* These are also made up of poly HEMA material, although in place of water retaining molecules these lens materials have lubricating additives coatings. These lubricating additives are usually present in packaging saline, used for storage of lens. For example, in case of SofLens daily disposable, a high water content material poloxamine is added in the saline solution which coats the lens surface and then slowly released into tear film when these contact lenses are inserted in the eye.

- *Lens made from polyvinyl alcohol (PVA):* PVA is a water-soluble non-toxic polymer, commonly used in lubricating eye drops and lens solutions. When these lenses are prepared using PVA, some of the PVA remains in unpolymerized (free) form in the matrix of contact lens. After wearing the lens due to blinking this free form of PVA is slowly released from the contact lens into the tear film. For example, Focus Dailies All Day Comfort (Nelfilcon A). Furthermore, addition of other substances like hydroxy propyl methylcellulose (HPMC) and polyethylene glycol (PEG), which are present in packaging saline, further maintain the release of PVA for a long period. For example, Focus Dailies Aqua Comfort Plus (Nelfilcon A Plus).

For daily wear disposable lenses, maximum wearing time suggested is summarized in Table 11.3.

These types of contact lenses are indicated particularly for daily disposable wear, hence should be discarded after removal from the eye. As these lenses are disposed of after every single daily use, risk of developing giant

Table 11.3: Wearing schedule of daily wear disposable contact lenses	
Day	Hours
1	4–6
2	7–8
3	9–10
4	11–12
5	12–14
6 and afterwards	All awakening hours

papillary conjunctivitis is reduced significantly. Daily disposable lenses provide more comfort in patient than other contact lenses which are worn for a long period especially, in those patients who feel discomfort and itching due to allergies.

Extended wear disposable contact lenses: These lenses are also disposed off, once removed from the eye, however, these lenses can be worn continuously for either six days (weekly) or thirty days (monthly), once inserted in the eye. Because of their longer duration of continuous wear, these lenses are called extended wear contact lenses. However, they differ from simple extended wear contact lenses which can be used again after removal from the eye.

Introduction of weekly replaced disposable lenses has resolved two major issues, i.e. corneal hypoxia and corneal edema. These lenses are worn for six continuous nights and then disposed, hence are referred as disposable extended wear lenses.

Disposable contact lenses are available for various wearing and disposing schedules such as they can be worn either on the daily basis or on extended wear basis. These lenses are available for daily, weekly, fortnightly or monthly disposable schedule. Generally wearing schedule is decided by the treating consultant, however, it vary a little for daily wear or extended wear disposable contact lenses.

Patients should be given following warnings related to extended contact lens wear:

- Eye discomfort
- Excessive tearing

Note

Several ocular problems including corneal ulcers may develop rapidly which can lead to visual loss.

- Eye redness
- Visual changes or diminution of vision

Extended wear disposable hydrogel contact lenses as compared to conventional non- disposable continuous wear lenses are found beneficial only in carefully selected patients with strict follow-up schedule. However, a significant hypoxia related adverse events and marked microbial keratitis is noted in many EW lens wearers as compared to conventional non-disposable continuous wear lenses.

Examples of disposable contact lenses are

- AVAIRA contact lenses exist in various lens designs form such as spheric, aspheric, toric and multifocal. These lenses are prepared using material comprising 46% water and 54% Enfilcon A (silicon containing hydrogel). A tint (phthalocyanine blue) has been added, so that the contact lens becomes more visible, hence can easily be handled. An additional UV absorbing monomer is also added in lens to block UV radiation.
- Various disposable lenses and their properties are summarized in Table 11.4.

Scleral RGP Lenses

RGP lenses when rest over sclera are termed scleral RGP lenses. These lenses cover the entire corneal surface and form a fluid vault for oxygenation of cornea. Majority of newer types of scleral contact lenses are made up of high oxygen permeable materials for better tolerance.

Scleral RGP lenses are grouped into following categories, depending upon overall diameter as

- Corneo-scleral (12.9 to 13.5 mm)
- Semi-scleral (13.6 to 14.9 mm)
- Mini-scleral (15.0 to 18.0 mm)
- Scleral (>18.0 mm)

Table 11.4: Various types of disposable contact lenses and their respective properties

Lens series	Lens material	Water content	Lens diameter
Precision UV	Varsurfilcon A	74 %	14.5 mm
Actifresh 400	MMA / VP	55%	14.3 mm
Proclear	Omafilcon A	62%	14.2 mm
Soflens 66	Alphafilcon A	66%	14.2 mm
Acuvue	Genfilcon	48%	14 mm
Dalies	Nelfilcon A	69%	13.8 mm

Indications

Corneal conditions:

Scleral lenses are indicated in cases of irregular cornea, diseased cornea and healthy cornea. Usually corneo-scleral lenses are used in irregular cornea and healthy cornea, whereas scleral lenses are used for scarred and severely pathological cornea.

Several conditions where scleral lens can be used are

- Naturally occurring ecstatic cornea: Like in young children and adults with keratoconus, pellucid marginal degeneration and forme frusta keratoconus.
- Secondary corneal ectasias: Post-surgery ectasias, post-corneal transplantation, post-infarcts corneal cross-linking.

Intolerance to corneal RGP or hydrogel lenses
is seen in the following conditions like

- Refractive conditions: Lens decentration in high refractive errors
- In dry eye
  - Due to ocular disease: Alkali burn, ocular pemphigoid, Steven Johnson syndrome, neurotrophic keratitis, Sjögren syndrome, filamentary keratitis.
  - Due to reduced tear meniscus, decreased tear production, conjunctival hyperemia— as seen in early or contact lens related dry eye.

Scleral Contact Lens Fitting Technique

Insertion technique

- To check lens fitting, fill the lens completely with isotonic, non-preserved artificial tears and add one drop of fluorescein from a strip.
- Scleral lens is either supported on a large DMV scleral suction cup or a tripod made by using thumb, middle, and index finger, as shown in Fig. 11.1A.
- Retract upper and lower eyelids as shown in Fig. 11.1B with the help of thumb and index finger of other hand while keeping the face parallel to the ground.
- Slowly raise the contact lens onto the eye in one continuous motion, then slowly release the eyelids before lowering the supporting suction cup.
- Suppose a large air bubble is seen underneath lens, either the lens was not inserted in one continuous motion or the lens cup was not completely filled with solution.
- Remove the lens and reinsert as shown in Fig. 11.1B.

Lens removal technique

- Scleral lenses are generally held by the force of suction so always loosen these lenses before removal.
- Put a few drops of rewetting solution and then inferior peripheral portion of lens is gently pushed in repeated motions for some seconds.
- Keep the upper eyelid in steady position and lower eyelid is used to raise the lower portion of contact lens, away from the eye. Otherwise, a medium DMV suction cup can be placed over the lower peripheral portion of contact lens, slowly pull the cup in downward and outward direction with force directed perpendicular to the lens surface.

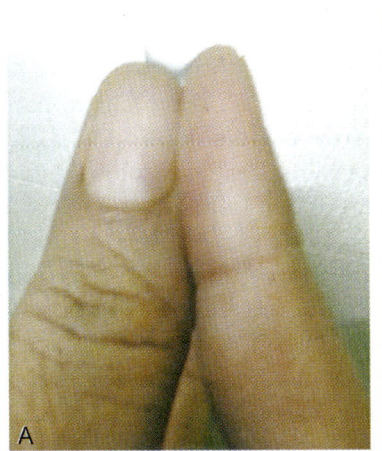 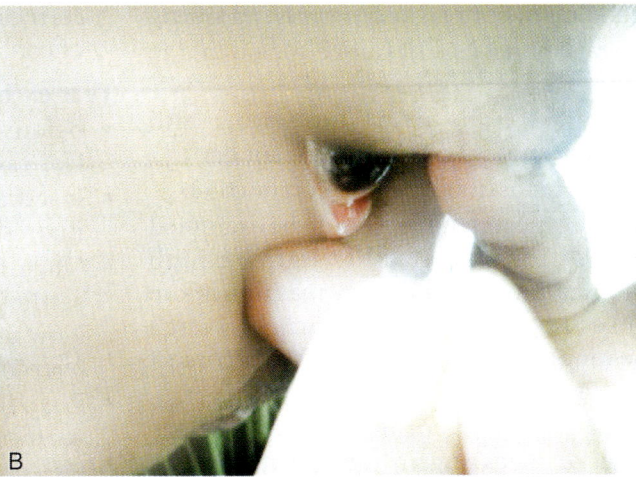

Fig. 11.1: A. Tripod of fingers; B. Insertion technique of scleral contact lens

Fitting principles: Most important principle for scleral lens fitting is that lens should vault the cornea entirely while lens is aligned to the bulbar conjunctiva. To achieve this fit following parameters need to be checked

Overall diameter

- Generally, lenses with large diameter can retain more fluid in the corneal chamber thus allow more clearance over the cornea, hence are more convenient for the user, whereas lenses smaller in diameter vault the cornea more strongly thus they require more accurate central fit.

- In case of irregular corneas, always choose a lens of larger diameter, although some lens manufacturers provide guidelines for selecting an overall diameter based on HVID.

Initial trial lens

- We can follow the lens manufacturer's fitting guide to select a trial lens, however, a simple clinical approach can be tried to assess the trial lens base curve.

- Stand on the side of the patient while examining shape and profile of the cornea. Suppose cornea appears very steep, select a steeper base curve similarly, if cornea appears flat then select a flatter base curve. For an average profile cornea, select an average base curve.

- Scleral lenses are fit on the basis of sagittal height, hence clinical assessment is an effective method when properly done.

Corneal fit examination

- On slit lamp optical section is made using white light and then in high illumination with medium magnification, examine the central corneal clearance.

- Various layers can be observed in cross section, the outermost band of dark black color is due to scleral contact lens. This dark area is surrounded by two thin reflections from the front and back surface of contact lens. Now, compare the thickness of this black layer with the green layer of tear lens.

- Suppose, if thickness of black layer (trial lens) is 300 microns and on examination the green layer is appearing approximately of half thickness than black band, then it tells that lens is vaulting the cornea by 125–150 microns which is considered an ideal clearance for a non- fenestrated lens design. Different trial lens are tried until a proper central corneal clearance value is not obtained.

- Usually all types of scleral lenses take 30–40 minutes time to settle into the conjunctiva. Scleral trial lenses showing gross excessive vaulting should be removed and replaced with a flatter base curve lens.

Correlation of corneal and peripheral fitting

- Scleral contact lens fit can be considered in two parts
  - Central fit is over the cornea and commonly called "corneal chamber"
  - Peripheral fit is over the conjunctiva.
- Entire corneal chamber should be examined with diffuse cobalt blue light in high illumination and medium magnification. Observe areas of lens-corneal touch (bearing) as in case of a corneal RGP contact lens.
- In an irregular cornea, commonly we observe a bearing in mid-peripheral or peripheral regions of cornea however, it is acceptable once central corneal clearance is present. In such a situation an additional clearance is produced in peripheral area, without increasing the central corneal clearance.
- An excessive lens movement or bubble formation underneath lens indicates that peripheral curves are too loose. To correct this condition simply tighten the peripheral curve by choosing scleral lens of an appropriate base curve.

An ideal scleral contact lens fit

An ideal scleral contact lens fit is expressed by the following factors:

- Centered lens
- Minimum 2 mm larger than limbus
- Minimum corneal vault
- No touch or bearing
- Good coverage to limbus
- Edge alignment
- No movement of lens

Over topography

- Many a times it is useful to perform a computerized topography, keeping the scleral contact lens in place, once it had settled for about 15–20 minutes. Topography will show any kind of lens flexure, if present.
- Toricity of >0.5 D may be clinically significant and may affect the vision. It can be corrected by increasing the central thickness of contact lens.

Tear exchange evaluation

- Before dispensing a scleral lens to patient, tear exchange evaluation is done.
- Insert a sterile scleral lens without adding fluorescein dye in filling media.
- Once lens is properly placed, wait for settling period of about 10–15 minutes. Now instill fluorescein dye with a dye strip over the lens surface.
- Periodic examination of tear lens is done to see the presence of dye which moves behind the contact lens into the corneal chamber.
- In ideal conditions, after 20–30 minutes a small amount of dye should be seen in the corneal chamber. Although tear exchange underneath contact lens is not so rapid, but it is significant for a proper lens fit.
- Suppose on examination after sufficient waiting period of 30–40 minutes, no fluorescein dye is observed in the corneal chamber; means it is a steep fit, hence to correct it either peripheral fit must be flattened or overall diameter should be increased.

Therapeutic Contact Lenses

Introduction

Therapeutic contact lenses (TCL) or bandage lenses have emerged as an effective alternative for the management of various eye diseases especially, in recalcitrant cases which show poor response to other treatment modalities. Although TCL is not used as first line treatment in majority of ophthalmic disorders but it can work as an effective adjunctive treatment in various ophthalmic disorders. Due to higher risk of development of microbial infections with TLC, the decision to use these types of lens should be taken with great precautions.

The most important purposes of prescribing the therapeutic contact lenses are

1. To provide relief and comfort from eye pain due to corneal disorders
2. To assist in healing of corneal wound

3. To provide mechanical support and protection to cornea
4. To maintain proper hydration of corneal epithelial surface
5. Also used as drug delivery system

Types of TCL: Therapeutic contact lenses made from both hard and soft lens materials are available, although hydrogels types TLC are more used. Silicon rubber and copolymers are also used to produce specific types of TLC, having good oxygen permeability.

TLC can be classified as

1. Soft hydrogel lens
   - Low water content (38–45%)
   - Mid-water content (45–55%)
   - High water content (67–80%)
2. Hard (PMMA) and gas permeable scleral lenses
3. Hard scleral rings
4. Silicon rubber and silicon hydrogels (38%)
5. Collagen shields having Dk/L = 63% water content soft lens.

Various commercially available therapeutic contact lenses are summarized in Table 11.5.

Choice of TCL from available TCLs will depend on main purpose for use (as discussed above) and on the physiological requirement of a pathological cornea, etc.

Fitting of a TCL: Fitting of a TCL is very simple if following guidelines are follows which are chiefly for soft TCL because these are most commonly used TCLs in various ocular conditions.

- Keratometry is usually of very little help because due to associated underlying corneal pathology there may be formation of irregular mires. Thus, a trial lens fitting is suggested. However, keratometry readings of other normal eye may be helpful.
- During fitting the use of topical anesthetics (except in a few conditions) should be avoided because it will mask the pain arising due to poor lens fit.
- Ideally, to check the dehydration effects on lens, the fitting must be evaluated at an interval of 20 and 60 minutes.

TCL fit should be assessed on slit lamp both in terms of central fit and peripheral fit.

- An ideal central fit TCL will provide good corneal coverage with proper mobility characteristics.
- Similarly, peripheral lens fit is also necessary to check because flared edges of lens may give rise to discomfort to patient and adhered edges indicate tight lens fit.
- It is recommended to keep several lens designs with similar parameters available

Lens type	Lens material	Water content	Total diameter (mm)
Hydrogels			
Plano	HEMA	38.6%	14
Plano	Polymacon	38.6%	13.5 /14.5
Plano ES 70	MMA / VP	70%	15
Troy		85%	15–20
Igel	Igel 67/ 77	67% / 77%	14.5
Collagen shields			
Bio-Cor type I	Porcine		
Chiron type I	Bovine		
Silicon rubber			
Silflex	Polysiloxane		11.7–13.7
Scleral lenses	Scleral sealed		~ 22

Table 11.5: Various types of commercially available therapeutic contact lenses and their properties

at time of insertion because if one particular lens design fails to produce desired lens fit, then another lens design may fit well.

- Generally, the excessive steep or flat lens should not be used for fitting. However, in some conditions like corneal edema or cornea epithelium defects, a TCL of flatter fitting may be preferred. On the other hand, steeper fitting TLC may be used in patients having irregular corneal topography.

Indications for use of therapeutic contact lenses: Therapeutic contact lenses are used in various diseases of cornea. In treatment of various ocular conditions which cause abnormalities in epithelium of cornea, the relief from pain is the most common and important part of treatment and these lenses can be used to relieve the pain effectively in these conditions.

Bullous Keratopathy: Use of TCL in following patients of intractable bullous keratopathy is very useful

- Patient of bullous keratopathy presenting with a painful blind eye.
- Patient is not fit for graft surgery.
- As a temporary relief measure in those patient who are waiting for penetrating keratoplasty.

These patients should be prescribed with TCL as early as possible. Use of TCL in these patients is associated with relief in pain as well as some improvement in vision. Relief in pain is probably due to protection of nerves by TCL which are exposed due to rupture of bullae. In some patients vision is also improved as irregular cornea is covered by regular surface of contact lens. In bullous keratopathy patients the movement of lens should be minimal but must be sufficient enough to allow adequate tear flow beneath the TCL. Hydrogel TCL of large diameter having high water content (Duragel 75, Plano ES70, etc.) can be used which maintain maximum oxygen permeability for constant wear. For temporary purposes, a thin high water content TCL can

be used to decrease the risk of corneal vascularization.

Thygeson's superficial punctate keratitis: It is a recurrent and chronic disorder described by presence of small and oval punctate corneal opacities of grey white color on cornea. Exact cause is not known but may be viral or immunological in origin. Corneal opacities cause warpage of corneal epithelial surface and reduced visual acuity. High water content extended-wear TCL (sometimes low water content) can be used for treatment of severe cases. The lens acts as a pressure bandage and improves symptoms of pain and foreign body sensation by covering the corneal lesions and nerves.

Superior limbic keratoconjunctivitis: It is a chronic inflammatory disease involving conjunctiva (superior bulbar), limbus and upper part of cornea, characterized by foreign body sensation, photophobia, and ocular pain. Along with other therapeutic modatilities soft TCL especially of large diameter are very effective in relieving the severe pain and symptoms associated with superior limbic keratoconjunctivitis cases. TCL with relatively large TD is used till symptoms and signs are disappeared.

Filamentary keratitis: It is a disease of eye in which filaments of mucus and degenerated epithelial cells get deposit on surface of cornea, usually it is self-limiting in most of the cases. The treatment includes topical therapy with artificial tears and lubricants. Cases which do not respond to lubricants alone, low water content disposable TCLs can be used along with steroids, topical antibiotics and atropine. Filaments get resolved usually in 4–5 days and within 2–3 weeks a complete disappearance of filaments may be seen; however filaments may recur after some time.

TCL are also effectively used for corneal healing in various recalcitrant cases which are poorly responding to routine medical treatment like in the following conditions.

Recurrent corneal erosion: Disturbance of corneal epithelial basement membrane due to anterior membrane dystrophies (Map dot finger dystrophy or Cogan dystrophy) or trauma may result in recurrent breakdown of corneal epithelium causing damage of corneal surface (corneal erosions). Majority of patients usually remain asymptomatic throughout their life but nearly 10–15% may develop recurrent erosion syndrome manifesting in form of pain and photophobia and foreign body sensations. Most patients of recurrent erosions are treated with lubricants and hypertonic saline, however, a disposable bandage contact lens (usually thick, high water content extended wear type preferred) can be used as an extended wear lens for 2, 3 or even 6 months duration, as per requirement. Before placing TCL, the affected area of corneal epithelium should be debride completely and irrigate with saline. Ultra thin TCL are not indicated due to possible chances of buckling of lens. Corneal abrasion (<5 mm) due to trauma can be managed by topical eye drops and eye pad. If the size of abrasion is more than 5 mm, then it can be treated by the use of TCL, because epithelium heals more quickly with disposable TCL as compared to conventional methods of treatment.

Persistent epithelial defects of cornea: When an epithelial defect of cornea does not heal or remain persistent for more than two weeks, the cornea get highly vulnerable to infection, ulceration, perforation and scarring. Soft disposables TCL are very useful as they protect corneal surface from mechanical trauma by eyelids and gives time to newly formed epithelial to get attach to newly secreted basement membrane. Soft contact lenses with high oxygen permeability are more preferred to reduce chances of corneal edema and neovascularization. Collagen shields hydrated with acidic fibroblast growth factor (FGF) can be also used to promote healing of epithelial defects.

Chemical injuries: Chemical injuries to eye result in breakdown of collagen leading to widespread damage to cornea, epithelial surfaces, etc. and formation of stromal ulcer. The purpose of TCL is to prevent the further progression of ulcer formation by preventing transfer of photolytic enzymes from tear fluid to corneal stroma. Due to presence of chemosis and epithelium defect, TCLs of small total diameter (~12 mm) are first choice of treatment. Hydrophilic lens with high oxygen permeability are more preferred because they help in epithelial migration and promote epithelial stromal adhesion. Scleral lens can also be prescribed if lids are also involved in injuries. In case of corneal melting due to injury cyanoacrylate tissue adhesive can be applied and then covered with TCL.

Epithelial disorders following surgical procedures: Temporary corneal epithelial defects may occur after many surgical procedures on eyes like vitrectomy, cataract extraction, post-penetrating keratoplasty, epikeratoplasty, kerato-refractive procedures (PRK, LASIK), etc. Soft and/or collagen TCL can be used to decrease the chances of epithelial trauma after surgery which promotes rapid epithelial healing.

Penetrating keratoplasty: In case of perforation of an existing corneal graft the silicon rubber TCL can be used. TCL can also be used if epithelial healing is delayed, epithelial filaments are formed or loose sutures are present after PK procedure.

TCL, in various designs and of different materials can also be used to provide mechanical protection and support like in cases of corneal thinning, perforation or corneal trauma so that the need of immediate surgery or corneal grafting is delayed or minimized. Various types of lens like hydrophilic TCL, scleral lenses or rings and silicon rubber lenses can be used to provide mechanical support to cornea.

Corneal perforation: Use of a TCL gives structural support and maintains integrity of an eye if applied in case of small corneal perforation (<2 mm) with no loss of tissue.

Healing rate is faster if lesions are small and noninfected. In addition, lacerations or perforations which lie adjacent to limbus and in well vascularized area respond faster on TCL application. As compared to suturing the small corneal perforations heal better and with very less degree of resultant astigmatism. Thin, low water content soft contact lenses are usually first choice.

Corneal wound leakage: Anterior segment wound leakage may occur secondary to surgery like post-cataract surgery and penetrating keratoplasty, trabeculectomy etc. Majority of leaks are mild and self healing. In moderate wound leakage thin low water content soft TCL can be placed. The lens will help in the wound healing by decreasing flow of aqueous to wound and promotes re-epithelialization and vascularization. Sometimes, even collagen shields can be placed in the eye at the time of surgery and then hydrophilic TCL after 24 hours of surgery. Post-trabeculectomy a leaking drainage bleb may form either just after procedure or after several days or weeks. TCL of large size (TD = 20 mm) with high water content (e.g. Mega soft 76.5%) can be placed which compress over the leaking bleb to prevent excessive drainage.

Thinning of cornea: Patients with a thin cornea have very high chance of perforation and usually present with a descemetocele. In such cases, hydrophilic TCL can be prescribed which act as a corneal splint and slows down the rate of corneal thinning and ultimately prevent corneal perforation. If corneal thinning is due to dry eyes, then silicon rubber lenses are better choice.

Protection of the cornea: In various conditions of eyes like entropion, trichiasis, eye exposure due to lid deformities, cranial nerve palsies, etc. epithelium of cornea can easily damage due to trivial trauma, hence TCL are used to protect the cornea. TCLs especially scleral lenses, are very useful to provide protection to cornea and comfort in cases of trigeminal or facial nerve palsy.

Various ocular pathologies can lead to dehydration of cornea which ultimately leads to corneal blindness, hence TCL are used to maintain corneal hydration in various conditions as follows

Cicatrizing conjunctival disease: Cicatrization of conjunctiva with involvement of cornea may occur in diseases such as Stevens-Johnson syndrome, ocular pemphigoid, chemical burns, trachoma and dry eye. In Stevens-Johnson syndrome, a thick TCL of low or medium water content having large TD (15–20 mm) can be used to prevent formation of adhesions, however, scleral lenses are more useful. Alternatively, a silicon rubber lens can also be effective in selective recalcitrant cases. Chemical burns due to strong alkali lead to severe ocular damage. The TCL can be prescribed in the later phase of treatment to promote epithelial healing and to protect the fornix from mechanical forces of eyelids. TCLs like Mega soft bicurve TCLs or scleral lenses or scleral rings can be placed to prevent symblepharon reformation.

Dry eye: It is most commonly encountered clinical problem in ophthalmology. Dry eyes occurring as a result of secondary causes like keratoconjunctivits siccca, Stevens-Johnson syndrome, ocular pemphigoid, etc. can be prescribed lens specially silicon rubber lenses which provide hydration to the cornea.

TCL as drug delivery devices: TCL can be used as drug delivery devices for treatment of some ocular diseases. Hydrogel soft lens impregnated with medications when placed on the cornea usually delivers high levels of medication in eyes as compared to topical eye drops. Several drugs such as pilocarpine, corticosteroids, antibiotics, antifungal and antiviral, etc. can be delivered through contact lens for treatment of glaucoma, herpes simplex infections, fungal ulcers, etc. The thickness and water content of lens and molecular weight may affect delivery of drug through contact lens. The use of TCL for drug delivery for prolonged time may be associated with increased risks of harmful reactions due to direct contact of cornea with drugs.

General instructions to patients: Proper care as per following guidelines of therapeutic contact lenses is must to achieve the best results.

- Cleaning and disinfection of TCL are done at least once in every 15 days.
- Proper size and adequate water content are prerequisite for good outcome; hence TD and water content are kept as per the requirement in a particular ocular condition.
- Specific suitable prophylactic topical antibiotic drops are used to prevent secondary infections.
- Never use a TCL for more than 6 months duration, however, some TCL requires to be changed even at 1 or 2 months intervals.
- Never apply certain topical drops such as fluorescein, hypotonic saline, phenylephrine or gels over TCL.
- In case of severe burning, irritation, chemosis or enhancement of symptoms report immediately to ophthalmologist.
- Always consult before insertion or removal of a therapeutic contact lens.

Complications of therapeutic contact lenses: Although, complications related to TCL are similar to those seen with an extended wear contact lens. Several complications related to therapeutic contact lens wear are

- Microbial keratitis is most serious complication.
- Ulcers induced by TCL wear.
- Giant papillary conjunctivitis (GPC).
- Neovascularisation.

For prevention of complications prophylactic antibiotics with TCL can be beneficial in short term, although role of antibiotic is highly controversial.

Colored Contact Lenses

Introduction

Colored contact lenses can be used for cosmetic, therapeutic, occupational or prosthetic purposes. Although, by many practitioners, all colored contact lenses are considered as cosmetic contact lens but soft hydrogel contact lenses are colored for various clinical indications also. Generally, hard or rigid contact lenses are not colored because it is difficult to center them on the cornea and are small in size, hence they do not serve the desired purpose. Several lens manufacturers have developed colored soft hydrogel contact lenses for cosmetic or prosthetic purposes. These lenses are also available in various refractive powers and thus can be used as an alternative to the regular soft contact lenses.

Various desirable properties in an ideal colored contact lens are

- Clarity and purity
- Quality and safety
- Color stability
- Reproducibility
- Variable lens designs
- Biocompatibility
- Heat tolerance

Indications: Colored lenses can be used in various ocular and non-ocular conditions

Ocular conditions: As a prosthetic colored contact lenses either to treat or as an adjuvant treatment modality can be used in the following ocular conditions

- Corneal pathologies like disfigured cornea or scarred cornea, either due to disease or trauma. In patients having leucocoria or white opacity with no light perception, these dark colored lenses are used to produce cosmetic relief.

- Visual problems due to photophobia or diplopia need colored contact lenses as treatment modality. Conditions like albinism, aniridia, fixed pupil causes excessive light entry and macular complications; here black colored contact lenses with small clear central pupillary area are needed. Similarly, amblyopia and diplopia due to any reason need an occluder contact lens having black pupillary area.

- Heterochromia is a condition where color of iris is different in both eyes. These patients need colored contact lenses to match the color of both the eyes.
- In young children, colored lenses can be used for the treatment of strabismus and amblyopia as occlusion therapy. These lenses have black pupil and iris pattern with a clear periphery, so that light does not pass through these lenses.
- Specific type of custom colored tinted lenses are used as low visual aid where central pupillary area is tinted with a specific material to reduce the glare, hence patients having poor vision due to macular pathologies or retinopathies gets benefit by these lenses.
- X chrome colored lenses are used in color deficiency patients which support in identification of colors. ChromaGen tinted color lenses are used to assist in color identification especially, in cases of deuteranopes.
- Colored contact lenses with power can be used in young persons with refractive errors, especially during festive seasons and social gatherings to enhance the looks.

Non-ocular conditions: Colored lenses are used by many persons to enhance the look or for occupational requirements

- Sports persons use colored contact lenses to decrease the glare while driving or playing games.
- Similarly, cinema or television actors need to change the color of eyes according to the demand of role they are performing, hence several colored lens designs are used for this purpose like having black pupil with white iris or different shape large pupils with colored iris patterns.
- Many persons use colored lenses to enhance their looks by wearing various iris patterned contact lenses. These lenses have clear pupil with different iris patterns and tints with a clear periphery.

Sometimes power is also incorporated in these lenses if person has associated refractive error.
- ChromaGen custom tinted contact lenses are useful in patients having learning disorders such as dyslexia.

Fitting methods: Fitting guidelines for color lenses are similar to those of a soft hydrogel contact lens.

- Initially a trial soft lens is tried to record the fitting parameters; once the lens fitting is checked as per guidelines, same type of soft lenses with same parameters, material and design are ordered to get tinted as per requirement of patient.
- Commercially several lens manufactures are providing these tinted colored lens in series of power and lens parameters in terms of thickness, total diameter and color pattern.
- In majority of cases where colored lenses are indicated as prosthetic lens to cover up the corneal deformities. The iris size, color and pattern of normal eye should be taken as standard to decide the required lens for deformed eye.
- Ideal fitting of color lens is decided not only by the type of fit, i.e. steep or flat, rather the color comparison between the two eyes is also important.

To summarize the fitting requirements of colored lenses are:

- Measure the pupil size in normal illumination
- Perform keratometry readings and obtain base curve by using a trial lens.
- Measure HVID, if not possible of diseased eye, then of normal eye.
- Get photographs of patient for color matching of lens.

Types of colored CL: Various types of colored lenses have been designed for cosmetic, prosthetic, and occupational purposes. These lenses can be grouped on the basis of colored patterns as follows

- Black pupil with clear mid-periphery and periphery (star burst, Fig. 11.2A): These lenses are mainly used to occlude the entry of light in cases such as amblyopia and diplopia. Sometimes, also used for cosmetic purposes in cases such as inoperable mature cataract, subluxated lens or in film industry. Generally, lenses are available with pupil size in the range of 2–5 mm and total diameter of 11–14 mm.

- Black pupil with iris pattern and clear periphery (iris pattern, Fig. 11.2B): These types of lens are also available in wide range of pupil size with various iris patterns to meet the requirement of different conditions. Mainly, used for cosmetic purpose in disfigured ocular conditions.
- Clear pupil with iris pattern and clear periphery (limbal rings, Fig. 11.2C): These types of lens are available in power (ranging from +6 D to –10 D) as these lenses are mainly used by patients (having refractive errors) during social gathering or special occasions to change the colors of eyes. Lenses are available, in various iris patterns and colors such as blue, hazel, brown, green, etc. according to different requirements. This type of lens can also be used as prosthetic lenses in conditions such as aniridia, heterochromia, albinism, polyocoria, post-iridectomy, and fixed pupil. These lenses have a clear pupil size in the range of 2.5–4.5 mm with iris pattern diameter from 9 to 11.5 mm, having a total diameter up to 15 mm with a clear peripheral zone.
- Clear pupil with dark periphery (under print, Fig. 11.2D): These lenses are mainly used to cover up the white cornea or disfigured cornea as in cases of leucomatous corneal opacities or phthiscical conditions for cosmetic purposes.

Complications of colored CL: Several complications related to colored contact lenses are similar to those encountered with use soft contact lenses like:

Corneal edema: May be due to decreased oxygen permeability, which in turn is because of excessive thickness of colored lenses as compared to the normal soft hydrogel lenses. In colored lens, the color coating is done in between the two layers of polymer to reduce the dissociation of dye in surrounding tissue, hence the two layers of polymers lead to increase in the thickness and decrease in the oxygen permeability of colored lens. Although in a large number of patients, the ocular condition is severely compromised, hence corneal edema is not a major issue to handle, however, in selected cases these colored lenses needs to be discontinued, if corneal edema occurs.

Protein and lipid deposition: Like all other contact lenses there may be protein and lipids depositions on colored lenses also, rather chances are more of depositions because these lenses are used as prosthetic lenses for longer duration than routine lenses. Chemical treatment can be done to deproteinize these lenses as done for other soft contact lenses.

Similar to soft lenses there may be belching of vessels or discomfort due to tight fit, hence lenses should be changed with a proper fit lenses.

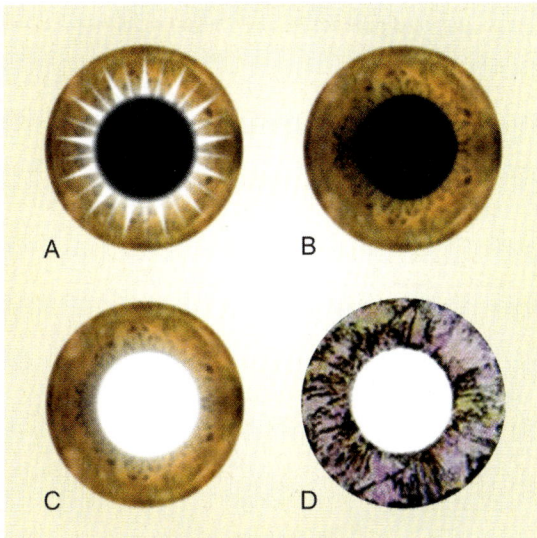

Fig. 11.2: Various types of colored contact lenses. A. Star burst; B. Iris pattern; C. Limbal ring; D. Under print

In addition, because of color tinting, many other complications can also occur with these cosmetic lenses such as

Toxic effects: These lenses are colored by using various types of dyes or chemicals to produce the tints and patterns, however, some of these may react with ocular or surrounding tissues to produce the toxic effect. There may be water soluble dye which is poorly hold by polymers and thus slowly dissociates into the surrounding tissues.

Discoloration of lens is another common problem encountered. In most of these colored lenses, water soluble dye is used which slowly dissociate with time and thus clear pupil and/or periphery of lens becomes discolor with time. Strict follow up and timely changing of lens is must to avoid these problems.

Care of colored CL: Care and handling of colored contact lenses are similar to those of a soft contact lens. These lenses are quite stable and heat tolerable, hence can be worn safely. Lens color withstands the chemical disinfectant and enzyme cleaning, hence can safely be cleaned like regular soft lenses. The tints of lenses are quite UV tolerant, so can be worn in hot climate without any additional problem.

Regular follow up and timely cleaning of lenses is the key to a successful wearing of colored contact lenses. Regular follow-up schedule is similar to those of a soft contact lens. In case any problem like red eye, pain, blurring of vision or intolerable foreign body sensation is felt, report immediately to an ophthalmologist.

Contact Lenses in Special Conditions

INTRODUCTION

High Myopia

Contact lens prescribed in the patients of high myopia (>–8 D) not only provide optical benefit (retinal image is larger and normal than glasses) but also helpful for cosmetic purposes. However, contact lens fitting in high myopes needs special attention due to two reasons

- Contact lenses usually ride high due to larger diameter and thick edges.
- Contact lenses base curve should be relatively flatter for proper fit.

As the degree of myopia increases, the edge thickness of contact lens will increase due to increase in the power of contact lens. As a result, thick edges create a base-up wedge effect and lens is pulled up by upper eyelid and lens tends to rise high. It can be reduced by reducing the peripheral thickness and by using lenticular or aspherical lens design. These lens design will decrease the irritation of lids and will prevent tugging of upper eyelid on lens. To minimize the flatness a smaller diameter lens can be used with better fitting, so that flatter edges will not create any problem. Hence, RGP lenses and lenticular design lenses are preferred choice of contact lenses in case of high myopes.

Aphakia

Aphakia means absence of crystalline lens, either due to surgical removal or any congenital condition. In surgical extraction placing an intra-ocular lens at the time of surgery is an ideal option, however, sometimes in very young children or with some associated conditions surgical implantation of intra-ocular lens is not possible. To have a clear vision these patients are dependent either on spectacles or contact lenses.

Contact lenses gives far better quality vision as compared to spectacle in case of aphakia because spectacles in an aphakic patient can produce the following problems

- Magnification of retinal image by 20–25%
- Reduced field of view and poor eccentric acuity
- Presence of a ring scotoma due to prismatic effect
- Pin cushion effect due to spherical aberrations
- Increased demand on convergence

These problems are eliminated by use of contact lenses, hence are very useful in pediatrics and adult patients. Aphakic contact lenses are specially used in monocular aphakic patients with good results. Both RGP and soft contact lenses are used in aphakics with variable results. Majority of aphakic contact lenses are made with a tint to prevent excessive light entry and thus reduce glare. Usually a grey color tint is given which act as a density filter and protects from UV rays.

Soft Contact Lenses in Aphakia

For correction of aphakia by contact lens, both daily wear and extended wear type soft contact lenses can be used. The aphakic contact lenses are rarely used in adult because of availability of newer intraocular lens implant techniques, however, in pediatric and elderly patients these contact lenses are still used with variable results.

- In young children, an extended wear lens is better choice than daily wear lens, because it is difficult to teach them the insertion and removal techniques of lens.
- In infants, the contact lenses should be prescribed immediately after cataract extraction because of potential risk of developing amblyopia, however, in adults it is advised to wait for at least two months after surgery, so that corneal topography and keratometry gets stabilized.
- There is an increased risk of neovascularisation and infection with use of extended wear contact lenses, hence daily wear lenses should be preferred wherever possible.
- Soft aphakic contact lenses are relatively thick and pose discomfort, hence lathe cut lenticular design lenses are used to increase the comfort and wearing time.
- For fitting these lenses in pediatric patients select the appropriate power, usually +1–1.5 D more than refraction value in children more than 2 years and +2 D more in children younger than 2 years age.
- Try for a steeper fit with good tear exchange as compared to flatter fit to minimize the lens loss.

RGP Contact Lenses in Aphakia

Rigid gas permeable contact lenses has following advantages over soft contact lenses in aphakic patients

- Oxygen transmissibility is high

- Optically better as compared to hydrogel and/or silicon lenses
- Flexibility in design
- Economical
- Easy to handle: Can be insert and remove easily
- High safety profile: Chances of bacterial infection and protein adherence are less

RGP lenses of excellent optical property are used in aphakia because in aphakic person strong plus power lenses are required and an unwanted cylindrical error may present with these high spherical powers which is not corrected by soft contact lenses. Mainly following lens designs are suitable for aphakic patients such as

- Single cut lens design
- Lenticular design

Fitting of RGP in children

- *Total diameter:* It is usually kept 1–2 mm smaller than the corneal diameter but relatively larger than adult TD to prevent loss of lens.
- *Power:* Based on the trial lens and over refraction, also correct for vertex distance. For example, suppose spectacle power is +20 D, then give +26.3 D contact lens. Similarly, if spectacle power is –15 D then give –12.75 D contact lens. In high power more than 10 D we also need to correct for tear layer, usually in the range of 2–3 D lacrimal lens.
- *Base curve:* Fit steeper than usual to prevent the loss of contact lens.
- *Material:* Usually material having high or hyper Dk is used for long-term results.

RGP lenses prescribed for aphakia usually ride low because RGP lenses have more central thickness (due to increase plus power) which creates a base down edge effect and the lens is forced down below by upper lids because of more weight and central thickness. To eliminate this problem a small lens with steeper fit is preferred. The single cut lens design RGP lenses have a diameter of 7.5–8.5 mm.

However, in spite of small size the centration of these lenses are poor; hence lenticular design lenses having an anterior central optical zone with a minus power carrier (peripheral zone) can be prescribed which has better centration.

Although RGP lenses have several advantages, but a few disadvantages of these lenses are

- More adaptation time
- Poor comfort of wearing
- Needs higher skill to fit
- High chances of lens loss or dislocation
- Increased possibility of self trauma

Presbyopia

Contact lenses for presbyopia correction may be considered an effective alternative to spectacles because they offer faster visual adaptation and more freedom of movement as well as increase in the quality of vision than ophthalmic lenses. Before prescribing contact lens it is essential to know the lifestyle, working distances, etc. of patient so that proper lens design can be selected for every patient depending on the information. For correction of presbyopia, multifocal contact lenses which contain distance and near vision in the same lens are used. There are several contact lens options which can be given to presbyopes including full monovision, modified monovision and bifocal or multifocal contact lenses of gas permeable or hydrogel or silicon-hydrogel materials.

One piece back surface hard bifocal contact lenses are most commonly used to correct presbyopia. In these bifocal lenses the power of addition is equal to the difference between the back surface interface powers in two portions of contact lens as shown in Fig. 12.1.

Broadly, three classes of lens design can be used to fit in presbyopes such as

- Non-rotational design lenses
- Rotational design lenses
- Simultaneous vision design lenses

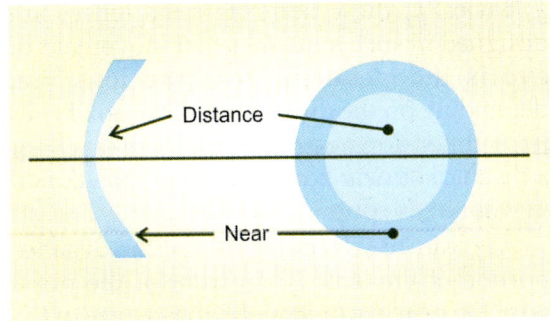

Fig. 12.1: One piece back surface bifocal contact lens

Non-rotational lens designs: Non-rotational contact lenses are similar to multifocal spectacle lenses, consist of a distance optic segment in the upper portion and a near optic segment in lower portion and are developed to move vertically on the eye. In addition, trifocal non-rotational lens design in which half of the add power is incorporated in the intermediate zone have been also designed which moves vertically on the eye. These lenses are manufactured using RGP material and are in the solid form (Fig. 12.2).

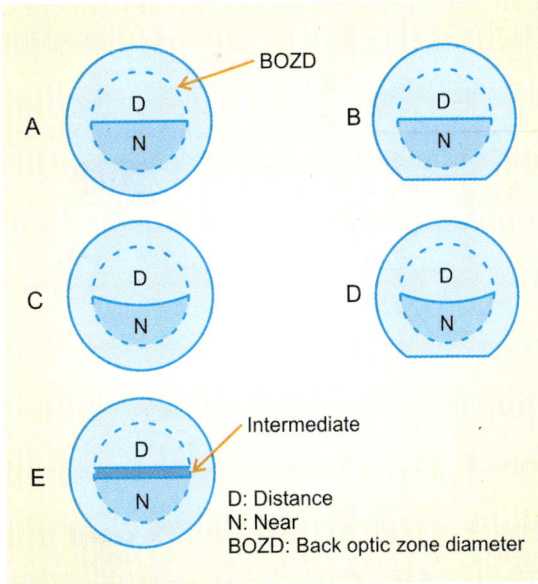

Fig. 12.2A to E: Various non-rotational multifocal contact lens design. A. Straight top non-truncated; B. Straight top truncated; C. Crescent non-truncated; D. Crescent truncated; E. Trifocal

Basically, these non-rotational lenses are designed in such a manner that movement of eye is independent from the lens, i.e. depending on the direction of fixation of eyes (straight or downward gaze) of person either a distance or near zone of lens are positioned in front of the pupil.

As it can be seen in Fig. 12.3A, the distance portion of the lens lies in front of the pupil with the primary or straight ahead gaze of the eyes, whereas near portion comes in front of the pupil with the downward gaze of the eyes (Fig. 12.3B). As the gaze is shifted in downward direction, the lower eyelid pushes the contact lens upwards. Due to this effect the lower portion of contact lens (having near addition) gets aligns with the pupil. Non-rotational contact lens design are similar to spectacles, i.e. allow an independent movement with simultaneous alignment with lower eyelids. Base-down prism is usually added in the lower portion of the lens so that thickness of lower portion of lens is increased as well as center of gravity of the lens is lowered. As a result, lens remains in a lower position on the eye and lens rotation also not occurs.

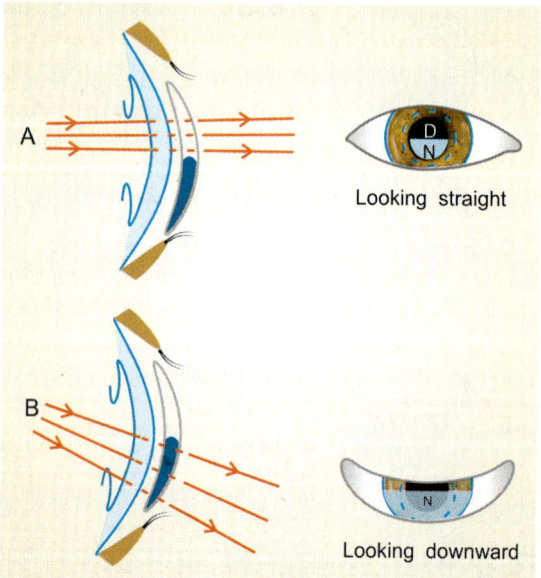

Fig. 12.3: Position of non-rotational design contact lens in various gaze. A. Straight gaze; B. Downward gaze

Sometimes, base-down prism alone is insufficient to control the lens rotation and its position, hence truncating a lens design along with lower edge of prism base, enhances the effect of base-down prism by increasing the area of contact between contact lens edge and lower eyelid so that lower lid can push the lens up during downward gaze.

For example, routine non-rotational contact lens parameters are lens diameter (8.7–10.5 mm), BOZR (6.0–9.4 mm), distance power (±20 D), add power(+0.75 D to +4.5 D), stabilization prism (1 to 3Δ), stabilization height (1 mm above to 2 mm below the geometric center) and truncation (0.4–0.6 mm).

Non-rotational lens designs are more preferred in presbyopes who are having

- Lower eyelid is just at or above the lower limbus with moderate to tight lower eyelid tensions.
- Flat corneal topography.
- Pupil of small size with normal illumination.
- Persons who need larger optical zones or back toric or bitoric lenses.
- Persons having residual astigmatism, with front toric designs.
- If add requirement is higher (>+3.00 D) means in case of advanced presbyope or who do frequent close work.

Rotational lens designs: Rotational lenses for presbyopes are designed in such a manner that distance or near segments of the contact lens remain in correct position even when the lens rotates. These lenses have concentric optical zones, hence rotation of the lens over the eye has no effect. Like non-rotational lenses, mostly these are also RGP lenses, where the concentric optical zones may be spherical or aspheric as shown in Fig. 12.4.

In these lens designs, when the individual's gaze is focused straight ahead then he/she will observe the distance objects through the center of the lens, whereas when his/her gaze shifts for reading (downward gaze) then the near

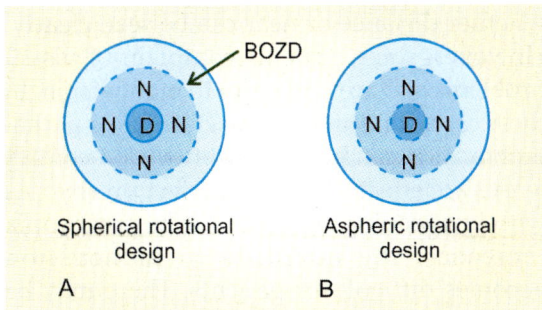

Fig 12.4: Rotational bifocal contact lens design

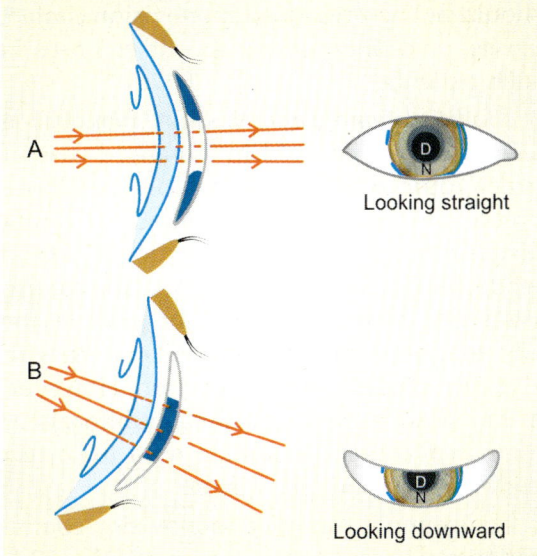

Fig 12.5: Position of rotational design contact lens in various gaze. A. Straight gaze; B. Downward gaze

vision will be observed through a surrounding annulus as shown in Fig. 12.5A and B, respectively.

Unlike non-rotational lens, with rotational lenses there is no need of incorporation of prism or truncation to stabilize the lens rather these lenses can rotate due to blinking, but still gives continuous optic power for distance as well as for near vision.

Concentric optical zones in a rotational lens may have

- Spherical design in front or back surface
- Aspherical design in back surface, or on both surfaces

Spherical design: Normally in spherical design on the front surface of lens, a central distance zone is present which is surrounded by a transition zone followed by a spherical near zone. The back surface of lens has a normal tricurve lens design or an aspheric design.

Aspherical design: In aspheric design lens the curvature of back surface changes progressively so that the add power remains limited. If additional add power is required, then it can be obtained by changing the front surface of these lenses.

> **Note**
>
> Smaller the distance zone, higher the add power; and steeper the lens must be fit.

Rotational lens designs are preferred in those who are

- Low adds presbyopes
- High myopes
- High hypermetropes
- Having steeper corneal geometries (especially aspherical rotational designs are used)

Simultaneous vision design lenses: These are the lens designs where both the distance and near light rays enter the pupil simultaneously, i.e. both distance and near vision are presented to the eyes at the same instant. The distance or near image is then selected by the brain of the observer depending on his or her visual requirements which further depends on the ability of the brain to distinguish between the blur and clear image. Contact lenses designed on this basis may be either center based (center-distance or center-near) monovision or modified monovision designs

Centration based designs: While prescribing simultaneous lens designs it is important to maintain lens centration with minimal lens movement because decentration of lens may result in visual symptoms. Simultaneously, too tight fit has to be avoided to maintain the proper corneal metabolism. Centration based design is mainly used for soft lenses. The lens designs may be

- *Center-near (CN) designs*: In center-near design, most of the plus power exists at the lens center while most negative power at the periphery as shown in Fig. 12.6A. It means the central portion of lens design focuses near objects while peripheral portion focuses distance objects. The center-near based bifocal and aspheric lens designs have been developed mainly to deal with problem of contraction of pupil occurring while working at near.
- *Center-distance designs*: In this lens design the central part is for the correction of distance vision while the peripheral part is for near vision correction as shown in Fig. 12.6B. This lens designs are mainly suggested for initial stage of presbyopia, requiring add up to +1.25 D.

Monovision: Monovision contact lenses means where in one eye (usually dominant eye) the full correction is given for distance vision, whereas the fellow eye (usually non-dominant eye) is corrected for near vision, using RGP or soft hydrogel contact lenses of bifocal or multifocal lens designs. Thus, in monovision the distance and near images are presented simultaneously to the brain or visual system. After a period of adaptation, the brain becomes versed to suppress the blurred image and thus the object of interest whether distance or near can be seen clearly. However, some patients complain of visual problems and are intolerant to monovision. In these cases, multifocal contact lenses or partial monovision can be tried. Monovision contact lenses are effective way to correct presbyopia with low reading addition. As the presbyopia increases, the adaption to monovision becomes difficult for patients. There may be loss of stereopsis as well as patient experience more difficulty to carry out distance and near tasks. Furthermore, patients having amblyopia should not be prescribed monovision contact lenses, prescribe multifocal contact lenses in such patients.

Modified monovision: Modified monovision technique can be used in advanced case of presbyopia where monovision may pose problem to patient. In this method, the center distance lens design is used for dominant eye while center near design is used for contralateral eye. Modified monovision provides the advantages of monovision while along with keeping some multifocal function. However, in modified monovision usually bifocals or multifocal contact lenses are used to correct both distance and near vision.

For example, modified monovision combination can be as done as shown in Table 12.1.

Diagnostic criteria to judge regarding whether to prescribe monovision, modified monovision or multifocal lenses can be done by performing this simple test. First do an assessment to know which eye is dominant eye, now try to give over plus lenses in non-dominant eye which are just enough for good

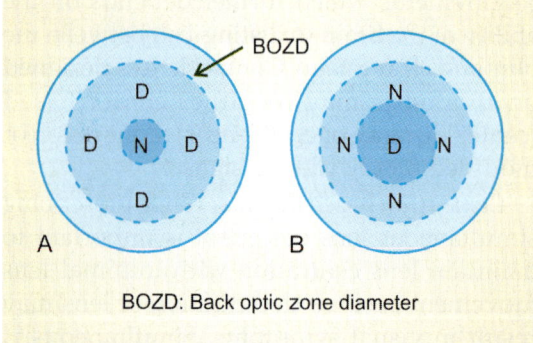

BOZD: Back optic zone diameter

Fig. 12.6: Rotational center based aspherical contact lens design. A. Center near; B. Center distance

Table 12.1: Various modified monovision combinations

Dominant eye	Non-dominant eye
Rotational multifocal (center distance)	Simultaneous multifocal (center near)
Rotational multifocal (center distance)	Near single vision lens
Distance single vision lens	Simultaneous multifocal (center near)

near vision. Suppose patient develops no symptoms and is comfortable in near vision, then he/she is a good candidate for prescribing monovision. On contrary, if the patient feels dizziness or an imbalance with significant difference in clarity of vision between two eyes, then avoid monovision and prefer binocular bifocals or multifocal lenses.

Contact Lens Fitting in Presbyopes

Fitting of rotational lens designs

- Examination of the patient to find out the lens related parameters
  - Lens diameter: Size of palpebral aperture (PA) and/or HVID can be used to calculate the diameter of lens. It is recommended that a lens with slightly larger diameter should be used to avoid discomfort to patient except if PA is extremely narrow in the size. The estimation of lens diameter on the basis of PA and HVID can be understood by Table 12.2.
  - Back optical zone radius (base curve): Corneal topography/keratometry readings are used, to select the suitable BOZR of the lens as per the manufacturer's instructions. Rotational lens with front surface spherical design usually has a tricurve shaped back surface and BOZR is fit to achieve an alignment fitting relationship. However, rotational lens with back surface aspheric design, BOZR is kept steeper than flat K (about 0.15–0.80 mm) depending upon the total add power required (e.g. for high add reading it is more steeper).
  - Calculation of distance power: Distance power is calculated according to change in BOZR, e.g. for every 0.05 mm change of BOZR, 0.25 D is added.
  - Calculation of near power: Calculate as per requirement of patient.
- Select the diagnostic contact lens according to BOZR, calculated power, near/reading add and total diameter. Insert this contact lens and allow it to settle for 15–30 minutes.
- Evaluation of lens fit: Assess position of contact lens and assess near vision in following terms
  - Lens centration and diameter: Ensure the centration of lens.
  - Lens movement with blink: 1–2 mm of lens movement is perfect.
  - Fluorescein pattern: In spherical rotational lens, the fluorescein pattern should appear centrally with optimal edge clearance (0.5 mm). For aspheric rotational lens, slightly high riding, with some central pooling and a wide band of peripheral edge clearance should be seen.
- Accuracy of lens prescription is checked by doing a binocular over refraction for distance and then for near, with the patient holding reading material under normal illumination.

Fitting of non-rotational lens designs: Fitting of non-rotational lenses is considered more difficult than rotational lenses as more parameters are taken into consideration for optimal visual performance.

First lens related parameters are calculated
- Assessment of lens parameters
  - Diameter of lens: Palpebral aperture (PA) size and/or HVID are used to calculate the lens diameter as summarized in Table 12.3. Like rotational lenses, lens

Table 12.2: Estimation of lens diameter according to palpebral aperture (PA) and horizontal visible iris diameter (HVID) in rotational lens design

Lens diameter (mm)	PA (mm)	HVID (mm)
9.0–9.3	<8	10–11
9.4–9.6	8–11	11.5–12.5
9.7–10.0	>11	>12.5

Table 12.3: Estimation of lens diameter according to palpebral aperture (PA) and horizontal visible iris diameter (HVID) in non-rotational lens design

Lens diameter (mm)	PA (mm)	HVID (mm)
9.0–9.3	<8	10–11
9.4–9.6	8–11	11.5–12.5
9.7–10.0	>11	>12.5

with slightly larger diameter should be used to avoid discomfort to patient except if PA is extremely narrow in the size.

- Proper BOZR should be selected for fit alignment. The BOZR should be modified according to corneal astigmatism, as the corneal astigmatism increased, select steeper BOZR. If cornea is spherical, then BOZR can be taken equal to flattest keratometry reading.
- Measurement of segment height: Determine the distance between lower edge of lens (or lower eyelid) and lower margin of pupil. Otherwise, segment height is kept 1 mm lower than the geometric center of contact lens.

- Stabilization using prism: In the absence of truncation, start stabilization with prism of 1 Δ in case of minus prescription lens and start with a prism of 1.5 Δ in case of plus prescription.

- Prism axis: Initially start with prism axis at 90°. Suppose there is a nasal rotation of 5–10°, then balance the prism axis, clockwise for right eye and counter-clockwise for left eye, means to 95° or 100°, respectively. Suppose the position of inferior prism marking is rotated towards examiner's left, then add same degree of rotation to prism axis. On the other hand, if rotated to right then subtract the same degree of rotation from the prism axis (LARS principle means left add, right subtract).

- Assess distance power: Using diagnostic lens, perform binocular over refraction to calculate distance power.

- Assess near power: Keeping distance over refraction in position, add an additional power for reading. Make sure that patient's head is tilted slightly downward, with eyes set at a down gaze which ensure upward translation of contact lens.

- Truncation: If upward translation of contact lens does not happen, then truncation is necessary to avoid lower eyelid from sliding over the inferior part of lens.

- After evaluating lens parameters order of lens can be done and then check the lens fit and assessment of ordered lens
  - *Lens centration and diameter:* Lens should be well centered or slightly low
  - *Lens movement with blink:* 1–2 mm of lens movement is ideal
  - *Lens translation on down gaze:* 2 mm of lens translation is ideal; which enables the near segment of lens to translate over the pupil.
  - *Lens rotation:* Usually 5–10° generally nasally, for both distance and near gaze
  - *Near segment position:* Near segment top should be present, at or just above lower pupillary margin.
  - *Fluorescein pattern:* An aligned fluorescein pattern should be seen; which indicates perfect lens centration, lens translation and movement of lens.
  - *Distance/near vision:* Should be optimal at working distances.

Fitting of center near designs: In these designs, centration and minimal lens movement is necessity to attain a good lens fit; because objective is to offer both distance and near vision, simultaneously. The lens fitting steps are similar to other lenses, i.e. evaluate the lens parameters and select the lens according to parameters. To get an ideal fit the lens diameter can be increased and steepening of optical zone can be done, i.e. either steepen BOZR or increase BOZD and reducing the axial edge lift.

Ideal lens fit of center near lens is checked by

- Lens centration and diameter: Lens should be well centered with good corneal coverage.
- Lens movement with blink: About 1 mm of lens movement is required.
- Fluorescein pattern: Should show centered lens with an adequate edge clearance.

Follow-up: On follow-up visits, if required alteration in parameters can be done if essential for comfortable visual performance like

- If too much lens movement is there, then TD can be increased or BOZR steepening is done.
- Ensure that a balance exist between distance and near vision requirements because on adding more minus power to improve the distance vision will affect the near vision on contrary, adding of more plus to improve the near vision will affect distance vision.

High Astigmatism

Correction of astigmatism by contact lens, especially of high degree, needs proper selection of contact lens design which may vary with each case.

Elements responsible for production of astigmatism are

- Cornea (mainly)
- Crystalline lens
- Retina (rare)

Cornea is considered major refracting surface of the human eye. Even a minor change in the curvature or radius of the corneal surface can induce change in the refractive power of the eye. Different types of astigmatisms usually appear due to toricity of the anterior corneal surface. Astigmatisms can also be induced by the crystalline lens (lenticular astigmatism) and retina and is termed internal astigmatism, however, still clinically most significant astigmatism is contributed by corneal surface.

The sum of corneal and lenticular astigmatism is termed total refractive astigmatism. Hence, for correction of astigmatism by contact lenses, both types of ocular astigmatisms should be taken into consideration. As we know that most of the astigmatism is contributed due to cornea but if there is large difference between corneal and total refractive astigmatism, it indicates presence of significant amount of lenticular astigmatism in that individual. For example, if in a case having higher refractive astigmatism as compared to corneal astigmatism and when a spherical rigid gas permeable (RGP) contact lens is prescribed to this case, then a significant amount of residual astigmatism (lenticular astigmatism) will remain uncorrected which will affect visual acuity. These types of cases require fitting of a RGP contact lens having toric design or alternately a toric soft contact lens can also be used.

Types of astigmatism: Depending on the angle between two principal meridians astigmatisms are classified clinically in two different types. The corneal surface can be assessed by performing keratometry and corneal topography. Keratometer is commonly used for measurements of corneal curvature. Corneal topography is an advance method for corneal assessment which does complete corneal examination.

Corneal topography is a useful method to assess and classify corneal astigmatisms. Broadly, astigmatism can be divided as

- Regular
- Irregular

Regular astigmatism: Astigmatism is said to be regular when corneal meridians representing maximum and minimum refractive powers are perpendicular to each other. Further regular astigmatisms can grouped as with the rule, against the rule oblique astigmatism. In regular astigmatis, corneal topography appears like a tie, having two perpendicular main meridians as shown in Fig. 12.7.

Irregular astigmatism: When the principal meridians do not lie perpendicular to each other and the meridians representing maximum and minimum refractive powers are not separated by an angle of 90°, it is called irregular astigmatism. Irregular astigmatism is more commonly seen with keratoconus, after surgical procedures or in scarred cornea. In irregular astigmatism, corneal topography

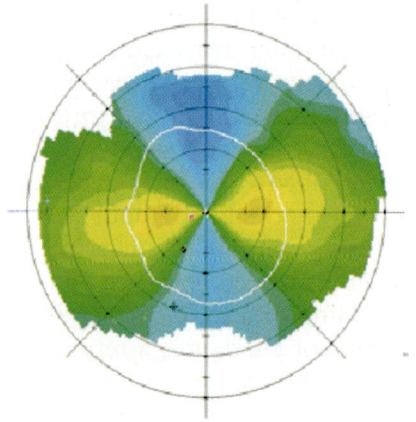

Fig. 12.7: Corneal topography showing regular astigmatism

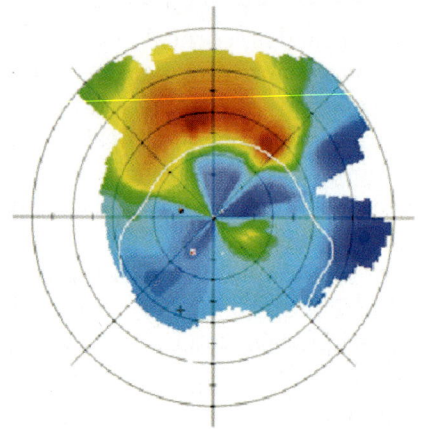

Fig. 12.8: Corneal topography showing irregular astigmatism

will show that two principal meridians which are not perpendicular to each other as shown in Fig. 12.8.

Contact lens for astigmatism: Various types of contact lens designs can be used to correct astigmatism, however, to avoid rotation of lens during blinking, different systems in the form of prism ballast, truncation, or thin zones are provided.

Correction of Regular Astigmatism

General rule for selection of a contact lens is that lens choice mainly depends on the amount of refractive astigmatism as summarized in Table 12.4 and shown in Fig. 12.9.

Table 12.4: Choice of type of contact lens on the basis of degree of astigmatism

Degree of astigmatism	Lens of choice
< 1.00 D	Soft or RGP spherical lens
1.00 to 4.00 D	Soft toric lens or RGP spherical lens
> 4.00 D	RGP toric lens or custom soft toric lens

Soft contact lens correction

- *Spherical soft contact lenses:* Spherical soft contact lens is the first choice to correct astigmatism in cases having astigmatic error up to 1 D and less than 1/3 of the spherical error. If visual acuity remains poor with spherical soft contact lenses, then soft toric or spherical RGP contact lens should be used. Generally, improvement in the visual acuity is observed better with use of spherical RGP lenses as compared to soft contact lenses in astigmatism. For example, a patient having refractive error as –6 DS × –1.25 DC, can be corrected with an equivalent soft spherical contact lens, and patient remains comfortable with fair amount of visual acuity. Whereas, a patient having refractive error as –2.5 DS × –1.25 DC will be uncomfortable with an equivalent spherical soft contact lenses.

- *Toric soft contact lenses:* Patients having astigmatic error more than 1.25 DC need toric soft lenses. In these cases, soft spherical lenses are unable to rectify the error and RGP lenses may be intolerable, hence soft toric contact lenses having different radii are used. These lenses are fitted as per the guidelines provided by the lens manufacturer; however, fitter should make sure that the patients refractive error should correctly match with contact lens parameters.

Soft toric lenses are available as

- *Standard lenses:* Consist of low cylinder amount and are available easily on order.

- *Custom lenses:* These lenses have high cylinder amount or nonstandard diameters

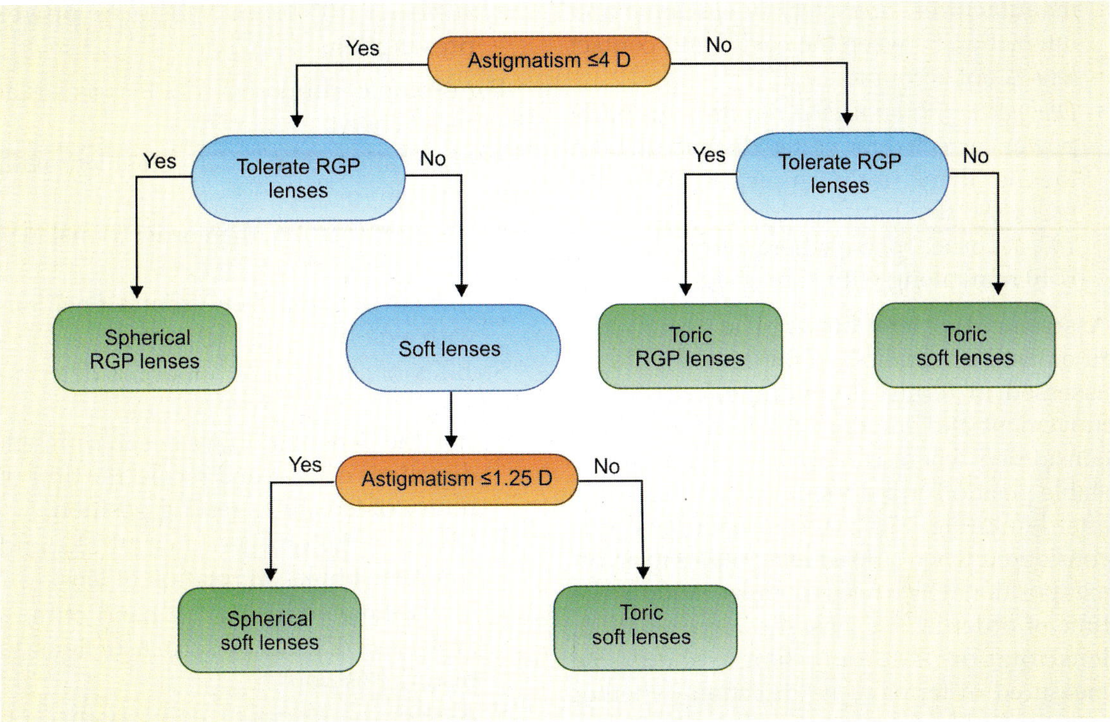

Fig. 12.9: Selection cascade for contact lenses in regular astigmatism

and usually require long time duration to receive from the laboratory.

Soft toric contact lens design

- Back surface toric (most common, good for toric cornea)
- Front surface toric (better for spherical cornea)

Stabilization: The soft toric lenses need to be stabilized, so that rotation of lens does not occur during blinking. Stabilization can be done by various methods

- *By using prism ballast,* i.e. in the inferior portion of lens additional material is added, generally 0.75 – 2 Δ of ballast added.
- *Prism ballast with truncation* (usually used in custom designs).
- *Truncation,* i.e. bottom of the lens is removed.
- *By making thin zones* (top and bottom of lens are thinned).

Systems generally used to stabilize soft toric lenses are, either thin zones or prism ballast; these designs can correct astigmatism up to 8 D as shown in Fig. 12.10.

Contact lens fitting methods are

- *Empirical fitting method* requires spectacle power and K readings adjusted by using type of guaranteed fitting program provided by

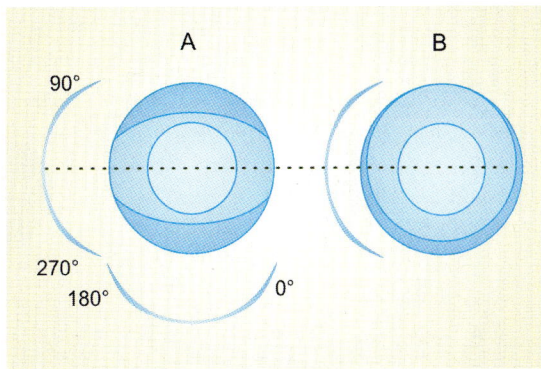

Fig. 12.10: Soft toric contact lens design. A. Thin zone toric stabilization system; B. Prismatic stabilization system

manufacturer, however, eyelid force and interaction between the eyelid and contact lens is not accounted.

- *Diagnostic fitting method* requires spectacle power corrected for vertex distance in both the meridians (for example, –4 DS × –2.5 DC × 180 will become –3.5 DS × –2 DC × 180, at corneal plane where vertex distance is 10 mm) along with K reading.

Assessment of lens fitting: The overall lens fit as well as rotation of the lens should be assessed in terms of coverage, centration, movement and rotation. An ideal lens fit is considered where contact lens remains in a stable position and does not rotate markedly after blink (Fig. 12.11A). Improper lens fit is considered when contact lens rotates to an off axis position which needs compensation at the time of ordering the lens. If on examination, lens rotation is found, then it should be measured in terms of its direction (whether rotated clockwise or counterclockwise from 6 o'clock position) and magnitude (means its degree of displacement from expected position).

In this case, during ordering of lens, LARS method should be used to compensate the misrotation of lens.

- Similarly, if trial lens base rotates to left of observer in 10° (Fig. 12.11B), then add 10° to spectacle power prescription.
- Suppose if trial lens base rotates to right of observer in 10° (Fig. 12.11C), then

subtract 10° from spectacle power prescription.

For example, suppose a trial lens axis is at 180° and it shows

- No rotation, then order a final lens with axis 180°
- 10° right rotation, then order a final lens with axis 170°.
- 10° left rotation, then order a final lens with axis 10°.

Stability of contact lens rotation is determined by

- Ask the patient to move eye in different directions of gaze and record the time of return of lens to its resting position.
- Observe the effect of fast blinks and complete blinks on rotation of lens.
- Move the contact lens by hand off axis and record time of return of lens to resting position.
- Assess the effect of convergence on rotation of lens.

Rigid gas permeable (RGP) contact lens

RGP contact lenses offer useful choices to correct regular astigmatism with high quality of visual acuity. Various RGP lens design can be used depending upon patient's astigmatism. Generally, in cases having low degree of astigmatism, spherical RGP contact lenses are recommended, however, with high degree of astigmatism, a toric RGP lens is recommended to correct astigmatism. Toric RGP contact

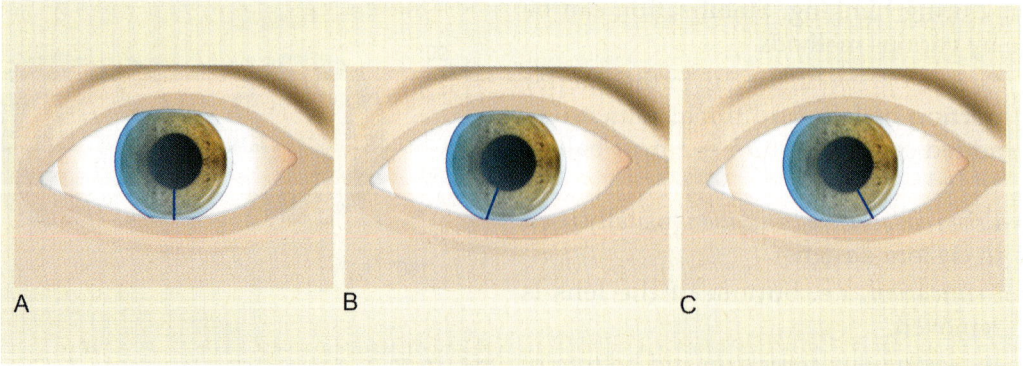

Fig. 12.11: Assessment of soft toric contact lens fit. A. No rotation, B. Left rotation, C. Right rotation

lenses can also be required for correction of astigmatism in cases of lenticular astigmatism.

- *Spherical RGP contact lens:* Primarily used to correct low degree astigmatism, means up to ≤4 D. These lenses are not useful in correction of moderate to high degree astigmatic refractive errors. Patients having corneal astigmatism to the tune of 4 D can be corrected by spherical RGP contact lenses, although these lenses are made with diameter 0.2–0.3 mm smaller than usual diameter.

- *Toric RGP contact lenses:* To correct moderate to high degree astigmatism mainly toric RGP lenses are used. These lenses are available in various designs to fit in different types of refractive errors.

RGP toric contact lens designs are available as

- Front surface toric RGP lenses
- Back surface toric RGP lenses
- Toric RGP lenses with peripheral curves
- Bitoric RGP lenses

Note

Generally in RGP toric lenses stabilization is done by creating back toric surfaces, although RGP front toric lenses needs an additional stabilization system.

Front surface toric RGP lenses: Front surface toric RGP lenses are used to correct high degree residual astigmatism or lenticular astigmatism in patients having spherical cornea. Stabilization in these types of lenses is done by an additional system such as prism blast or truncation method. In blast method usually a base down 2 D prism is added on the front surface during manufacturing of contact lens, however, sometimes more dioptre prisms may be required to center a very high degree minus power contact lens.

In truncation method contact lens diameter is reduced in one meridian, usually by cutting (nearly 0.5–1 mm) an entire edge of contact lens.

Back surface toric RGP lenses: Usually stabilization of toric RGP lenses is done by creating back surface as toric. These lenses are usually used to correct low degree astigmatism. Usually Keratometry reading are used for a proper lens fit of posterior curves of contact lens, accurately with corneal curvature.

Toric RGP lenses with peripheral curves: Similar to back surface toric lenses, these lenses are also used to correct low degree (2–3 D) astigmatism. In these cases of astigmatism a spherical RGP lens will fit improperly, because edge of lens will lift over steepest meridian of cornea; which may cause decentration and loss of contact lens. Hence, to correct this problem additional steeper peripheral curves are made in steepest corneal meridians, whereas standard lens curves are fitted along the flatter corneal meridian.

Bitoric RGP contact lens: Bitoric RGP contact lens is used in patients who are presented with moderate degree astigmatism along with a residual astigmatism. Usually, a RGP contact lens is fitted with a posterior curve, same as that of keratometry reading however, when this toric back surface RGP lens is placed on the cornea the interface between contact lens and tear film forms a toric surface. This newly formed toric surface causes a state of an induced astigmatism and to correct this condition, an additional anterior surface toricity is created which forms a bitoric RGP contact lens.

Correction of irregular astigmatism: Correction of an irregular astigmatism using RGP contact lenses provides a considerable enhancement of visual acuity than spectacle correction. Hence, RGP contact lenses became the first choice of management, in some corneal pathology having an irregular cornea such as keratoconus, post-keratoplasty, complicated refractive surgery, corneal trauma and post-herpetic keratitis.

Contact Lens Fitting in Primary Corneal Ectasias

Keratoconus is one of the most common types of primary corneal ectasias seen in clinical practice. Others less common are keratoglobus and pellucid marginal degeneration. Keratoconus is characterized by thinning of cornea and ectasias resulting in varying degrees of irregular astigmatism.

Spectacles can be used for management of initial stages of keratoconus, while surgical procedure (most commonly penetrating keratoplasty) is done only when other available treatment have failed or there is significant reduction in visual acuity. Majority of keratoconus cases can be managed by prescribing contact lenses.

Classification of degree and type of keratoconus is important in making the decision about type of contact lens fitting method. Position and size of cone in the eye affect the selection of contact lens fitting method, hence it is advised to do computerized corneal topography to identify the type of cone. Basically there may be three types of cones as follows

1. *Nipple cones:* Mostly these cones are located below the visual axis (sometimes central), small in size with variable conicity.
2. *Oval cones:* These cones are also located below the visual axis having larger inferior conical area.
3. *Globus cones:* These cones are rarely seen, where about 75% of cornea gets affected and clinically Munson's sign is present in majority of cases.

Ideal fit in keratoconus: Keratoconic patients or other primary corneal ectasias patients require high levels of comfort, because they need to wear contact lenses for longer duration, hence appropriate lens materials should be chosen. Cases where steep high minus lenses are required, lens material having high dimensional stability should be prescribed so that chances of the contact lens distortion are less.

Contact lens of different Dk/t (moderate to high values for large or flatter lenses, low value for stability and wetting purpose) can be used.

Rigid contact lens fitting: Rigid gas permeable (RGP) contact lenses for correction of keratoconus are the most common and most successful method which provides a new anterior surface to cornea. Several contact lens designs are available and can be fitted accordingly at different stages of keratoconus and cone types. Various fitting methods of RGP lenses are summarized as follows:

Apical clearance method: In this method the contact lens rest on the paracentral cornea and vaults the cone. Central cornea is not covered, hence chances of trauma and scarring of central cornea is reduced. These types of lens are of small diameter, having less back optic zone diameter which may result in significant flare and glare problems. In addition, there may be corneal edema, decreased tear exchange, air bubbles under contact lens (may creep into central optic zone, causing poor visual acuity).

Apical touch flat fitting method: In this method nearly entire weight of contact lens lies on the cone, with wide edge standoff. The lens remains in position due to top lid. Due to apical touch better visual acuity is obtained and improvement in visual acuity is noticed immediately probably because of corneal molding by RGP contact lens. These contact lenses can cause to development or progression of apical changes and/or abrasions and scarring of cornea. It is more successful in early keratoconus cases, but still can be used in certain cases where corneal apices are displaced.

Three-point touch method: It is most commonly used fitted design for keratoconus especially for multicurve contact lens designs. The main principle used is to distribute the weight of contact lens uniformally between the cone and peripheral cornea. Hence, a three-point touch fitted lens will show an apical contact area of about 2–3 mm and an annulus rim of mid peripheral contact zone. The area and shape of the contact zones may vary due to cone asymmetry, e.g. mid-peripheral contact zone may assume more crescent shape, if cone is vertically asymmetrical.

Contact lens designs for primary corneal ectasias: Various lens designs are used to correct and improve visual acuity in patients having keratoconus and other corneal ectasias. These lens designs are broadly grouped as

- Multicurve design contact lenses
- Aspheric/elliptical design contact lenses
- Large diameter contact lenses
- Combination or Piggy back lenses

Multicurve lenses Standard form of multicurve lens designs may be used in persons having early keratoconus, however, for advanced stage of disease more specific lens designs are available to use like Woodward multicurve lens design. Most important advantage with these lenses is that practitioner knows all the parameters of this type of lens design which are already provided by manufacturer, hence any modifications in lens can easily be ordered by practitioner. The multicurve lenses are designed on the basis of the fact that in early or moderate keratoconus the periphery of cornea is not much changed, thus multicurve lenses have normal curves in the periphery, but steeper base optical zone radius (BOZR).

Central keratometry decides the selection of cone radius and for each cone radius a number of peripheries with different diameters are available. For example

- Shepherd NLK (Northern Lenses) also called acuity lenses
- Profile lenses (Jack Allen)
- Rose K system

Among these lenses the most widely used is Rose K system, which is mainly useful in cases having central cone, however, in cases having inferiorly displaced cones, Rose K is not very useful.

- *Rose K system:* On the basis of statistical data collected from keratoconus patient by Dr Paul Rose of New Zealand, these contact lens designs were developed having complex computer generated peripheral curves. The important characteristic of these lenses are
  1. To obtain an ideal edge lift of 0.8 mm, these contact lenses include triple peripheral curve system, i.e. standard, flat and steep.
  2. Rose K design lenses are existing in wide range of base curve (4.75–8 mm) and diameters (7.9–10.2 mm). As the steeping of base curve increases, the optic zone diameter of lens decreases.
  3. Toric curves are available on all surfaces of lens, i.e. front, back and periphery. Traditionally, Rose K lenses are made from Boston ES material, however, Boston XO material was also used by some laboratories to increase oxygen permeability property.

Aspheric/elliptic lenses are the one in which lens flatten in curvature progressively from the center to the periphery. Many aspheric lenses designs like Quasar K No 7 lens, Jack Allen KD lens, and Persecon Elliptical K lens are available for early keratoconus cases. These lenses have large optic zones thus very useful in patients having large pupils and/or oval type cones. Aspheric lenses are available in wide variety of materials, and can be made in specific material on order.

Large diameter lenses: These contact lenses are large in diameter (up to 14.5 mm) having bicurve or multicurve and are available in a number of lens designs such as

- *Soper cone design:* These contact lenses are of bicurve design having two posterior curves, one curve is fitted on the central cone and the second curve is fitted on the normal peripheral cornea (like a hat on the head). Lens has small diameter and fixed back optic zone. As the base curve is decreased for a given diameter, the vaulting effect of lens get increase.

- *McGuire lenses:* It is a modification of Soper cone lens design and consists of four peripheral curves (primary, secondary, tertiary and quaternary) instead of two which are blended together. These four peripheral curves are 3, 6, 8 and 10 D more flatter than the base curve of the lens. This lens system contains three diagnostic lens sets, i.e. nipple, oval or globus types of cones. Fitting principle is to achieve a three-point touch which in turn is dependent on the size of optic zone in relation to cone size. The optic zone sizes differ from 6 mm for the nipple cone to 6.5 mm for the oval cone, and 7 mm for the globus.

- *Dyna Intra Limbal (DIL):* These large diameter lenses are specifically designed for cases having inferiorly displaced keratoconus, pellucid marginal degeneration and post-keratoplasty where stability of lens is difficult to attain by using smaller diameter lenses. These lenses are mainly used to provide stability. These lenses are available in various diameters ranging from 10.8 mm to 12.5 mm, diameter range. Ideally, the total diameter of lens is kept 0.2 mm smaller than that of corneal diameter because it allows a lens movement of approximately 0.5–1 mm. Epithelial/stromal scarring may occur with lens due to 'settle back' tendency of these lens. Usually materials having high DK/t are recommended for manufacturing of these lenses.

- *S-Lim lenses (Jack Allen):* These semi-scleral contact lenses mainly remain on the limbus with very little movement. These lenses are mainly designed to vault the corneal grafts by changing the sag depth according to requirement. For exchange of tears, 2–4 fenestrations are present in the lens.

- *Kerasoft lenses (Ultra vision):* Normally soft lenses, e.g. hydrogels or silicon hydrogels are not preferred for correction of irregular cornea as these lenses have propensity to drape on the surface of cornea, hence soft lens, e.g. Kerasoft have been specially manufactured for treatment of keratoconus which does not drape over the cornea. Kerasoft lenses (58% water content terpolymer) has a back surface cylindrical design and are available as lens series called A, B and C with total lens diameters of 14 mm, 14.5 mm and 15 mm respectively. Among these lenses series B lenses are most commonly used and has flatter fit as compared to series A lens. Kerasoft lenses are mainly used for early keratoconus and for those patients who have difficulty in wearing RGP lens. These lenses offer more comfort and prolonged wearing time in patients who cannot tolerate RGP corneal lenses.

- *Hybrid soft perm lenses:* These lenses are manufactured by using RGP material for the center portion of lens and soft 25% water content HEMA in the periphery. The total diameter of lens is about 14.3 mm with 8.0 mm of central portion. These lens provide good centration, better visual acuity and less discomfort as compared to RGP lens, hence are preferred in RGP intolerant patients. However, these lenses have very less oxygen transmissibility (Dk/t), chances of giant papillary conjunctivitis and corneal neovascularisation are more. Research and advancement in lens manufacturing are coming up with newer versions which give higher oxygen permeability (Dk 100–105) and 40–45% water content HEMA skirt.

Combination or Piggy back lenses As we know that soft contact lenses are recommended in cases where patient is sensitive to RGP lenses or excessive lid sensation to RGP lenses are present. However, good visual acuity is difficult to attain with use of only soft contact lenses. Hence, a concept of combination or piggy back lenses means fitting a RGP lens over a soft lens (silicon hydrogels) gained popularity so that same level of visual acuity can be obtained as with a single lens. Generally, silicon hydrogel with the steepest base curve is preferred for piggy banking lens manufacture especially in cases of early keratoconus and irregular astigmatism. As compared to conventional soft lens, silicon hydrogels have more oxygen transmissibility and rigidity. However, in severe cases of keratoconus particularly in inferiorly displaced cones, a piggyback combination is not so successful because silicon hydrogels tend to pucker and do not fit well. Fitting of RGP lens should be done first and an apical touch of slight larger area is tolerable.

Problems arising due to lens fitting in keratoconus

- *Peripheral staining:* Staining in the form of 3 and 9 o'clock may occur. It usually develops due to dryness in the areas surrounding the contact lens. It can be managed by using lenses of large diameter, decrease lens edge lift, performing blinking exercises and instillation of ocular lubricants.
- *Vortex staining:* This type of staining is more common with flat fitting contact lenses which may damage corneal epithelium. Recommended measures are steepening of contact lens (causes reduction in pressure over the cone), and increasing Dk/t of lens material.
- *Dimpling:* Air bubbles trapped under contact lens which acts like smooth foreign bodies causes dimpling. Usually this happens when normal GP lens designs are used in early keratoconic cases or when an excessive apical clearance is present. In case of dimpling, reduction of BOZD and addition of peripheral curve by using a different multicurve design will help to correct the situation.

- *Stromal scarring:* It is usual in advanced stages of keratoconus which can affect visual acuity. In cases of significantly decreased visual acuity, graft surgery is indicated.
- *Thinning:* Corneal thinning may occur which can be managed in a similar manner to stromal scarring. In cases of severe thinning graft surgery is required.
- *Giant papillary conjunctivitis:* As keratoconus is generally associated with atopic disease, hence GPC is commonly seen in patient with keratoconus. If develops can be managed by preservative free eye drops, mast cell stabilizers (e.g. sodium cromoglycate) in the initial stages, however, in severe conditions steroids are used to control the situation.
- *Neovascularisation:* Most commonly associated with use of Softperms and PMMA scleral contact lenses. It is recommended that development of neovascularisation should not be allowed in any case because this will seriously affect the success rate of corneal graft surgery to be done in the future.
- *Nebulae:* Nebulae means a small raised area of scarring developed in the superficial corneal stroma due to wearing of flat fitting contact lens leading to discomfort and decreased wearing time. It can be debrided by mechanical means (using a scalpel blade) or by an excimer laser (phototherapeutic keratectomy).

Contact lens fitting in keratoconus
Before fit assessment
- Fleischer's ring and Vogt's striae are hallmark signs of keratoconus.
- In cases of keratoconus, on doing corneal topography the steepest area of cornea usually measures more than 48 D. Furthermore, if eccentricity value ≥ 0.8, then it is more likely to be because of keratoconus.
- In absence of corneal topography facility, patients having moderate to advance

keratoconus can be assessed by clinical examination. When a +1.25 D trial lens is placed over patient's side of keratometer, then the range of value extends about 8 D in case of keratoconus.

Contact lens fitting

- In centrally located cone having relatively small apex, usually small diameter RGP lenses are used.
- Cases having large oval or globus cone and inferiorly decentered apex: hybrid design lenses, intra-limbal, scleral, or piggyback lenses are successful.
- However, most of the lens designs used for keratoconus needs minimal apical clearance or mild touch; because excessive apical bearing can cause corneal staining and probable corneal scarring while excessive apical clearance can cause peripheral seal off.
- Sometimes, when patient is prescribed RGP lens and there is poor centration, discomfort to patient or scarring then piggyback combination can be tried. For example, soft silicon hydrogel contact lens of very low power (0.5 D) is placed under RGP lens, however, in combination the GP material of hyper Dk (>100) should be used. Sometimes, soft contact lens of moderate plus power (+6 D) having thicker center can also be used with RGP lens if positioning of RGP lens over soft contact lens is low due to presence of low corneal apex.

Orthokeratology

Orthokeratology or ortho-K is reversible, non-invasive method used as an alternative to refractive surgery for correction of visual acuity in low to moderate degree of myopic cases. This approach was known since many years, however, its clinical applications have increased in recent years because of availability of lens materials having high oxygen transmissibility and availability of better contact lens manufacturing technology.

Principle of orthokeratology is that reshaping (change in curvature) of corneal surface occurs due to constant wearing of a specially designed RGP contact lens, for longer period of time. These types of lenses are worn overnight or on alternate nights, then removed in the morning and not worn during the day. By orthokeratology there is flattening of the cornea so that overall refractive power of the eye is reduced, however, effects on the shape of cornea are temporary and cornea regains its original shape on discontinuation of lens. Sometimes, due to compromised corneal epithelium, serious complications can occur. Orthokeratology does not affect shape of posterior cornea or depth of the anterior chamber. Reverse geometry design lens have been designed to improve centration and refractive effect which consist of central optic zone more flat relative to cornea while surrounded peripheral zones are more steeper with reverse curves.

Assessment before lens fit

- Ideal candidates for this technique are
  - Myopic having refractive error less than 5 D.
  - Cylindrical error of ≤ 1.50 D, in case of with the rule astigmatism or ≤ 0.50 D in case of against the rule astigmatism.
  - Pupillary diameter less than 6 mm.
- Important screening tests to be done are refraction, slit lamp examination and corneal topography. Topography provides values of corneal eccentricity and also helps to rule out those patients which are having irregular cornea.

Lens fitting Process

- Base curve radius of RGP lens is determined by using "Jessen formula", which uses FAP (flat add plus) tear lens factor. This results in a final contact lens power of +0.75 D, which permits regression of corneal surface during daytime. For example, suppose patient has a refractive error of −3 DS × −0.75 DC × 180 with keratometry values

44.00 D at 180°/horizontal meridian and 44.75 D at 90°/vertical meridian. Base curve of contact lens should be, equal to flatter by 3.75 D (3.00 D + 0.75 D) than K (44 D), which becomes 40.25 D (44 D–3.75 D).

- Selection of initial diagnostic lens is based on achievement of bull's eye fluorescein pattern (means there is central and mid-peripheral bearing with narrow tear circulation zone and slight peripheral edge lift).
- Before evaluating lens fit it is advised to wait for 10–15 minutes. Ideally, during evaluation there must be good centration of contact lens with a minimum ≤ 1 mm lag during blinking.
- Again patient must be examined in the morning as follows
  - Check the fitting relationship of lens and cornea; remove contact lens for assessment of corneal integrity.
  - If on examination, a consolidated staining of cornea is observed, then it indicates that contact lens is too flat in central portion.
  - Do corneal topography which should show bull's eye pattern (central flattening with paracentral steepening) in ideal fit. If there is flattening in superior part with an steepening of inferior arc (smiley face pattern) then it indicates that lens is too flat in fit. If, there is presence of slight central steepening (central island pattern) then it indicates that lens is too

steep. Cases where no obvious topography patterns noticed during examination, then patients are advised to wear contact lenses for another 2–3 days, then again re-evaluate the fitting.

- On an average, the favorable results are obtained in about 10 days of lens wear although, duration may vary with degree of myopia, i.e. less for lower myopic and more for moderate to severe myopic patients.
- During treatment period, daily disposable lenses of progressively decreasing power should be prescribed to patient and then re-evaluate after one week time.
- Once treatment period is over, these contact lenses are worn on a retainer basis; which is every night for severe myopic patients and once a week for low myopic patients. These patients can self-monitor their retainer wear time, whenever patients notice blurring of vision for distance they can wear contact lenses overnight.

Precautions during lens wear

- To obtain optimal lens centration and to decrease corneal staining it is recommended to use highly viscous artificial tear drops before insertion of contact lens.
- Lens should not be removed immediately after awakening. Rewetting drops should be applied before removal of contact lens.
- To break the suction (if present), lower eyelid margin can be used to gently push the lower lens edge.

Complications and Maintenance of Contact Lenses

INTRODUCTION

Contact lenses can cause a wide range of changes in eye and complications related to contact lens include inflammatory, mechanical, or metabolic changes. Although risk of complications is low, but poor hygiene and improper handling of contact lenses can cause several complications. Majority of lens related problems are insignificant and without any consequences, however, sometimes serious ocular and vision threatening complications can occur. Recent advancements in contact lens materials and multipurpose cleaning solutions have reduced several risks related to extended wear but some problems still exist today.

Risk Factors Related to Complications with Contact Lens Wear

Factors related to contact lens itself

- *Materials used for contact lens:* Generally complications are more frequent in soft contact lens wearer as compared to RGP contact lens users. However, hydrogel and silicon hydrogel lenses are commonly used as daily wearer or monthly/three monthly disposable lens. As compared to other soft lenses silicon lenses have less chance to develop limbal injections, protein deposition, corneal neovascularisation and less damage to epithelium and its functions.

- *Various deposition and risk of contamination:* A large number of proteins and lipids present in the tear film can deposit on the surface of contact lenses, although on silicon hydrogel materials proteins deposition is least as compared to other materials. The deposition starts as soon as lens is placed in the eye and increases with time of wear. Deposition of proteins on surface of lens appears as thin hazy layer, and it is mostly due to deposition of denatured lysozyme, sometimes due to albumin and gamma globulin. Lipids deposition on surface appears as oily appearance on the lens surface. Sometimes excessive deposition of lipids and mucin as jelly bumps may elicit immunological reaction in conjunctiva. In daily wear lenses the quantity of deposition on lens also depends on factors like water content, chemical and ionic characteristics of hydrogel lens materials. Generally lenses with low water content show less deposition than high water content lens. Similarly, deposition of proteins is more with ionic lenses as compared to non-ionic lenses. In addition, the environmental contaminations and pollutants such as oils, dirt, lotions, make-up, powders, smoke, aerosols like perfumes and hair sprays can also deposit and contaminate the lens.

There may be deposition of bacteria, such as *Pseudomonas aeruginosa* and *Staphylococcus epidermidis*, along with several fungi and protozoa on lens surface. Bacterial infection lead to formation of a bio film on lens surface and can penetrate into lens material, especially in high water content lens, leading to increase risk of development of bacterial keratitis.

- *Deformation and damage of contact lens:* Contact lens warpage may occur due to change in various parameters of lens which can be confirmed by using a spherometer. Change in parameters of lens is indicated by bad lens fit and increased or decreased lens movement on the cornea, which further lead to injury of corneal epithelium and other complications.
- *Cleaning and care solutions for contact lens:* Complication may occur due to improper cleaning of lens. Multi-purpose solutions used to clean contact lenses, must have cleaning agents, disinfectants, preservatives and polymers or softeners to make contact lenses wearing more comfortable. Regular and proper cleaning of contact lens is must, however, improper handling of lens or solution can lead to contamination of solution itself; which gives continuous problems because patients do not change the multipurpose solution regularly.

Factors related with contact lens wearer

- *Ocular pathology:* Many eye related conditions such as vernal conjunctivitis seasonal and constant allergic conjunctivitis, atypical keratoconjunctivitis, dry eye syndrome or keratoconjunctivitis sicca, systemic diseases like thyroid diseases and dermatological conditions related to meibomian glands dysfunction act as limiting factors for contact lens wearing because the risk of complication due to contact lens wearing is increased in compromised ocular state.

- *Blinking pattern:* Chances of dryness of lens and deposition on lens are increased with less frequent blinking or incomplete blinking. There is diminution of tear exchange between contact lens and cornea which may cause retinal hypoxia. To prevent these complications it is essential to achieve full blinking by blinking exercises.
- *Intake of medicines:* Medicines like diuretics, anticholinergics, antihistamines, and antipsychotic may increase dryness of eye surface by decreasing production of tears. Constant use of steroids and other immunosuppressant drugs is associated with alteration in body defense mechanism leading to increases risk of infections in contact lens.
- *Smoking:* Due to smoking there is change in the stability of tear film as well as sensitivity of conjunctiva and cornea is reduced because due to smoking lipid layer of precorneal tear film is damaged.
- *Wearing schedule of contact lens:* Generally, contact lens wearing is associated with some physiological changes like thinning of epithelium and decrease rate of epithelium cell exchange in the eye which is further increased with use of continuous wear or extended wear contact lenses. Silicon hydrogel lens which have high oxygen transmissibility may also produce these changes but in lesser frequency. Furthermore, wearing of contact lens during night is also associated with increased risk of complications and it is assumed that silicon hydrogel lens can be prescribed for night wear if required, because of their high oxygen transmissibility.
- *Frequency of replacement of contact lens:* With continuous wearing there is ageing of polymers material of lens and chances of deposits over lens increased which are not removed completely with regular cleaning

and disinfection of lens. Nowadays, although lens with better materials are available which show less deposit formation but it is advised to prefer disposable or daily wear contact lenses causing less complications.

- *Contact lenses wearing without professional advice:* Many wearers buy contact lenses without a prescription through internet and use them irregularly with improper handling. Due to poor compliance and without professional control a large number of complications related to contact lens wear may arise.
- *Maintenance of lens in hygiene conditions:* Appropriate hygiene is very necessary for proper maintenance of contact lenses, lens cases, and cleaning solution bottles so that chances of contamination decreased. Occasionally, contact lens wearers do not follow hygiene during insertion and removal of contact lens and predisposed to infections.

Complications and Diseases Related with Contact Lens Wear

Contact lens related complications are declining gradually because of better lens material, wetting solution, awareness among wearer, and better sterility maintenance. In spite of these factors some amount of insult to ocular tissue is caused by regular wearing of contact lenses.

Problems occurring due to contact lens wear in relation to various ocular structures are summarized in Table 13.1.

Problems related to eyelids

- **Unusual blinking pattern:** Blinking abnormality may already be present in contact lens wearer however, it may precipitate due to lens wearing. Blinking abnormalities may be in the form of forced blink, partial blink, inadequate number of blinks, and dry eye. These abnormalities may lead to drying of ocular surface, lens deposits, accumulation of tears behind

Eyelid	Tear film	Conjunctiva	limbus	Cornea			
				Epithelium	Corneal stroma		Endothelium
Unusual blinking pattern	Dry eye	Conjunctival congestion	Limbal redness	Epithelial erosions	Edema of corneal stroma	CLPU (CL peripheral ulcer)	Endothelial bubbles
Ptosis	Mucin balls	Papillary conjunctivitis	Vascularized limbal keratitis	Corneal microcysts	Thinning of corneal stroma	CLARE (CL induced acute red eye)	Polymegathism/Pleomorphism
Meibomian glands dysfunction			Superiorlimbal keratoconjunctivitis	Epithelial edema	Corneal neovascularization	Infiltrative keratitis	
External hordeolum				Vacuoles	Deep stromal neovascularization	Acanthamoeba keratitis	
Internal hordeolum					Corneal stromal pannus		
Squamous blepharitis							

Table 13.1: Contact lens wear complications related to various ocular structures

contact lens, corneal hypoxia or hyper-capnia, epithelial erosions specifically at 3 and 9 o'clock positions, reduction in tear break up time. Blinking training or exercise will help to improve blinking and thus reduction in signs and symptoms.

- **Ptosis:** It is commonly seen in RGP lens wearers, there may be reduction of palpebral aperture due to edema of ocular tissue. Edema may occur due to injury obtained during frequent insertion and removal of contact lenses. Other factors which may predispose it are forced pressing of eyelids, extension of lateral eyelid, papillary conjunctivitis (GPC) and blepharospasm. To treat these conditions RGP lenses should not be wear for up to three months, treat GPC with proper anti-allergic and lubricants, use soft contact lenses and in very severe cases eyelid surgery shall be performed.

- **Dysfunction of Meibomian glands:** It is due to mechanical blockage of Meibomian glands ducts leading to collection of yellowish creamy secretions and drying of eye. Contact lens does not receive sufficient hydration, hence causing dry eye and intolerance to contact lens. This condition can be treated by applying warm compressions over eyelids, using lubricants eye drops, improvement of eyelid hygiene. In severe cases antibiotics therapy and eyelid scrubbing can be done.

- **External hordeolum:** Commonly known as stye. It is characterized by an inflammation of eyelash root tissue or sometimes associated with inflammation of gland of Zeis or Moll. It is an acute infection caused by Staphylococcus common in those having associated staphylococcal squamous blepharitis. It manifests as infectious swelling of external lid edge and cause discomfort and pain. Treatment includes removal of eyelash related to that gland along with hot compressions which facilitates the spontaneous drainage of abscesses outside. Topical and systemic antibiotics are also prescribed for 5–7 days period along with other symptomatic drugs. Use of contact lens should be avoided during acute phase, usually about 7–10 days.

- **Internal hordeolum:** An acute staphylococcal infection of meibomian gland is called internal hordeolum and it is also frequently associated with staphylococcal squamous blepharitis. Patient presents with lid swelling with eyelid edge inversion and discomfort, pain and intolerance to contact lenses. General treatment includes application of hot compressions and antibiotics for 5–7 days, along with other symptomatic drugs. Contact lens wearing is not recommended during this acute phase, usually about seven days.

- **Squamous blepharitis:** Infection by Staphylococcus may cause conjunctivitis, staphylococcal infection of follicles of eyelash and toxic punctal epitheliopathy. Patient will present with diffuse redness, scales at roots of eyelash, sticky eyelashes, along with feeling of warmth, intense itching, and photophobia with foreign body sensation leading to an intolerance of contact lenses. Treatment includes antibiotics, corticosteroids (as ointment), artificial tears, and improvement of eyelid hygiene. Contact lenses should not be worn during this acute phase, usually variable in duration, because of periods of remission and recurrence of this condition.

Problems related to tear film

- **Dry eye:** Dry eye in contact lens wearer may occur due to increased evaporation of tear film. In contact lens wearer the tear film remains compromised and there is limited mobility as well as exchange of lipid deposits on the surface of lens. As a result disintegration of lipids occurs at rapid rate leading to decrease in lubrication of lens. Other mechanisms proposed for dryness are decrease production of tears due to increase in osmolality, ocular surface inflammation and lack of biocompatibility of the lens surface. Treatment measures include change of contact lens thickness, material and design, along with solution used for caring of lenses. Artificial tear drops, control of tear evaporation, reduction of tear drainage and reduction in time of contact lens wear are other measures to be done to control the dry eye situations.

- **Mucins balls:** With contact lens wearing, the production of mucus may alter, leading to change in characteristics of tear film and lens surface. There may be accumulation of balls of mucin under the lens surface which appears as tiny grey points on slit lamp examination. Normal corneal defense mechanism of cornea and visual acuity may compromise due to mucin balls. Usually more common with use of silicon hydrogel contact lenses. This condition can be corrected by fitting of a flatter contact lens, contact lens must be replaced frequently along with change in lens material. Artificial tear drops along with mast cell stabilizers should be added. A drastic improvement in condition will occur soon after contact lens is taken out of eye.

Problems related to conjunctiva

- **Conjunctival congestion:** Due to presence of contact lens, toxicity of contact lens solution or change in pH may lead to irritation, immunologic reaction, hypoxia, hypercapnia and relaxation of smooth muscles, causing vasodilatation of conjunctival vessels. This condition is usually asymptomatic, however, sometimes itching, slight irritation along with feeling of hot or cold sensation may be seen. If severe redness occurs, then contact lenses should not be used until complete healing occurs.
- **Contact lens associated papillary conjunctivitis (CLAPC):** Due to immunological mechanism, deposits present on contact lens (especially proteins) act as allergen and causes thickening of conjunctiva. Patients

having allergic conditions like asthma, hay fever or general allergies are more prone for development of papillary conjunctivitis. Common symptoms are itching which is more intense at time of removal of lens because of more degranulation of mast cells due to handling on eyelids, more mucus discharge (especially in the morning), discomfort to contact lens and intense photophobia and slight blurring of vision. On examination, giant papillae on upper tarsal conjunctiva (like cobble stone) along with conjunctival oedema and hyperaemia are seen. Management includes removal of contact lens (until inflammation is over), reduction in time of lens wear, change of lens material, reduction in time of lens change, change of lens care solution and improvement of eye hygiene. Mast cell stabilizers like sodium cromoglycate and steroid eye drops are used to treat these papillae for nearly a period of 4–6 weeks. However, these giant papillae may remain for weeks, months, or even years, hence contact lenses can be worn with control of acute phase with all the precautions mentioned above.

Problems related to limbus

- **Limbal redness:** It is similar to conjunctival congestion and may be partial or complete. There is vasodilatation, contributed by hypoxia, hypercapnia, mechanical irritation, immunological reaction, infection, inflammation (acute red eye). Management includes removal of cause and fitting of a silicon hydrogel contact lens.
- **Vascularized limbal keratitis:** It is a complication usually seen in rigid contact lens wearer involving cornea, limbus and conjunctiva. On examination, an elevated vascularised epithelial lesion is seen at limbus along with conjunctival oedema and corneal vascularization. Corneal infiltrates are present near the limbus, with positive fluorescein staining around limbus. Common presentation is discomfort, lacrimation and photophobia. Management

includes shortening of contact lens wear time and changes in lens design, i.e reduce the overall diameter, increase edge lift and/or more flat base curve. Antibiotic, ocular lubricating and steroid eye drops are given for 5–7 days and RGP lenses should be removed during this phase; however, soft contact lenses can be fitted later on. Prognosis is usually good and condition heals within 1–2 weeks time.

- **Superior or upper limbal keratoconjunctivitis:** It is another contact lens related inflammatory condition, mainly occur due to hypersensitivity to preservatives of contact lens solution, especially thiomersol. Patients generally complain of foreign body sensation with redness, itching and photophobia. In case of extensive pannus there may be an associated diminution of visual acuity. On examination limbus, bulbar and tarsal conjunctiva, and cornea involvement seen in the form of redness on superior limbus with infiltrates, micro-pannus, and micro-erosions of cornea and/or conjunctiva are seen. Irregular superior cornea and epithelial and subepithelial infiltration of superior cornea along with hypertrophy of superior bulbar conjunctiva also found. Management includes immediate removal of lens and application of lubricating eye drops along with non-steroidal anti-inflammatory drugs until inflammation disappears. Usually redness disappears early but epithelium takes time to heal, hence treatment is continued for 3 weeks to a few months. Later on patient can be prescribed lens with different design or polymer which cause less mechanical irritation of limbus. Patients should also be instructed about change of lens care solution, reduction in time of lens wear and use of preservative free contact lens.

Problems related to cornea

Contact lens can affect epithelium, stroma and endothelium of cornea leading to various complications.

Effect on epithelium of cornea: Wearing of contact lens may cause erosion and edema of epithelium and formation of microcysts on epithelium of cornea.

- **Corneal epithelial erosions:** The surface defect of corneal epithelium or breakdown of epithelium in contact lens wearers may present as small lesions or large lesions with different shapes and locations. The lesions can be identified through fluorescein test as staining areas because fluorescein dye will enter in the inter-cellular space where epithelium is eroded. Healthy epithelium remains unstained with fluorescein. Small lesions affecting superficial layer of epithelium generally do not pose any problem to patient and can be treated by prescribing lubricating eye drops. Symptoms in the form of foreign body sensations, severe pain and rarely photophobia arise when there is involvement of large area and epithelium is affected up to deeper extent. Erosions may be seen at different areas of cornea

1. *Erosions at three and nine o'clock position:* Usually more common in persons using RGP type contact lens and appears mainly due to interruption of tear flow leading to local dehydration and death of epithelial cells. Lesions are mainly present laterally and inferiorly on the cornea, the sites where upper and lower lids are in contact during blinking. Thus, insufficient or incomplete blinking and elevations of lids (due to thick edge of lens) so that a gap is created adjacent to lens edge leading to drying of tissue. To prevent this it is advised to patient to perform blinking exercises with tears supplements. Fitting of contact lens having small diameter or reduced thickness can be considered.

2. *Superior epithelial arcuate lesion (SEAL):* More commonly seen in silicon hydrogel lens users, wearing lens of improper design and elasticity. The upper lid creates an inward pressure on the contact

lens and results in excessive mechanical friction pressure on the epithelium and ultimately its disruption. The lesions involve the full thickness of epithelium and seen in that area which is covered by upper eyelid, i.e. within 2 to 3 mm of superior limbus and parallel to it. Patient usually remains asymptomatic, however, sometimes may complaint of slight discomfort in wearing contact lenses for longer duration. To manage this contact lens of either less elastic material or a hard RGP lens, should be chosen.

3. *Inferior epithelial arcuate lesions:* The arc-shaped lesion (smile stain) is present parallel to the inferior limbus, usually associated with soft contact lens with less mobility. It also results from insufficient blinking causing drying out of contact lens and consequent necrosis of epithelium. Management includes changing the contact lens with more thickness with better movability on corneal surface. Material of soft contact lens is changed or select a hard RGP lens.

4. *Central corneal epithelium erosions:* More common in extended hydrogel lens wearer. There is complete loss of epithelium from large area of cornea, seen as circular staining with fluorescein. Exposure of epithelium to hypoxia for prolonged time results in loss of its function and ultimately epithelium get completely detached when lens is removed. It is advised to remove the lens for recovery of epithelium which may take 7–10 days. Contact lens having high oxygen transmissibility should be prescribed later on.

Sometimes, any foreign body entrapped beneath hard contact lens can also damage the corneal epithelial surface, seen as irregular lines with fluorescein stain. Management includes removal and thorough rinsing of contact lens in multipurpose solution and then reinsertion.

- **Corneal microcysts or microbullae:** Microcysts are small (15–50 micrometer diameter) circular or oval-shaped points scattered on the cornea. Usually common with extended hydrogel contact lens wearers. The microcysts formation occurs due to chronic hypoxia, trauma or mechanical irritation caused by lens, poor movement of lens and accumulation of debris in intercellular spaces. Microcysts in small number are well tolerated and do not need treatment. If present in large numbers and causing discomfort and decreased vision, then use silicon hydrogel or hard RGP contact lenses instead of extended hydrogels. After discontinuation of contact lens, the number of microcysts are increased in the first few days due to increased metabolic activity, however, then they start to decrease and completely disappear within two months.

- **Epithelial edema:** During adaptive phase of lens wear especially of hard contact lens there is reflex tearing which results in decrease tonicity of precorneal tear fluid. Due to this hypotoncity of precorneal tear film, water get enter in the epithelial cells of cornea. Commonly this condition is asymptomatic, however, halo effects can be seen in a few cases. Management includes changing the adaptation regime for hard contact lens.

- **Vacuoles:** Like microcysts these are also small (5–30 micrometer diameter) circular scattered points filled with clear fluid. These vacuoles differ from microcysts in a manner that their shadow is formed opposite to the direction of light as compared to formation of shadow in the same direction of light in case of microcysts. Vacuoles are formed due to hypoxia and are usually asymptomatic. Usually no treatment is required for vacuoles because they disappear soon after removal of contact lenses.

Effect on stroma of cornea: Change in thickness and transparency of corneal stroma may occur due to chronic hypoxia induced by contact lens wearing. Various changes observed in stroma of cornea due to contact lens wear can be grouped as

- **Edema of corneal stroma:** Accumulation of fluid into corneal stroma leads to increase in the thickness and distortion of the cornea. The main factor responsible for stromal edema is chronic hypoxia. Due to hypoxic stress (anaerobic respiration in stroma) there is increased production of lactates in the stroma causing elevation of osmotic pressure within the stroma and ultimately tissue swelling or edema. Other factors like hypotonic characteristic of tears, hyper-capnia and low temperatures also contribute in edema. Percentage increase in the thickness of cornea is correlated with amount of edema. Up to 2% increase in the thickness of cornea is not associated with significant damage and hence no treatment is needed. Thickening of cornea up to 8% due to edema is dangerous and on examination striae and folds are seen in posterior stroma. To manage this condition, contact lenses with materials having higher oxygen transmissi-bility, thinner design and better movement on the cornea should be fitted. In severe edema it is recommended to remove contact lenses for longer duration (3–4 months).

- **Thinning of corneal stroma:** Edema of corneal stroma for prolonged period results in decrease of stromal mass which ultimately become visible as stromal thinning (measured by Pachymetry after disappearance of the edema). It is important to treat the cause of stromal edema for prevention of stromal thinning. This tissue loss is irreversible and corneal thickness remains permanently the same which cannot be recovered to original state before onset of stromal edema. Management includes removal of contact lens perma-nently, if not possible, then use contact lenses having high oxygen transmissibility.

- **Corneal surface neovascularization:** Surface neovascularization may occur due to chronic hypoxia or release of inflammatory mediators from damaged epithelium. Due to hypoxia, accumulation of lactates promotes softening of stroma which further induces in growth of new vessels. Release of inflammatory mediators also promotes migration of inflammatory cells which stimulate growth of vessels in stroma of cornea by releasing vaso-proliferative agents. Usually, in mild to moderate cases the person remain asymptomatic. In severe case if central cornea is involved, then loss of vision may occur. In severe corneal neovascularisation, the use of contact lenses should be stopped permanently. However, in mild to moderate cases contact lens can be used with proper care and maintenance, contact lens with higher oxygen transmissi-bility, i.e. more gas permeable lens should be used and daily wearing time of lens should be reduced.

- **Deep stromal neovascularisation:** Deep neovascularisation can develop in deeper layers of stroma, but it is slow in onset. Corneal hypoxia induced by lens especially by low oxygen permeable lens and thick lens results in softening of stroma due to edema. Furthermore, neovascularisation can also be precipitated by infection and toxic reactions due to lens solutions. In mild case progression of neovascularisation can be stopped by improving the handling of contact lenses, using lens of high dK/L value, reduction in schedule of daily lens wear and careful monitoring of condition. In severe cases, wearing of lens should be completely stopped.

- **Corneal vascular pannus:** Corneal pannus means growth of fibrovascular limbal tissue and fine blood vessels on the surface of cornea. Hypoxia induced by lens wearing (causing stromal edema) and damage of epithelium of cornea due to infection are important precipitating factors for formation of pannus. Generally, it does not cause difficulty to patient, but in extreme cases it can cause reduction of visual acuity. In mild cases, replace lens material with better oxygen transmissibility, reduce schedule time of daily lens wearing and careful monitoring of pannus progression. In cases of severe pannus, contact lens wearing should be permanently stopped and pannus is treated surgically.

- **Contact lens peripheral ulcer (CLPU):** It is rare with daily wear, more commonly seen with extended contact lens wear. A small (0.5–1.0 mm), distinctive circular ulcer or infiltrate with clear defined margin appears at periphery of the cornea. It is noninfectious and usually develops due to action of toxins on hypoxic cornea released from gram-positive bacteria. There is redness of eyes, pain, foreign body sensation and mild photophobia. Management includes removal of contact lens, start appropriate antibiotics, analgesics and steroids in topical and systemic form as per severity of condition.

- **Contact lens induced acute red eye (CLARE) or tight lens syndrome:** It is an acute inflammatory reaction affecting cornea and conjunctiva, presents in early morning when patient use an extended wear contact lens for overnight and eyes remain closed for long period. There is hyperaemia of conjunctiva and periphery of cornea. It occurs due to release of endotoxins from gram-negative bacteria contaminating beneath lens or in lens care solution. Symptoms are characterized by severe pain, excessive lacrimation, severe photophobia and severe conjunctival injection. On examination, punctal and diffuse infiltrates are seen in corneal periphery along with signs of inflammation. Management includes immediate removal of contact lenses, antibiotic treatment and anti-inflammatory drugs. Once the red eye is completely settled, contact lenses with high Dk/t for daily wear use can be fitted.

- **Infectious keratitis (IK):** A unilateral inflammatory reaction in anterior corneal stroma is seen where numerous small infiltrates of irregular shape are present in peripheral area along with bulbar redness. It occurs due to infection of corneal epithelium and stroma by microbes mainly pseudomonas, leading to inflammatory reaction and necrosis of tissue. There is loss of corneal epithelium with stromal infiltration and corneal ulcer. Patient presents with extreme red eye with surrounding swollen and inflamed ocular tissue, severe pain, irritation, excessive lacrimation, photophobia, purulent discharge diminished visual acuity. The incidence of infectious keratitis is more with extended hydrogel lens than daily wear RGP lens. Other predisposing factors are warm climate, poor hygiene, non-compliance with contact lens wear and care instructions, swimming with contact lenses, hypoxia, mechanical trauma, dry eye, smoking, diabetes. Treatment includes immediate removal of contact lens, proper antibiotics and anti-inflammatory drugs.

- **Acanthamoeba keratitis:** Infection by protozoa acanthamoeba is not so common in contact lens wearer usually persons having poor immunologic response are more affected. Infection can occur with any type of lens but more common with soft type of lens. Early signs of acanthamoeba keratitis appear as dendriform keratitis, subepithelial infiltrates and diffuse coarse punctate epithelial keratopathy. Later on, it can invade the stroma also. Treatment includes removal of contact lenses and application of topical neomycin and propamidine isethionate with or without oral ketoconazole. After recovery the RGP lenses with high Dk/t can be fitted with the instructions regarding the wearing and handling of contact lenses.

Effect on endothelium of cornea: The endothelium of cornea has important role in preventing the excessive swelling of stroma. The various changes may occur in endothelium by all types of contact lens but these are more common with the use of low gas permeable lens.

- **Endothelial bubbles (blebs) response:** The bleb response (focal, circumscribed defects in endothelium) occurs due to edema of endothelium which is precipitated by acidic pH change caused by corneal hypoxia. It may appear within a few minutes after insertion of contact lens and is subsides rapidly after removal of lens (i.e. reversible). Endothelial blebs usually do not require any treatment but development of blebs indicates presence of hypoxia in the eye due to lens wearing. Occasionally, blebs are in large numbers, then a contact lens with higher *Dk/t* should be prescribed.

- **Endothelial cells polymegathism and pleomorphism:** Endothelial polymegathism (i.e. significant variation in the size of endothelial cells) and pleomorphism (i.e. variation in shape of endothelial cells) may occur due to use of lens of poor oxygen transmissibility (PMMA wearers or extended wear lens) for a long period. Chronic hypoxic stress and hypercapnia due to contact lens wearing lead to weakening of junctions between endothelial cells followed by change in their shape and size. The cornea in presence of polymegathism swells at faster rate than normal cornea. Wearers will complaint of discomfort and intolerance with lens. Management includes fitting of contact lenses with high oxygen transmissibility and reduction in duration of daily lens wear.

MAINTENANCE AND CARE OF CONTACT LENSES

Introduction

Maintenance and care of contact lenses by its wearer is most critical step to decide the success rate and satisfaction in contact lens wearer patients. Different regimen can be used for care of lens and choice of regimen will depend on many factors including type of lens and its material, specific patient needs, lifestyle or wearing schedule of contact lens. Triad of prescribed good contact lens, patient compliance for lens and monitoring by professional at periodic interval decide the outcome of safe and effective contact lens wear.

Aims of care and maintenance of contact lens are

- Provide comfortable lens wear
- Minimize and/or prevent contamination by microbes
- Decrease deposits formation on contact lens
- Maintain availability of contact lenses in ready wear status

To achieve these aims, various maintenance products are used, which serve following functions to keep the contact lens in wearable state

- Keep the lens clean
- Maintain wetting/re-wetting of lens
- Prevention of infection
- Removal of protein deposits
- Maintain physical and chemical state of contact lens

Elements of maintenance and care: The maintenance and care system of contact lenses consists of following elements to deliver an effective result

- Personal care
- Contact lens solutions
- Disinfecting agents
- Preservative agents
- Protein removal process
- Lens storage system

Personal Care

Personal hygiene of contact lens wearer remains the most important first step in maintenance and care of contact lens. Person using contact lenses should keep his/her nails properly trimmed and hands should be washed thoroughly with soap and water prior to using contact lenses. Then, dry the hands and use antimicrobial rubs, if possible before removal of lenses from lens case. Use of any oil-based solutions like cream or ointments before handling the contact lenses should be avoided because, it may cause deposition of lipids over lens surfaces. Hence, foremost important aspect of a good contact lens wear outcome starts with a proper handling and caring of contact lens during insertion or removal.

Contact Lens Solutions

Various solutions are used for care and to maintain contact lens in good condition and for comfortable wear. These solutions are routinely used by the contact lens wearer and purchased by users along with lenses. For convenience of understanding we can group these contact lens care solutions as

- Cleaning agents
- Rinsing solutions
- Wetting and lubricating drops
- Multipurpose solution

Cleaning agents or solution: Lens surface can be cleaned manually by rubbing and rinsing with saline or by using cleaning solutions on daily basis. These cleaning solutions generally consist of surfactants which act on the contact lens surface to remove most loosely attached foreign substances like lipids, residues, dirt, mucus, proteins, microbes or other deposits. Cleaning of lens is very important step to remove the cysts and trophozoites of acanthamoeba from surface of lens. The cleaners may be available in a separate bottle or may be combined with disinfecting/soaking solution in one bottle. Along with surfactants other agents can be added in cleaning agent like

- Different non-ionic or ionic chemical substances, added to decrease contact between lens and the solution
- Agents acting against microbes are also added in daily cleaner
- Agents which maintains osmolality
- Buffer system to regulate the pH
- Chelating agents for removal of contaminants from lens

- Abrasive material as adjunct to remove adherent substances or muco-proteinaceous deposits from surface of lens which cannot be removed by surfactant itself. However, use of abrasive material or excessive rubbing can lead to scratches and may induce change in power to contact lenses.
- Agents like polyvinyl alcohol or methylcellulose as viscosity enhancers
- Alcohol to remove lipids

The cleaning agents may be of two types

Surfactant cleaners: These agents have detergent like action and by reducing surface tension act as surface active agent. Surfactants have both hydrophobic and hydrophilic components and molecules of surfactant combine with different type of debris or residues and deposits on lens, as a result, a layer of surfactant molecules is formed over contaminant (micelles formation), surface tension get decrease and it causes dispersion of contaminant from contact lens surface which get suspend in surrounding liquid and finally removed by rinsing. Some common examples of surfactants are isopropyl alcohol, hexylene glycol, polyvinyl alcohol, poloxamine, poloxamer-407, octylphenoxy ethanol, etc. Surfactants are able to remove lipid, inorganic deposits, mucus, etc. however, they are not much effective for removal of proteins.

Enzymatic cleaners: As surfactants cannot remove protein effectively, hence enzymatic cleaners can be used which contain proteolytic enzymes to break down proteins from surface of lens. However, use of these cleaners is not obligatory and not used on daily basis. Enzyme cleaners are usually used for types of lens which are not replaced frequently and are nondisposable.

Cleaning procedure: Principle is Rub and Rinse of lens. Contact lenses should be cleaned every time before insertion and after removal to get a complication free result. Following steps are done for cleaning of lenses

- Thoroughly wash hands and dry them (avoid moisturizing cream/perfumed soaps before cleaning).

- Place the contact lens in palm of hand.
- Pour 4–5 drops of cleaning agent on each surface of contact lens.
- Gently rub contact lens using pulp of forefinger, for about 15–20 seconds per side in a circular motion. Slowly roll forefinger in both directions to clean periphery of lens.
- Rinse well using rinsing solution.

Process of rubbing and rinsing is important because it significantly helps in removal of loose debris and many microbes from contact lens surface. Cleaning should be done on daily basis for all types of contact lenses including disposable lenses.

Rinsing solutions: Cleaning of lens is followed by rinsing. The purpose of rinsing is to remove surfactant cleaners, microorganisms and suspended residues from the surface of lens completely, irrespective of the type of cleaning agent. It is advised to rinse all types of contact lenses and before and after overnight soak. Various types of solutions which can be used for rinsing are

- Unpreserved saline
- Preserved saline
- Multi-purpose solutions.

Rinsing should not be done with tap water due to increase risk of infection with acanthamoeba.

Buffering agents are also added in rinsing solution and usually buffered isotonic saline is more preferred as compared to un-buffered saline.

Wetting and Lubricant drops: These drops are used, while contact lens is in the eye and before insertion of lens in eye where these agents provide lubrication and rewetting of contact lens surface. Standard wetting drops contain following components in a proportionate amount, to increase the comfort and duration of contact lens wear.

- Non-ionic surfactant in very low concentrations to promote cleaning of lens
- Polymer for lubricating the lens surface
- Buffering agents to compile pH of tears

- Viscosity agents to reduce friction
- Preservatives for maintaining the sterility of drops.

In patients, who use extended wear or continuous wear contact lenses, use of these wetting and lubricant drops are very helpful for wearers, although drops can also be used with daily wear lenses. These are especially indicated on those patients who have relative tear deficiency and use contact lens during sleeping also, who work in dry atmosphere and work for prolonged period on computers, etc. These wetting and lubricants prevent the contact lens from dryness due to wind exposure, low humidity and high temperatures. Patients facing difficulty in removing soft hydrogel lenses because of dehydration or the one who frequently damages his/her lenses on removal will also be benefited by use of lubricants.

Wetting and lubricating drops are also formulated with various viscosity enhancing agents like

- Polyvinyl alcohol
- Methylcellulose and hydroxyl methylcellulose
- Hydroxy propyl methylcellulose (HPMC)
- Polyethylene glycol
- Polysorbate 80

Presence of viscous agents in lubricants helps to increase the contact of solution with lens and also help to decrease the friction. These viscosity agents help to maintain the relative density of cleaners, soaking solution and lubricants. Usually, cleaners are kept more viscous than lubricants while lubricants kept more viscous than soaking agents.

Note

Viscosity order: Cleaners > lubricants > soaking agents.

Multi-purpose solutions: Most widely used solution for maintenance and care of contact lenses is multipurpose solution. As name suggests this single solution performs functions of several components of lens care system, hence reduces the requirement of actual number of lens care solutions.

For patient convenience and ease of utilization, this multi-purpose solution performs a combined function of cleaning, rinsing and disinfection. Moreover, in newer solutions even protein remover agents are also added to enhance efficacy of solution and reduce another maintenance step in contact lens care.

Disinfecting Agents for Care of Contact Lens

Disinfection means removal and/or killing of microorganisms (microbes, fungi and viruses) from contact lenses and is important step to be followed after daily cleaning and rinsing of lens. In contact lens wearer the natural defence mechanism of eye remains compromised, i.e. protective barrier function of corneal epithelium affected and there are more chances of infection by microorganisms. Thus, disinfecting contact lens care solutions are used to minimize or kill potentially harmful micro-organisms (bacteria, viruses, amoebas, fungi) along with maintenance of contact lens hydration. By disinfection the living or vegetative microorganisms are destroyed but not the spores of microorganisms. Sterilization is a process which kills all life form of microorganisms including their spores and it is impossible to achieve sterilization with normal lens care solutions.

The disinfection for contact lens can be done mainly by two techniques

- Disinfection based on heat (thermal disinfection)
- Disinfection based on chemical methods (chemical disinfection)

Disinfection based on heat: As the name indicates heat is used to deactivate or kills most of living contaminants from contact lens. Normally sterile thiomersol, persevered (with potassium sorbate) saline or unpreserved saline are used as medium to boil the lens. Boiling of lens can be done by keeping it in a bowl filled with saline and boiled for 10–15 min in range of 70–90°C. A saline-based solution containing thiomersol with EDTA can also be used, where EDTA helps in removal of calcium from contact lens surface. Thermal disinfection method should not be used with high water content lens.

Advantages

- Very effective method for disinfection
- No associated allergic reactions or discomfort

Disadvantages

- Decreased life span of lens due to alteration in property of lens
- Discoloration of lens with time due to heating
- Reduction in water content of lens especially high water content lens
- Change in optical and physical properties of lens due to exposure to heat
- Warpage of lens due to denaturation of proteins

Chemical-based disinfection systems: Wide varieties of chemical-based disinfection systems are present for disinfection of contact lenses that can grouped as follows

- Conventional cold chemical disinfectant-based solution
- Hydrogen peroxide-based system
- Chlorine system

Conventional cold chemical disinfectant-based solutions: Ideal characteristics required in chemical disinfectants are

- Non-toxicity
- Non-irritating
- Compatible with other ingredients
- Stable over time
- Effective against a wide range of micro-organisms

Many chemical agents such as chlorhexidine, benzalkonium chloride, thiomersol, and sorbic acid are used as disinfectant solution, although with caution because they may cause sensitivity reactions.

- *Chlorhexidine gluconate (CHG):* It is a biguanide antimicrobial agent, mainly effective against bacteria. It has no antifungal activity. It can be used as preservative and disinfectant with thiomersol for both soft and hard contact lenses. It can bind with lens materials and with protein deposits and cause allergic reactions. Its breakdown product may cause yellowish discoloration of lens.

- *Benzalkonium chloride (BAK):* It is a quaternary ammonium compound and can be used as disinfectant and preservative with ophthalmic solution for PMMA lenses. It acts as cidal agent against many bacteria and fungi. BAK is not used in solution for hydrogel lens (e.g. silicon acrylate and fluorosilicon acrylate) because it binds with lens materials, lens being gas permeable also absorb BAK which can accumulate to toxic levels and may cause eye injury. Additionally, BAK also increases hydrophobicity of lens surface, chances of deposit formation increased. Normal concentration of BAK in contact lens care solution is 0.001–0.01% and it is more active at alkaline medium (pH = 8). It shows synergistic action with EDTA and require in low dose when combined with it.

- *Thimerosal:* It is a mercurial compound having bacteriocidal activity against many bacteria and fungi. It can be used both as a preservative (0.001%) and as a disinfectant (0.0005%) and acts by inhibiting the activity of cellular enzymes leading to killing of micro-organism. Its activity is maximal at neutral or slightly alkaline pH and usually used in the concentration of 0.001–0.2% in the solution. It is comparatively nontoxic but in some patients it may cause allergic reactions especially in persons wearing hydrophilic contact lens. It should not be combined with EDTA because its activity is reduced with EDTA. When compared with BAK, it shows less activity against some gram-positive and gram-negative micro-organism than BAK. To achieve effective antimicrobial action it can be combined with other preservatives like chlorhexidine, etc.

- *Sorbic acid:* Sorbates or sorbic acid act as antibacterial and antifungal agent and is added in contact lens saline as enhancing agent. When used alone it usually does not cause any allergic reactions but in formulation with other compound it may cause burning sensations due to change in the pH of solution (as it is acidic in nature). It may cause yellow or brown discolouration of contact lenses by reacting with amino acids present in tear proteins.

Hydrogen peroxide-based system: In this system, microorganisms are exposed to oxidative atmosphere by using 3% peroxide concentration with an acidic pH of 3–4. Hydrogen peroxide is effective against majority of all microbes responsible for infection in contact lens wearer. Residual hydrogen peroxide on lens after disinfection process may cause irritation on eyes, hence it is necessary to do neutralization of peroxide by using substances like sodium pyruvate, sodium bicarbonate, sodium thiosulphite, and catalase. The hydrogen peroxide get decompose into saline and oxygen. Disinfection by hydrogen peroxide for bacteria and viruses requires its exposure for about 10–15 minutes (45 minutes for fungi, 2–3 hours for acanthoemaba) followed by neutralization for about 30 min–3 hours.

The disinfecting solutions based on hydrogen peroxide may contain preservative or may be preservative free. Depending on the method adopted to neutralize the peroxide, two types of peroxide lens care systems can be used for disinfection with hydrogen peroxide

- One-step disinfecting system
- Two-step disinfecting system

One-step system: These systems are formulated in such a manner that both disinfection and neutralization of hydrogen peroxides is done in a recommended time period (30–60 minutes). This is very simple to use and usually most of the hydrogen peroxide get neutralize in first 30–60 minutes. These systems are either tablet using systems or a disc-based system. In tablet using systems delay period is done during neutralization phase, whereas in disc-based systems no delay is done during neutralization phase. The effectiveness of this system can be improved by controlling the rate of neutralization of hydrogen peroxide.

Two-step system: System where neutralization of contact lens is done as a separate step is called two-step disinfecting system. Thus in this system the neutralizing agent in the form of tablets is added separately during disinfection process. These tablets release catalase enzyme to neutralize the hydrogen peroxide so that it reaches to safe residual level. The main advantage with this system is that the neutralization of hydrogen peroxide can be delayed according to requirement so that high peroxide concentration remains maintained for a long time which will enhance the antimicrobial effect of solution compared to one-step system. Recommended method for two-step system disinfection is that contact lenses are kept in hydrogen peroxide solution overnight, then neutralize the lenses just before their usage.

Advantages of hydrogen peroxide system

- Rapidly kill most types of micro-organisms in large numbers
- Takes very short time period, usually a soaking time of 10–20 minutes.
- High anti-microbial efficacy
- Decomposition products (oxygen and water) are non-toxic in nature.

Disadvantages of hydrogen peroxide system

- If not neutralized properly, it can cause irritation to eyes

> **Note**
>
> Multi-step hydrogen peroxide systems although available; but are very complex and can confuse patients.

- Once completely neutralized, has no antimicrobial activity
- Occasionally not compatible with contact lenses such as high water content, ionic contact lenses; where this system can alter (reversibly) lens parameters and water content.

Chlorine Systems: For disinfection of soft contact lenses anhydrous effervescent tablets of either stabilized halane or halazone benzoic acid are used in convenient blister pack, where both these tablets differ in amount of available chlorine (4–8 ppm).

These chlorine releasing tablets are dissolved in unpreserved saline (~10 ml), which forms a disinfecting solution having pH in range of 5.5–7.5. Recommended exposure time is usually four hours, however, concentration of undissociated hypochlorous acid decides the effectiveness of antimicrobial activity. Contact lenses should be rinsed thoroughly before insertion into eyes.

Dissociated hypochlorous acid produces hypochlorite and chlorine which also act as bleaching agents, hence contact lenses tinted with reactive dyes may change color.

Preservative Systems

Preservatives are used usually with other chemical agents. These are used to either kill or inhibit the growth of microorganisms. An ideal preservative present in contact lens solution

1. Should provide effective degree of disinfection in the existing environment
2. Should be nontoxic
3. Should be compatible with lens material and tear film, i.e. no effect on wettability and parameters of lens

Commonly used preservatives are

- Benzalkonium chloride
- Chlorhexidine

- Thiomerosal
- Chlorbutanol
- Benzyl alcohol
- EDTA
- PAPB and PHMB
- Quaternary ammonium compounds

Chlorbutanol: It is an unstable volatile preservative with a characteristic smell. Basically, it is used as chlorinated alcohol (0.5%) along with other preservatives. Although it has broad spectrum action on bacteria in acidic pH, however, it acts slowly. Initially, it was used to disinfect PMMA lenses, but now it is rarely used. It remains stable at low pH, at high pH it get break into hydrocarbons and HCl.

Benzyl Alcohol: It can be used both as a preservative and disinfectant. Pure benzyl alcohol because of its physio-chemical properties is considered as ideal preservative. It has low molecular weight and can enter easily into intermolecular spaces of lens polymers. Being bipolar molecule it has low polarity. It is more stable than chlorbutanol, water soluble and can be used to disinfect and preserve RGP and PMMA lenses. Benzyl alcohol is not suitable for hydrophilic materials because it can interact with contact lens and may cause irritation and toxicity to eye. It is converted into aldehydes, leading to hardening and discoloration of soft contact lens. It is effective against both bacteria and virus but not active against *Pseudomonas aeruginosa*.

EDTA (Ethylene diamine tetra acetic acid): EDTA *per se* is not a true preservative rather it acts as a chelating agent, preservative enhancers and potentiator. It has no antimicrobial action but it potentiates the antibacterial action of other quaternary ammonium preservatives against gram-negative micro-organisms especially pseudomonas. In addition, because of chelating property it binds with divalent cations like calcium and magnesium present in solutions or on the cell walls of gram-negative organisms which is necessary to prevent cell growth of microbes. EDTA does not interact with lens material and is used in combination with BAK and other preservatives in most contact lens solution.

Poly aminopropyl biguanide (PAPB) and Poly hexamethlene biguanide (PHMB): PAPB and PHMB both are high molecular weight preservatives, specially developed to avoid the problem of ocular irritation and hypersensitivity occurring due to previous preservatives. PHMB is used in the concentration of 0.001% and show broad spectrum antimicrobial action and less toxicity.

PAPB which is also known as Dymed contains positively charged biguanide group which selectively bind to negatively charged phospholipids of membrane of micro-organisms, leading to disintegration of micro-organism. It is nonirritating, nonsensitive and has more antimicrobial effect as compared to chlorhexidine. It can be used as preservative and disinfectant in very low concentration of 0.00005–0.0005%.

Quaternary ammonium compound (Polyquad): These high molecular weight cationic polymers like poly quaternium-1, polidromium chloride, Onamer M are effective antibacterial but show less antifungal activity. Polyquad in the concentrations of 0.001–0.005% can be used as disinfectant and preservative for both rigid and soft lenses. Quaternary ammonium compound being large in molecular structure cannot adhere and enter into lens material, thus chances of ocular reactions are less.

Note

Opti-Free and Opti-Free Express (Alcon): contain Poly quaternium-1.

Protein removal process or enzymatic cleaners: Enzymatic cleaners contain proteolytic enzymes like papaine, pancreatin, lipase, subtilisin, etc. and are included in lens care systems for removal of proteins from surfaces of contact lens. The enzyme cleaners can be used once a week or more frequently depending on the length of lens wear, for example: Disposable lens usually do not require treatment with enzymatic cleaners while soft and some RGP lenses require it because they are not replaced frequently. Papaine containing cleaners are not compatible with hydrogen peroxide and thermal disinfection.

For protein removal, the enzyme tablets are dissolved in saline or distilled water and lens is placed in this solution for 4–6 hrs. Lens should be cleaned and rinsed before and after process of protein removal. This mechanism of enzyme tablets only loosens the proteins hence patients are advised to clean and rub their contact lenses after completion of deproteinization process.

Lens Storage System

Storage system for soft lenses and RGP lenses is slightly different because soft lenses are stored in a hydrated state, while RGP lenses are stored in a dry state.

All soft contact lenses once removed from their sterile packing are kept in a lens case (filled with rinsing or multipurpose solution) in such a manner that entire lens is merged in solution. Normally lenses are removed from the case and cleaned with cleaners before inserting in the eye. Similarly after removal from the eyes, lenses are rinsed and kept back in the lens case containing multipurpose solution. However, these lenses need to be treated chemically at least once a week to prevent contamination and to remove debris and proteins.

RGP lenses are stored in dry state in a simple shape (usually flat), fitted inside a lens case which can be kept in purse or pocket. After removal from the case these lenses are cleaned and rinsed before inserting in the eye. Similarly, after removal from the eyes these lenses are cleaned and rinsed with multipurpose solution before keeping them inside the lens case.

Care of Lens Cases

Improper care and maintenance of contact lens case may cause contamination of contact lenses by various microorganisms by formation of a biofilm or glycocalyx on its surface. Contamination may occur by pathogens like *Pseudomonas aeruginosa* and Serratia marcereens which in turn can produce biofilms. The glycocalyx formed on lens surface protect bacterial cells from action of chemical disinfectants or preservative and also helps in trapping of nutrient particles for micro-organism growth. To avoid chances of contamination it is necessary to rinse the lens case after every use and to discard all used solution from lens case. Thereafter, lens should be stored in fresh solution so that disinfecting efficacy of solution remains maintained which might loss due to mixing of fresh solution with used solutions. Lens cases should be scrubbed with a toothbrush preferably with oil-free soaps or detergents, usually on weekly basis. Then rinse with hot water and rub thoroughly with clean and dry tissue. Colonization of microorganisms like protozoa can be prevented by keeping lens case dry, because protozoa needs moist or wet environment for their growth.

CIBA vision has introduced a unique lens case called Pro Guard. In this lens case an anti-microbial agent is already incorporated which prevent contamination of case by micro-organisms. This type of case comprises electrically charged silver ions which help to reduce the chances of contamination up to 40%.

> **Note**
>
> Ideally, the lens case should be replaced at regular intervals.

Maintenance and Lens Care Methods

Newer approach for better lens care is to simplify the cleaning, storing and disinfecting systems required for maintenance and care of contact lenses which can easily be understood by patients and they can comfortably adopt them. Various lens care methods for better outcome that are recommended for RGP and soft contact lens wearers and also for allergy sufferer patients are as follows

Simplified RGP lens regimens: RGP contact lens solutions usually used are in a sequence initially for cleaning followed by disinfecting, then wetting and lastly for conditioning and cushioning purposes. Most of the commercially available solutions serve all these function in one solution, however, if patient is switching to a solution which serves purpose of cleaning, disinfection and conditioning but not of wetting and cushioning, then an additional solution should be added to the lens care regime.

Soft contact lens regimens: Most common approach adopted by majority of patients wearing soft contact lenses is to use one bottle lens care system. For example, commercially available soft lens care products like ReNu (Bausch and Lomb), Opti free and Opti one (Alcon) are very popular. These solutions have very low toxicity. Simply a digital cleaning with rinsing (use clean hands) followed by soaking of lens in a clean case is needed for maintenance and care a soft contact lens by these solutions. Although these solutions has very low toxicity and allergic reactions because they avoid use of preservatives like thimerosal, chlorhexidine and hydrogen peroxide exposure, better compliance and results are still doubtful with these solutions.

Sometimes one bottle lens care systems which contain surfactants can cause Sicca like syndrome. To prevent these patients are advised to adopt a saline rinse technique before insertion of contact lens, preferably with sterile saline which may be sorbic acid preserved or non-preserved.

Care regimes for allergy lens wearers: Patients suffering from allergies should use topical eye drops of either anti-histaminic or mast cell stabilizers or non steroidal anti-inflammatory drugs before and after lens wear to minimize the discomfort.

In a nutshell, care regimen is selected on the basis of patients wearing schedule, type of lens selected for wearing, ocular sensitivity, replacement schedule and patient's convenience. Patients are advised not to mix different types of solutions and brands and take advice from clinician before substituting any solution for lens care.

Radiuscope

Measurement of the base curve (i.e. radius of the curvature of back surface) of a contact lens is done by using an instrument called Radiuscope. In the year 1900 eminent scientist Drysdale described a principle which is used in all types of Radiuscope although they may vary from each other in design and method of displaying the readings.

Principle: When a parallel beam of light is directed on center of a concave reflecting surface, the light gets reflected along the same path as that of incident light. Now if this parallel beam of light is directed to the center of curvature of same concave reflecting surface; it will again reflect back along the same path, as that of incident light.

As both center of a concave reflecting surface and center of curvature of the same surface are reflecting incident light along its original path sometimes we call these points as self-reflecting points. It means that center of curvature and surface of the lens are two positions where the object and image coincide.

Thus the examiner needs to focus the Radiuscope upside and downwards until two clear images (one from center and second from center of curvature of contact lens) of the same target are seen at two different positions as shown in Fig. 13.1A and B. Radius of curvature of contact lens is the distance between the two positions of Radiuscope, where target images are focused clearly.

Main parts of Radiuscope are
- Compound microscope
- Internal illuminated target
- Half-silvered mirror

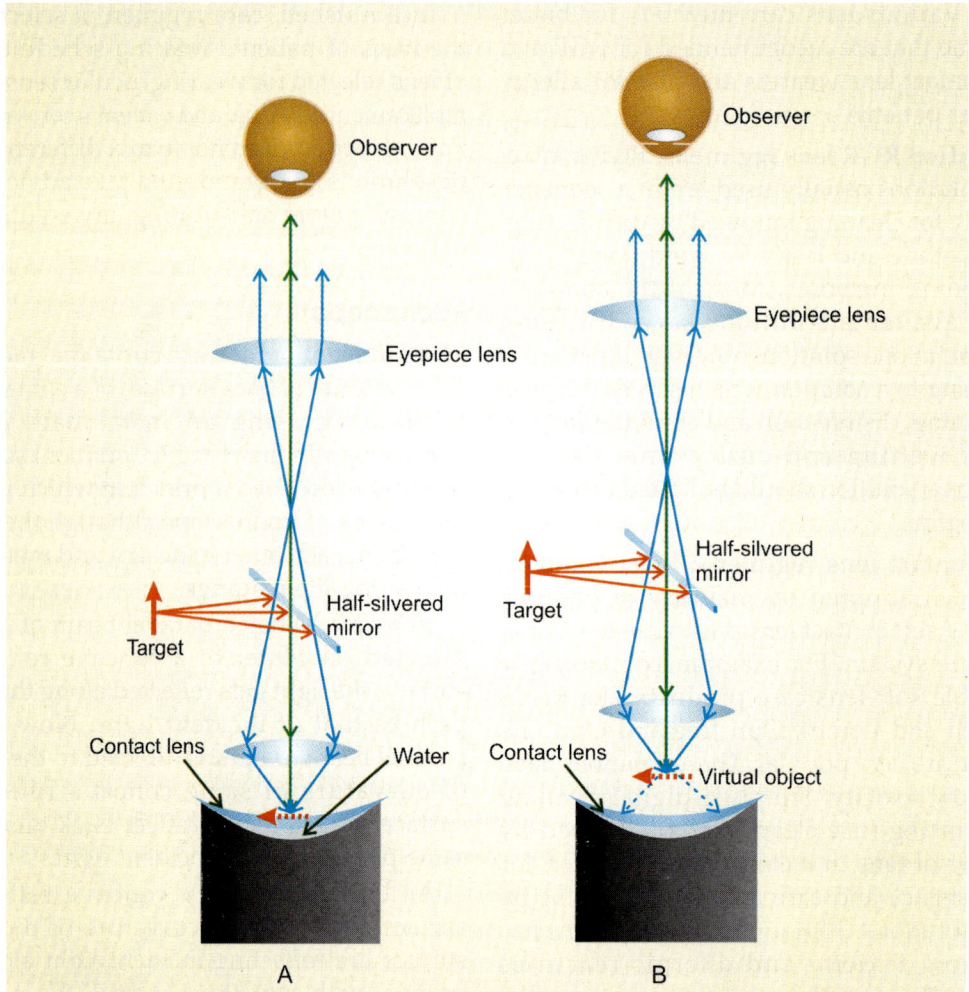

Fig. 13.1: Radiuscope; Zero position (First focus): When microscope objective focuses at back surface of contact lens. Final position (second focus): When microscope objective focuses at center of curvature, of back surface of contact lens

Radiuscope includes a compound microscope having an internally illuminated target, such as a radial line target (Fig. 13.1) which is projected along visual axis of Radiuscope in such a manner that image of target is seen clearly through an eyepiece by an observer. Half-silvered mirror is fitted above the microscope objective, which is set at an angle of 45°. When an object is focused (through Radiuscope), either on its concave reflecting surface or at its center of curvature image of this target is seen clearly in both the situations.

Procedure: To measure the back radius of a contact lens following steps are done

- Place the contact lens (keeping its concave surface upward) on the platform of Radiuscope, while convex surface of contact lens is kept in downward direction and float on fluid or wetting solution. The fluid helps to reduce the reflections from the lower (convex) surface of the lens when the reflections from upper (concave) surface of contact lens are observed.

- Slowly move the stage of Radiuscope so that illuminated target gets aligned with mirror and a real image is formed at working plane of objective lens from the light reflected through mirror.
- Once alignment is done, now move the microscope downward, toward contact lens surface, until working plane of microscope coincides with plane of back surface of contact lens.
- At this point reflected light (passing through half-silvered mirror) form an image in focal plane of microscope eyepiece, where it is seen clearly by the observer, as shown in Fig. 14.14A. This point is termed zero point and observer notices the reading on the scale of Radiuscope.
- Now slowly observer raise the microscope, until a second point is found where image of target is in finest focus; which occurs when working plane of objective lens align with center of curvature of back surface of contact lens.
- At this point concave surface of contact lens is again returning the light, along its own path. This point is called second focus point (Fig. 14.14B) and observer again notices the reading on the scale of Radiuscope.

Measure the distance covered by microscope between zero point and second focus point; where images were clearly focused. This distance denotes real length of radius of curvature of concave surface (base curve radius) of contact lens under examination.

Problem-based Learning

Problems Related to Refractive Errors and Presbyopia

MYOPIA

Problem 1: A young person aged 17 years, having mild asthenopic symptoms was presented to clinic. On examination, distance visual acuity was found relatively normal, however, on performing a subjective refraction patient is accepting minus spherical power of reasonable degree.

1. Why patient is accepting minus power?
2. How do you manage such cases?

Solution

1. While performing a subjective refraction it is very important to keep in mind that the patient should not be corrected with too much minus power. Many a times, young patients use accommodation during subjective refraction, hence they accept minus power lenses. Usually young patients prefer extra minus power because when compensated by accommodation, letters on acuity chart look smaller and darker which patient think as better vision.

2. For managing such situation following methods can be used during refraction
   - Patient must be trained to compare only the clarity of letters on vision chart. Inform the patient that if letters become smaller and darker, then they should be considered as same choice, not as better choice.

   - Fogging or astigmatic dial technique (Chapter 3, page 47) should be performed where patient begins with a choice from plus power lenses.
   - Duo chrome test (Chapter 3, page 48) should be done to know if more minus power is given or not.
   - Finally, if we are not satisfied with above mentioned methods then cycloplegic refraction or wet retinoscopy (Chapter 1, page 20) can be done to relax the accommodation. This gives us the accurate refractive status of this young patient who is accepting the significant degree of minus power.

> **Note**
>
> In young asymptomatic patients accepting minus power spheres for distance vision, always perform cycloplegic refraction specifically with atropine to know the correct refractive status.

Problem 2: A 60 years old lady presented with complain of fluctuation in distance vision since 3–4 years. She had a history of radial keratectomy done about 40 years back and since then she had problem of glare and poor contrast sensitivity. Recently, since 15 years her power of glasses for distance and near had increased regularly and abruptly.

1. What are the causes of symptoms and fluctuation in refractive error?
2. How would you manage this case?

Solution

1. Most probable cause of symptoms like glare and poor contrast sensitivity may be
   - Radial keratectomy (RK) especially, with smaller treatment zone and deeper incisions to correct higher degree myopia. Size of pupil plays an important role for manifestation of glare because if size of pupil is larger than optical zone (especially during nighttime) then glare will increase.
   - Formation of cataract is another possibility for increased glare at nighttime at the age of 60 years.
   - Fluctuation in refractive error may also be due to change in refractive status post-radial keratectomy because contraction of incisional wound usually causes refractive shift mostly towards hypermetropia.
   - Similarly, the corneal irregularities, scarring and smaller optical zone are causes for fluctuation in refractive errors. Moreover, formation of cataract especially nuclear sclerosis will also contribute to the change in refractive status.

2. Management of this case includes detail evaluation of
   - Pupil size in daylight and dim light
   - Status of cornea in terms of optical zone, scarring and keratometry
   - Cycloplegic refraction twice in daytime and evening
   - Assessment of cataract if present
   - Detailed fundus evaluation
   - Suppose the size of pupil is large, then advice the pharmacological treatment using pilocarpine to induce miosis which will reduce the glare, especially during nighttime. Perform meticulous cycloplegic refraction to know the amount and type of refractive error and prescribe glasses accordingly. Majority of these post-RK patients will have irregular type of astigmatic refractive errors, hence they may require refractive surgical procedures for correction of refractive error.

   - Hypermetropic refractive shift (due to radial keratectomy) and presbyopia (due to progressive age) will cause difficulty in near vision, hence she may require higher additional power than usual to see the near objects.
   - Suppose cataract is present, then decide according to the best corrected visual acuity with glasses, if BCVA is satisfactory, prescribe glasses and if not, then advice for cataract surgery with possible visual outcome.

Problem 3: An elderly person of age about 68 years presented to clinic with diminished distance vision with existing spectacles (fitted with two years old prescription). On examination, an additional –1.5 D change was found in each eye.

1. What are the probable causes for this acquired myopia?
2. How you will prescribe a new spectacle power in this case and what all possibilities you will consider in management of this case?

Solution

1. Probable causes for acquired myopia at an age of 68 years may be
   - Cataract (most probably nuclear sclerotic type)
   - Diabetes mellitus of recent onset or with poor glycemic control
   - Recent retinal detachment surgery (scleral buckling)
   - Medications (e.g. chloroquine, antidepressants, sulfa drugs, chlorthalidone, etc.)

2. Prescription of new spectacle power requires consideration of following possibilities
   - Suppose cause of acquired myopia is cataract, then patient must be described in details that change in power in spectacles will improve the vision but will not solve the problem of cataract.

- New prescription power should be placed in trial frame and shown to the patient binocularly to check the distance and near vision. Suppose there is an improvement in the distance visual acuity with new prescription power but the near vision get more adverse due to increased myopic shift, then more add power should be prescribed.

- Consult with the patient whether the change in prescription will allow them to carry out their daily activities adequately or not. Suppose outcome is that they can perform their daily activities comfortably with glasses, then offer new prescription. However, if they feel difficulty in performing daily activities with new prescription, then advice cataract surgery for vision improvement. When patient is unclear about outcome, then prescribe the new glasses and wait for the outcome in follow-up visits.

- If cause of acquired myopia is uncontrolled diabetes, then first it is necessary to stabilize the blood sugar level. Once the sugar level is stabilized, then do cycloplegic refraction again and prescribe new glasses.

- If cause of acquired myopia is exposure to medications, then first of all discontinuation of medications is required. In addition, also discuss with patient about the duration of exposure to medications which will decide whether patient requires change in prescription or not.

- Myopia secondary to retinal detachment surgery is usually astigmatic error and will improve when scleral buckle is removed after some time, however, until that period appropriate power glasses with prisms should be prescribed to maintain the visual acuity and avoid monocular diplopia.

Problem 4: An adult aged 38 years having moderate degree myopia appeared for routine eye checkup to the clinic. This patient was habitual of wearing contact lenses in office and outdoor activities. On examination, a small increase in the myopic correction was found.

1. What should be further course of management in prescribing new refractive power?
2. How will you reduce the accommodative demand and also increase the retinal image size in this 38 years old patient?

Solution

1. An ideal way to manage this case is that show the amount of change in vision quality to the patient, first by placing the older prescription and then the newer prescription. Now ask the patient whether he/she would like to wear a new pair of glasses (contact lenses) or not depending on the improvement in vision noticed by him/her during examination. This methodology (i.e. let the patient decide about the change) should be followed in every case presenting for any probable change in prescription.

2. To reduce the accommodative demand we will advice use of spectacles for correction of myopia because in myopes spectacle glasses not only increase the retinal image size but also reduce the efforts of accommodation, which is very useful in person approaching the age of presbyopia.

Note

As this patient is approaching the age of presbyopia any amount of increase in minus power will affect the near vision significantly, hence it is advisable to evaluate the patient both for distance and near vision if we are correcting the myopic error at this age.

Problem 5: A 40 years old male presented with diminished distance vision with monocular diplopia from left eye since one month. He had undergone an encirclage band buckle surgery in left eye for large retinal tear about one month back. The retinal tear was located in the periphery and was not involving the macular area. After scleral buckle surgery the unaided visual acuity was 6/6 in the right eye and 6/60 in the left eye, however, with pinhole the visual acuity in left eye improved to 6/9. On further evaluation left eye showed 12Δ exotropia with 4Δ hypertropia.

1. What are the causes for his symptoms?
2. Outline the effects of lenses on tropia.
3. How would you mange this case?

Solution

1. Scleral buckling causes myopic shift due to elongation of posterior segment of eye. This myopic shift leads to diminution of distance vision in this case. Simultaneously, the pressure effects and changes in corneal curvature after scleral buckling lead to irregular astigmatic error which causes monocular diplopia in some cases. These symptoms are more pronounced in those cases where encirclage buckle is applied compared to partial buckle.

2. As per the rule the minus lenses show more deviation than plus lenses, hence with minus lenses the tropia appears more and with plus lenses the tropia appears less. Simple formula 'percentage difference = 2.5 × deviation' can be used to calculate the prismatic effect of lenses on tropia.

3. As significant amount of increase in visual acuity is seen with pinhole test, the diminished distance vision and also the diplopia can be managed by correction of refractive error alone. Cycloplegic refraction is done to estimate the complete amount of refractive error and glasses are prescribed. To correct exotropia prisms (base in) are added, this will also eliminate the monocular double vision.

> **Note**
>
> If diplopia is not improved with correction of refractive error with glasses and prisms, then the cause of diplopia is probably muscular misalignment. This needs correction in scleral buckle or removal of buckle once retina is settled.

Problem 6: A 46 years aged person is reading book comfortably without using reading glasses or bifocals or progressive glasses at routine reading distance.

1. What are possible reasons for clear near vision at this age in this patient (normally we expect symptoms of presbyopia at this age)?
2. What sort of management is needed in this case?

Solution

1. Various possibilities of this patient reading comfortably without using glasses are
   - Patient may be having low degree myopia and not using glasses for distance vision.
   - Another possibility is that patient is wearing glasses for myopia, but almost certainly his/her myopic refractive error is not fully corrected.
   - Sometimes, a myopic person might be reading after taking off their spectacles, a condition called natural near sightedness.

2. Various possible modes of management in this patient are
   - Suppose patient is low degree myope and is satisfied with his/her distance and near vision, then there is no need to prescribe glasses either for distance or near vision.
   - In the situation where patient is wearing myopic glasses but is undercorrected, then the best way is not to prescribe an additional minus power to fully correct the distance refractive error because patient is not complaining about distance vision and also is comfortably seeing the near objects. Moreover, keeping them under-corrected allows them not to move for a bifocal or progressive addition lens immediately. However, correction of myopic prescription may be required along with addition of a bifocal or progressive addition lens if patient performance for distance is not satisfactory.
   - In case of natural near sightedness where patient is comfortable, then there is no

need to prescribe for a bifocal or progressive glasses because these patients are used to read from a nearer distance than normal reading distance and prescription of bifocals or progressive lenses will disturb their routine reading distance.

Problem 7: An elderly person aged 52 years having high degree myopia, wearing progressive glasses regularly arrived to clinic for eye check up with desire to remove heavy progressive glasses. Ocular examination reveals that spectacle power is accurate, needs no correction and eyes are also in good health.

1. What kind of advice we should give to this patient considering that he/she has no systemic illness?
2. What other alternatives we can offer to this patient to get rid of heavy glasses?

Solution

1. Considering the age of patient and high degree of myopia following advices can be given to this patient:
   - Usually high degree myopes have increased chances of development of posterior segment complications like lattice degenerations, retinal holes or tears and macular degenerations. In this patient a detailed fundus examination should be done to rule out any posterior segment lesion and the patient should be informed about potential complications of high degree myopia.
   - We must advice the patient to report immediately if he/she develops symptoms of retinal damage in the form of change in temporal vision, floaters or flashes.
   - On every regular follow-up visit including present visit a detail dilated fundus examination is done to rule out any pathological myopic changes. If changes are present an immediate treatment should be done to prevent any devastating outcome like retinal detachment.

2. Various alternatives to high power myopic glasses can be offered to this patient after performing the corneal keratometry and corneal topography
   - Suppose patient is fit for refractive surgery, then the best possible alternative to glasses is laser correction of myopic error. Considering the age of patient and degree of myopia, the best possible laser treatment is with Femtosecond Lasik surgery.
   - If the patient is not fit for refractive surgery, then other optical alternatives such as contact lenses of suitable designs (rotational non-spherical contact lenses) and aspherical high index lenses (reduces the weight and thickness of glasses) can be offered to this patient.

Problem 8: An adult aged 36 years having moderate degree myopia, presented with complaint of difficulty in reading while using existing glasses. However, the reading fluency is increased when glasses slides down on the patient's nose.

1. Can we consider this as presbyopia and what is the possible diagnosis for near vision problem?
2. How will you manage this case?

Solution

1. For an individual of 36 years of age, presbyopia is very unlikely diagnosis for difficulty in near vision. Most strong possibility is that patient was over corrected for myopic error with minus lenses for distance vision since starting of glasses wear. This is further confirmed by the fact that reading ability improves with sliding down the glasses on nose, because with increase in vertex distance the minus power decreases. At a younger age, the patient's accommodation power was able to compensate for this extra minus power prescribed in glasses. However, with advancing age (at 36 years) the accommodative ability is decreased gradually which

is now not sufficient to overcome the excessive minus power in the present glasses. So this myopic patient is not left with enough accommodation to be use for reading purposes and developed symptoms of near vision.

2. Best method to mange this patient is to perform a cycloplegic refraction (preferably using atropine) and estimate the accurate degree of myopia. Once the exact amount of myopic error is determined, then the patient may be prescribed with the new prescription, which most likely will have less minus power.

> **Note**
>
> It is necessary to advise patient that new glasses prescribed to him may take some time to adjust for distance vision because accommodative tone may take a little time to relax or to return to normal tone.

Problem 9: A 38 years old asymptomatic patient walked in clinic for routine eye check-up. He had never used spectacles for either distance or near vision and presently working comfortably on computers. However, after ocular examination and post-cycloplegic refraction, a small degree of myopia is revealed.

1. What should be our course of management in this case?

Solution

1. On discussion and examination, following advices can be given to this patient
   • If patient feels that his/her distance vision is adequate and on examination only a slight myopic correction is needed, then it is better for the patient to continue his/her routine work without distance glasses.
   • At the age of 38 years avoid any kind of near correction, especially when we found a small degree of myopia.
   • Manage this patient just by Counseling and advice of regular follow-up.

Problem 10: A 48 years old –2 DS myopic patient presented to clinic with the complain that he has to remove the distance vision glasses off and on to read the books or newspaper. Presently patient's near vision without glasses is satisfactory at routine reading distance, however, the patient desires to prescribe new glasses so that he needs not to remove the glasses either to see the distance or near targets.

1. Describe the problem with possible solutions.
2. Explain the various prismatic effects associated with bifocal or multifocal glasses.

Solution

1. The patient is presbyopic at the age of 48 years and his accommodation is completely exhausted. Hence he is unable to compensate for 2 dioptre myopia while reading a book so he needs to remove the myopic glasses to read the book comfortably. As patient does not want to remove his glasses to read, then the best option for him is to use either bifocal or multifocal glasses so that he can see both the distance and near targets without removing the glasses. Suppose patient works on computer, then options are trifocals, computer glasses or progressive glasses.

2. In case of bifocal lenses the common prismatic effects (discussed in Chapter 7, pages 108–109) are
   • Differential displacement at segment top (image jump): This image jump occurs due to near segment in bifocal lens and is more problematic than other prismatic effects of bifocal lens. When person sees suddenly from distance portion to near portion the image of the object appears as if jumped from its place, which take some time for adjustment.
   • Differential displacement at reading level (image displacement): This occurs due to the relative reading position in near segment and is minimum with straight top D bifocal lenses design.
   • Total displacement is the sum of both these prismatic effects and is dependent on the refractive power of distance and near addition portion.

Problem 11: A 40 years old office executive having moderate degree (–3.5 DS) myopia presented to clinic with a desire of corrective refractive surgery for myopia. There is history of wearing contact lenses during family functions or gatherings. No history of medical illness is present.

1. What advice would you give to this patient?
2. Compare refractive surgery and progressive glasses in relation to this case.

Solution

1. As this patient is approaching the presbyopic age and might not have been aware about the fact that refractive surgery will correct only distance refractive error in his case, our prime duty is to counsel this patient about the pros and cons of myopic corrective refractive surgery. Patient should be well informed that after surgery the distance vision will be alright and there is no need to wear optical correction for distance vision ever, however, as the person is nearing presbyopic age there will be requirement of reading glasses in coming years. The patient will also loose the advantages of natural near sightedness after laser surgery. Moreover, complications related to laser surgery should be explained in detail before performing the surgery.

2. Considering the age of patient and work profile, progressive glasses are also very good alternative for his problem because the patient can have quality vision with less accommodative demand in progressive glasses. For cosmetic reasons patient can occasionally use contact lenses of bifocal or multifocal design (Chapter 12, page 193). Post-LASIK surgery patient needs to wear glasses for near vision and moreover there

are chances that intermediate vision may also get affected after LASIK, hence progressive glasses are very good choice at age of 40 years.

Problem 12: 56 years old moderate degree (–2.75 DS) myopic patient presented to clinic with a desire of myopic corrective refractive surgery. Patient is already wearing progressive glasses since 14 years and having a vision of 6/6 and N6 in each eye with glasses. There is no history of medical illness or symptoms of cataract, however, grade one peripheral cortical lenticular changes are seen on dilated fundus examination.

1. How will you counsel the patient?
2. What is line of management in this case?

Solution

1. Before counseling the patient clinician must confirm about
   - Status of anterior segment specially cataract.
   - Posterior segment status
   - Corneal surface status and related problems like dry eye or scars.
   - Pupillary assessment in bright and dim light conditions

   Once these evaluations are recorded and found to be within normal limits, then explain the patient regarding their refractive status, stating that the patient needs refractive correction both for distance and near vision and counsel the patient with these options.

   - Suppose distance vision is corrected fully in both the eyes by refractive surgery, then he/she will need to wear glasses for near vision.
   - There is no option that only near vision gets corrected by refractive surgery.

- Rate of progression of cataract or any other ocular condition will not be affected by refractive surgery and patient will eventually require cataract surgery when it will mature.
- With gradual maturity of cataractous changes there will be slight changes in refractive status specifically for distance vision.

2. Management of this particular case is slightly on different line compared to routine refractive surgery case because practitioner needs to correct both the distance and near vision in an elderly patient by corneal refractive surgery. Following treatment options can be given to the patient
    - Monovision LASIK can be done which means one eye is corrected fully for distance vision and fellow eye will be fully corrected for near vision, so that no spectacles are required for both distance and near vision.
    - Multifocal LASIK is another good option to correct both distance and near vision simultaneously in both the eyes.
    - Alternately multifocal intraocular lenses can be advised in both the eyes one after the other.
    - Monovision with IOL, where in one eye the IOL of distance power correction and in fellow eye IOL of near power correction can also be done to correct both the distance and near vision.

☐ Note

In adult patients having 6/6 and N6 vision in each eye, the multifocal LASIK is good option for correction of refractive error.

HYPERMETROPIA

Problem 1: An elderly person aged 47 years presented in clinic with difficulty in distance vision, although there was no such complaint in the past. The patient is wearing half eye reading glasses for near work comfortably without a prescription since 10 years. Recently the power of half eye glasses was increased by the optician.

1. Describe the probable cause of difficulty in distance vision?
2. How will you manage the case?

Solution

1. The most probable cause of difficulty in distance vision at this age is uncorrected latent hypermetropia. The latent hypermetropia usually remains uncorrected because young healthy person does not experience any difficulty in distance vision since they have sufficient reserve of accommodation and can use his/her accommodative power to overcome the defect in distance vision. However, as the age advances, the ability of person to accommodate get deteriorate and no enough accommodation is left to overcome the latent hypermetropia, which ultimately will appear as manifest hypermetropia. In this case also prior to age of 47, the person used accommodation to correct distance vision and as the age increased his/her latent hypermetropia has now turn into manifest hypermetropia.

2. This patient requires correction for both the near and distance vision after performing the cycloplegic refraction. The correction can be given in the form of bifocal or progressive addition lenses or if the patient is comfortable with two pairs of glasses (used separately for distance and near), then it is another economical option. Moreover, over the counter available reading glasses can also be used if patient is having low and binocularly equal degree of hypermetropia without astigmatism. For example, +1 D pair for distance and +2.75 D pair for near.

☐ Note

In these types of cases it is mandatory to perform a cycloplegic refraction preferably using atropine drops to evaluate the exact degree of latent and manifest hypermetropia.

Problem 2: A 21 years old college student presented to clinic with history of ocular strain, frontal headache and brow ache since 2 years. His symptoms are exaggerated with continuous reading or studying in classroom. Past history revealed that he had been prescribed spectacles for distance and reading purposes about 3 years back, which he used off and on to relieve the symptoms of headache. Patient has no history of medical illness.

1. What all additional evaluation you would like to perform to reach the diagnosis in this case?

2. On cycloplegic refraction of this patient, the error found in right eye is +0.75 DS (6/6) and left eye is +0.25 DS (6/6), and orthoptic examination showed orthophoria for distance and 4Δ exophoria in near. Discuss the differential diagnosis of this case.

3. Outline the management strategies for this case.

Solution

1. To establish diagnosis in this case we should perform cycloplegic refraction, orthoptic assessments and measure the range and amplitude of accommodation. This additional information will help us to confirm the diagnosis like hypermetropia, and/or muscular imbalance in this young patient.

2. Various possible diagnoses in this patient are hypermetropia, convergence insufficiency or accommodation insufficiency. As for distance there was orthophoria and exophoria for near and the range and amplitude of accommodation was also normal, thus this case may be of low degree hypermetropia with convergence insufficiency.

3. Management of this patient is mainly done by advising orthoptic treatment of convergence insufficiency. Optical correction of low degree hypermetropia should not be recommended because it may worsen the asthenopic symptoms in case of convergence insufficiency. As the amount of exophoria is small there is no need of additional prism therapy in this case, however, sometimes for rapid and effective results base in prisms can be added. Surgical treatment of convergence insufficiency will not be required in this particular case.

Problem 3: Young adult male, aged 36 years wearing hypermetropic correction was having no problems with distance and near vision with prescribed glasses since last 12 years. Now this patient is presented to clinic with difficulty in near vision with his present glasses, however the distance vision with these glasses is comfortable and clear.

1. Whether this patient became presbyopic and if not, what is the likely diagnosis?

2. What sort of management is required to correct near vision problem?

Solution

1. The appearance of presbyopia at the age of 36 years is very unlikely. Most possible diagnosis is that the hypermetropia of this patient was not corrected completely with the glasses prescribed to him, i.e. latent hypermetropia persisted in spite of correction for hypermetropia. This latent hypermetropia was getting compensated by the excessive accommodation efforts of the patient till age of 36 years. As the age advanced the accommodation ability decreased gradually, as a result an inadequate amount of accommodation is left for reading so this patient experienced difficulty in near vision. Most likely diagnosis in this case is under corrected hypermetropia, where only the manifest part was corrected and latent part was not corrected by glasses.

2. Management strategies for this under-corrected hypermetropic patient are
   • The latent hypermetropia can be revealed by doing cycloplegic refraction or retinoscopy, i.e. testing refraction after

abolishing the tone of ciliary muscle so that hypermetropia cannot be overcome by accommodation of patient. If latent hypermetropia of high degree is detected on refraction with cycloplegia, then it is recommended to do post-cycloplegic refraction to confirm that the additional plus power prescribed to patient during cycloplegic refraction is adequate for patient without cycloplegia also, because as the accommodation tone of the eye returns to normal, the visual acuity may alter.

- On the other hand, a push plus technique can be performed during non-cycloplegic refraction to know the maximum plus power which the patient can tolerate. During testing, the plus spherical power is added progressively until the patient notices slight blurring or discomfort. This plus power indicates full hyper-metropic correction to be given and it should be corrected in stages to avoid intolerance because tone of ciliary muscle (accommodation) returns to normal gradually.

- Alternately, contact lenses can be prescri-bed to this patient, because the mechanism of relaxation of accommodation is much gradual and also the tolerance to high plus power is better.

Note

Many a times patients of younger age group having quite well distance and near vision without any glass may also complain the problem in near vision when they approaches the presbyopic age because of latent hypermetropia.

Problem 4: A 5 years old child having history of occasional mild deviation of eyes was brought by parents to the clinic for detailed evaluation. There is no past history of any systemic illness. On examination no manifest squint was seen, however, cycloplegic refraction has revealed a refractive error of +1.75D in both the eyes.

1. Explain the probable cause of deviation of eyes.
2. What should be the course of management?

Solution

1. Most probable causes of occasional deviation of the eyes in young child are mild degree of hypermetropia or muscular imbalance due to systemic illness. As there is no history of systemic illness in this child then the most probable diagnosis for deviation of eyes is hypermetropia.

2. There is no need of any optical correction in this case. Usually, young children presenting with low to moderate degree of hypermetropia, with no strabismus and no visual difficulty do not require any correction for refractive error because child has enough amount of accommodation to overcome the hypermetropia which is elicited without any conscious effort by the child, i.e. without any symptoms of eye strain. However, if hypermetropia is more than 3 D and child also having symptoms of eye strain then optical correction should be prescribed. If there is associated strabismus or amblyopia, then other therapies like occlusion therapy, etc. are also required with optical correction.

Problem 5: An elderly male aged 70 years wearing bifocals since 28 years is presented to clinic with recent onset of diminution of vision for distance and near. On examination, a change in refractive power suggestive of recent onset hypermetropic shift was found.

1. What are the possible causes for this recent onset hypermetropic shift?
2. How would you mange this case?

Solution

1. Diminution of both distance and near vision along with refractive shift towards hyper-metropia in this age may probably occur due to
   - Diabetes mellitus: Recent onset diabetic mellitus having poor glycemic control or

fluctuations in glucose levels due to long standing diabetes mellitus may cause hypermetropic shift.

- Cortical cataract in some cases may cause mild hyperopic shift in older age patients, however, majority of cortical cataract causes an associated astigmatic error which can lead to the difficulty in distance and near vision.
- Anterior shifting of retina due to retinal edema or central serous chorioretinopathy will lead to hyperopic shift because of the defective focusing of light rays on the retina.

2. The management of this patient includes detailed posterior segment evaluation and sometimes even assistance of advance diagnostic instruments like optical coherence topography, fundus angiography to establish the cause of hyperopic shift.

- If poorly controlled diabetes mellitus is the cause of change in refractive status, then the patient should be referred to physician for better control of blood sugar.
- In case of cataract if change in glasses gives satisfactory vision, then we can prescribe new power of glasses and if vision is not satisfactory with glasses then patient should be advised to undergo the cataract surgery.
- If posterior segment lesions are the cause of hyperopic shift, then treatment of the lesions is advised.

Problem 6: Parents of a 3½ years old child brought him with complaint of deviation of eyes and inattentiveness of surroundings while playing with toys. Parents noticed deviations of eyes when child tries to focus the near objects, however, the deviation was less marked when child watches the television. The birth history is normal and child is showing normal developmental milestones.
1. What is the probable diagnosis?
2. If on refraction moderate degree of hypermetropia found in the child, how will you manage the case?

Solution
1. Most probable cause of deviation of the eyes in young child having no other ocular abnormalities is uncorrected refractive error specially hypermetropia. To confirm the diagnosis cycloplegic refraction should be done using atropine ointment. Suppose the refractive error found in this case was moderate degree hypermetropia (say +6.5 DS in each eye). Thus, the diagnosis of this case is accommodative squint due to high degree hypermetropia with high AC/A ratio.

2. Management of the case includes correction of hypermetropia by plus power glasses. In this case the full correction is given in spectacle power and parents are advised to make sure that the child must wear the glasses regularly. Due to defective accommodation and high AC/A ratio the child may show deviation in near vision in spite of using hyperopic glasses. Suppose after full correction this child shows deviation of eyes (esotropia) in near vision, then the bifocal glasses are advised, where an add is given to compensate for high AC/A ratio. The power of bifocal lenses is gradually adjusted as the age of child advances, where add power is gradually decreased because accommodation efforts are slowly compensated with plus lenses. Follow-up of child should be done strictly at 6 months interval to evaluate the amount of visual acuity and deviation of eyes.

> **Note**
>
> Accommodative esotropia with high AC/A ratio remain the only ophthalmic condition where bifocal glasses are advised for very young child (2–8 years age group).

Problem 7: An asymptomatic young adult aged 24 years presented to clinic for routine ocular examination. On cycloplegic refraction and examination a diagnosis of latent hypermetropia was made for which plus power glasses were prescribed to the patient.

After a few days the patient again came to the clinic with complaints of intolerance to newly prescribed glasses to him.

1. What could be the causes of these symptoms?
2. How we should manage this case?

Solution

1. In this case the most probable causes of intolerance to the prescribed glasses may be
   - Imperfect cycloplegic refraction
   - Post-mydriatic test (PMT) was not performed

   Most probably the refraction performed was not correct (*see* the guidelines in Chapter 3 for refraction techniques) and either an overcorrection or undercorrection of hypermetropia has been done. In both these situations accommodation ability of patient will affect which lead to asthenopic symptoms or intolerance to glasses. Moreover, a post-mydriatic test was also not performed to assess the tolerance of the plus power lenses, because this patient was going to wear the plus power spectacles first time in his life. In these patients the ciliary muscle tone had been used to overcome the latent hypermetropia since long duration and this increased ciliary tone is difficult to get relaxed all of a sudden by use of plus power lenses.

2. To manage the condition of intolerance this patient should be advised to come for a repeat cycloplegic refraction to check the accuracy of prescription.
   - If cycloplegic refraction is found accurate and significant amount of plus sphere power is detected then advice the patient to come again for a post-mydriatic test. Post-cycloplegic refraction gives an accurate assessment of patient's tolerance of new plus power prescribed to him so it is mandatory to perform this test before writing the final prescription. In first prescription it is recommended

to prescribe less plus power lenses than the total power required to correct the entire hypermetropic error. Gradually, in subsequent follow up visits the plus power can be increased as the tolerance of patient increases to plus power spectacles.
   - Suppose the refraction was incorrect and an undercorrection or overcorrection had been done, then simply perform a PMT and write a new prescription with accurate power of lenses.

> **Note**
>
> Once the plus power lenses are started to be used by the patient then this increased ciliary muscle tone will gradually decline. Now gradually the power of plus lenses can be stepped up to correct the entire degree of hypermetropic error.

Problem 8: A 21 years old high hyperopic (+7 DS in each eye) female patient presented to the clinic with dissatisfaction of wearing thick lenses and she wants to get rid of her spectacles.

1. What all possible options are available for her to get rid of her glasses?
2. What best advice you will give to this patient?

Solution

1. The various possible options for this high hyperopic patient to get rid of glasses are
   - Contact lens wear: As the power of glasses is only spherical, she can comfortably wear contact lenses and get rid of glasses. Advantages of contact lenses are better cosmetic appearance and lesser spherical aberrations compared to the spectacles. Efforts on accommodation are also reduced due to decreased vertex distance in the contact lenses (Chapter 8, page 129).
   - Refractive surgery: Her hyperopia can be permanently corrected by refractive procedures specially C-LASIK or Femtosecond LASIK. Advantages of

refractive surgery are lifetime correction of refractive error, however, a few disadvantages are dry eye, glare and decreased contrast sensitivity.

2. Considering her age and amount of the refractive error the best possible advice for this young lady is to undergo the refractive procedure for correction of high degree hypermetropia. Using contact lenses for long period are very cumbersome and also not complication free, hence refractive surgery is a better choice in this case.

Problem 9: Young college student aged 25 years presented with difficulty in reading for some duration continuously. There is no history of wearing glasses and previous ocular examination. This student tries to read in installments and get relief when take rest in between reading.

1. Discuss the possible diagnosis in this case.
2. How will you manage the problem?

Solution

1. At 25 years of age presbyopia is not a diagnosis so reading difficulty might be due to these following situations
   - Latent hypermetropia: A large amount of latent hypermetropia may cause difficulty in near vision in young adult because at this age, the accommodation ability of person is unable to compensate the hypermetropic error and the hidden refractive error will manifest.
   - Convergence insufficiency: Patients having convergence insufficiency face difficulty in reading for longer duration and develops asthenopic symptoms. Normal near point of convergence should not be farther than 8 cm, however, a receding in NPA will cause reading difficulty.
   - Drugs: Several pharmacological agents used to treat condition like common cold, migraine, motion sickness or some central nervous system disorders may affect pupillary sphincters. This causes

faulty accommodation and leads to difficulty in reading. A detailed treatment history is must before concluding the cause of reading difficulty in a young adult.

2. Management of this case depends on the cause of near vision problem
   - Suppose the latent hypermetropia is the cause, then perform cycloplegic refraction and prescribe the full correction in first sitting.
   - Suppose convergence insufficiency is the cause of problem, then the convergence exercises are very effective in relieving the symptoms.
   - Suppose the patient is on any drug causing difficulty in near vision then the best option is refer the case to physician and ask the opinion about discontinuing the drug.

ASTIGMATISM

Problem 1: Young adult of age 20 years, having mixed myopic error came for routine follow-up visit. The patient is presently wearing a small cylindrical power lenses, whereas now on subjective refraction suddenly the patient was found to be accepting a larger degree of cylindrical power.

1. What could be the possible reasons for this change in cylindrical power?
2. How would you prescribe new power?

Solution

1. Various possible reasons for sudden acceptance of large cylindrical power in this case are
   - Firstly, the reason of increase cylindrical power may be increase in the astigmatic power of the patient. Though it is very unlikely that there is only increase in the astigmatic error of patient's present prescription; thus it becomes necessary to recheck for inaccuracy of earlier prescription.

- Another possibility is that the patient is using too much minus spherical power which will ultimately lead to increase in cylindrical power. In this case chances of over minusing are high, because for every half dioptre of over-minused prescription, the cylinder plus power needs an increase by one dioptre to maintain the spherical equivalent.

For example, suppose the exact refractive error of patient is: $-2 \times +1.0 \times 90°$; means the spherical equivalent is -1.5 D.

- If spherical power of this patient gets wrongly overcorrected by -0.50 dioptre sphere, then to maintain a spherical equivalent of -1.5 D an additional $+1.0$ D cylinder power is needed to equalize this spherical overcorrection. So the resultant final prescription will become $-2.5 \times +2.0 \times 90°$.

- Suppose this patient is overcorrected by -0.75 D spherical power then to maintain a spherical equivalent of -1.5 D, an additional $+1.5$ D cylinder power is needed to equalize this spherical overcorrection. So the resultant final prescription will become $-2.75 \times + 2.5 \times 90°$.

2. In this patient repeat cycloplegic refraction is done to know the exact power of spherical and cylindrical errors. Post-mydriatic test (PMT) is done to know the minimum power of minus sphere and maximum power of plus cylinders acceptance by the patient. After PMT the power must be prescribed for spectacle lenses.

Problem 2: Middle-aged patient having a mixed astigmatic refractive error was presented to clinic for routine follow-up. Previous prescription of glasses was -5.5 DS $\times + 1.5$ DC $\times 90°$ in both the eyes. After cycloplegic refraction the new glasses prescription came out to be -5.25 DS $\times + 2$ DC $\times 95°$ for right eye and -6 DS $\times + 2.75$ DC $\times 85°$ for left eye.

After wearing this new prescription for 2–3 days, this patient came back with a complaint of severe asthenopic symptoms like sloping of computer screen, and rising of ground on walking with nausea.

1. What could be the cause of these asthenopic symptoms?
2. How does the corneal topography will appear in this case?
3. How would you manage this case?

Solution

1. The strongest possibility of these asthenopic symptoms is the modification done in new prescription for improvement in refractive error. Among all types of refractive errors the most sensitive part of a prescription is corrections in the astigmatic portion of entire prescription. Usually a change in > 0.5 D power and >5 degree of axis in astigmatic error can cause asthenopic symptoms, especially in patients who are already wearing the astigmatic glasses with different power and axis of cylindrical lenses.

2. In this case the corneal topography will show a typical bow and tie appearance in vertical orientation. This patient has the regular with the rule type of astigmatism, where topography shows a plus astigmatic power in vertical direction.

3. This case can be managed by performing a trial screening of prescription before prescribing the final total correction in cylindrical power and axis. Initially place trial lenses of changed cylindrical power and axis in a trial frame and ask the patient to look around in the clinic or walk around wearing this trial frame. Suppose patient feels discomfort, then immediately remove the trial frame. Suppose the visual acuity is showing significant improvement with new prescription, then the change in cylindrical power is first prescribed. Once patient is adjusted to new power of cylinder, then gradually change in axis of cylinder is prescribed till the total power and axis of cylinder gets corrected.

Problem 3: In our routine village camp 26 years old person presented with complain of gradual diminution of vision for distance and associated frontal headache, since few years. This patient has no medical illness and also no history of wearing glasses in the past. In our camp set up there is no facility for retinoscopy or autorefraction.

1. What are the methods to determine an accurate astigmatic error (if present), without these facilities?

Solution

1. When a young adult presents with gradual diminution of vision for distance and we do not have facility of autorefraction or retinoscopy; perform accurate subjective refraction as per guidelines described in Chapter 3. Many a times young adults have uncorrected astigmatic errors of mild to moderate degree. As the accommodation gradually diminishes with age, these astigmatic errors produce symptoms of diminution of vision and asthenopia. After subjective refraction patient can be prescribed the glasses to be used constantly for distance and near work.

Problem 4: A young female aged 19 years undergraduate student of college presented with complain of difficulty in seeing the letters on whiteboard in classroom and also reading book for long duration, since a few months. There is history of associated frontal headache and brow ache off and on with occasional blurring of letters in book. She has no history of medical illness or wearing of glasses in the past.

1. Outline the evaluation method to reach the proper diagnosis.
2. How will you manage the case?

Solution

1. Complete anterior segment examination on slit lamp with unaided visual acuity is recorded. Fundus examination with optic disc evaluation is done to rule out retinal pathology and glaucoma. Cycloplegic refraction is done to assess the refractive status of the patient. Blood tests to rule out systemic conditions like anemia, thyroid disease or microelement deficiency (e.g. calcium) are ordered.

2. Suppose all the medical investigations and ocular examination came out to be normal; then probably the cause is refractive error. Cycloplegic refraction in these sorts of cases usually show a simple or mixed astigmatic error of mild to moderate degree. To manage the case complete amount of astigmatic error is recorded and initially glasses are prescribed after performing PMT, so that patient can tolerate the new prescription. Once the patient is comfortable with glasses, then complete amount of astigmatic error can be advised. After a few months of comfortable wear of glasses she can be advised to go for toric contact lenses. Once the refractive error becomes stable she can go for astigmatic refractive surgery to get rid of glasses or contact lenses.

Problem 5: An adult aged 44 years was presented with complaint of difficulty in reading small fonts since a few months. On examination along with signs of presbyopia he also had a plano-astigmatic error of $-0.75\,DC \times 180°$ for distance vision in each eye. There is no history of using distance vision glasses in the past and also the patient is asymptomatic till recently. On subjective refraction this patient is well accepting a $+1.5\,DS \times -0.5\,DC + 180°$ for near correction.

1. What is the probable diagnosis of this case?
2. What should be our prescription?

Solution

1. The most probable diagnosis of this case is recent onset presbyopia, because the small degree with the rule astigmatism is very common and produces no clinical symptoms. Usually these small degrees with the rule astigmatism require no correction for distance vision.

2. As per the past history patient was comfortably seeing at distance till now and would simply require correction for reading. A prescription of +1.25 D sphere is advised depending on the spherical equivalent calculated from the subjective refraction of +1.5 DS × –0.5 DC × 180°. In this particular patient there is no need to prescribe an additional astigmatism correction; however, astigmatic addition can be prescribed if patient feels an improvement in either reading or distance acuity with the addition of cylindrical power, or patient prefers to use bifocal or progressive additional glasses.

Problem 6: An 11 years old class 6th student was brought by the parents with complaint of difficulty in seeing the letters properly on blackboard. History revealed that child usually sits in front row in the class and never worn glasses; also there is no previous history of refraction done. Subjective refraction of this child is OD –1.75 DS (6/12), OS – 1.5 DS × + 0.75 DC × 70° (6/6).

On detail examination no ocular pathology was found, and VA in right eye was improving to 6/6 with pinhole.

1. What is the cause of low visual acuity in right eye?
2. How it should be managed?

Solution

1. Most probable cause of low visual acuity in right eye is improper refraction, because young children may have different degree of ciliary tone in each eye and hence subjective refraction may not give accurate amount of refractive error. Secondly, in majority of patients astigmatic correction is symmetrical, so it is better to search for this possibility.
2. To manage this case we need to perform a cycloplegic refraction with atropine eye drops. On PMT a complete symmetry in astigmatic error would have been indicated when refractive error for the right eye is –1.5 DS × + 0.75 × 110°, so a repeat subjective refraction for the right eye can be done considering this symmetrical prescription.

> **Note**
>
> When there is significant improvement is seen in visual acuity with pinhole and no ocular pathology is found on examination; then the most common cause of low visual acuity is inaccurate refraction.

Problem 7: A middle aged 52 years old patient presented with complain of diplopia since few days. Ophthalmic history revealed that the patient was wearing a sphero-cylindrical correction of moderate degree in each eye since many years. On clinical evaluation monocular diplopia was discovered in right eye; however there was no deviation of eyes and extraocular movements were free and full. There is no history of medical illness like diabetes mellitus, hypertension or thyroid disease.

1. Whether refractive error can cause this recent onset diplopia?
2. How will you investigate this case?
3. Outline the management of this problem.

Solution

1. Few selective refractive errors especially irregular astigmatism of moderate to high degree can cause severe blurring of vision with distortion of images; which occasionally can manifest as monocular diplopia. In this particular case the moderate degree astigmatic error was wrongly corrected either in terms of spherical power, cylindrical power or axis; hence the symptom of monocular double vision was appearing.
2. Any case of diplopia should be thoroughly investigated in terms of blood parameters (complete blood count, blood sugar, thyroid profile, lipid profile, etc.), MRI brain and ocular B-scan. Clinically a detail posterior segment evaluation is also necessary to rule out any intraocular lesion.
3. For the management of this case perform a meticulous cycloplegic refraction to determine the exact refractive power and cylindrical axis.

- Suppose new prescription eliminates the symptoms of diplopia, then the cause was established and patient will be alright in a few days after wearing the new glasses.
- However, if symptoms of monocular diplopia are still present and investigation data shows some deviations from normal, then search for other causes of monocular diplopia. Then the line of management is either medical or surgical.

> **Note**
>
> In cases of monocular double vision suppose pinhole test abolishes the diplopia, then the cause is either refractive error or cataract.

PRESBYOPIA

Problem 1: A 44 years old office employee started facing difficulty in performing the routine desk work. He has no difficulty in distance vision and was not wearing any glasses. On his own he purchased an over the counter reading glasses for near vision, but after advise from colleagues he presented to clinic for ocular evaluation. This patient asks following question during examination

1. Whether using over the counter reading glasses are correct for my eyes?
2. What are the advantages and disadvantages of over the counter reading glasses?
3. What is the problem with my vision and using over the counter glasses will affect my vision?
4. How would you treat me?

Solution

1. Usually when the patient of 44 years age are asymptomatic and have good distance vision without glasses, the near vision problem is due to presbyopia. For this usual presbyopic condition over the counter (OTC) glasses are good alternative, when given by trained ophthalmic personnel. In this particular case the OTC glasses were purchased by patient under no supervision, so chances of overcorrection or undercorrection are high.

2. Most common advantages of OTC glasses are economical, easily accessible and immediately available to use.
   Disadvantages of OTC glasses are
   - These glasses have equal power on both sides, however, majority of person have some amount of difference in refractive status of both the eyes.
   - OTC glasses are available in common size small frames, whereas facial anatomy of people are quite different; hence the optical center and reading center may not properly align in OTC glasses.
   - Quality of lenses used in OTC glasses is usually poor because of mass production; hence proper refractive correction is not possible.

> **Note**
>
> Indirect disadvantage of OTC glasses is that patient does not feel like visiting an ophthalmologist at presbyopic age; hence the chances of missing potentially blinding conditions like glaucoma and cataract increase.

3. Problem in this case is simple presbyopia due to decreased accommodation ability at 44 years of age. Using OTC glasses prescribed by ophthalmic personnel will not weaken the eyes, however, in this case the patient had purchased OTC glasses without any prescription so these glasses may not be correct for him. Many a times due to unproven concern of weakening of eyes, occasionally patients report that despite of having difficulty in reading they avoided using the recommended reading glasses; to keep their eyes strong.

4. To manage this case we will perform dry retinoscopy to evaluate any refractive error for distance and then check the near vision monocularly then binocularly. Suppose distance vision retinoscopy is normal, then near vision is corrected using plus power spherical lenses monocularly and then binocular balancing is done as discussed in Chapter 3, page 52.

Problem 2: A 50 years old presbyope using over the counter reading glasses since 8 years presented with difficulty in seeing the fine near objects. On examination it was found that patient needs an increase in the strength of the existing over the counter reading glasses. On declaring that patient needs to increase the power of their existing reading glasses the patient asked these routine questions:

1. Can I still use my old reading glasses which are less strong?
2. Will the old glasses harm my eyes?
3. Write an appropriate solution with explanation.

Solution

1. The patient can continue to use his/her old reading glasses as long as patient feels that the glasses are providing satisfactory vision for reading.
2. Suppose these old reading glasses are not causing any eyestrain; means they are also not doing any harm to patient's eyes, by using them. However if there is difficulty in seeing small objects or performing fine work, then change of glasses is recommended.
3. Best option for this patient is to perform a cycloplegic refraction to record the exact amount of refractive error. Suppose there is no refractive error for distance vision, then the power of near vision is determined and balancing is done as discussed in Chapter 3, page 52. It is always better to wear the glasses of exact power rather than OTC reading glasses for the reasons explained in the above solution. Suppose patient is an office employee and do computer work, then it is better to use the progressive glasses rather than OTC reading glasses.

Problem 3: A 55 years old moderately high myope successfully using progressive addition lenses for normal reading recently discovered that now she is facing difficulty in threading a needle. There is no history of medical illness and the power of her present glasses is nearly one and a half year old.

1. What might be the cause of her problem?
2. How will you solve the situation?

Solution

1. The most probable cause of her difficulty are
   - Change in refractive power.
   - Beginning of cataractous changes.
   - Power of addition used since beginning was less (means just sufficient to read).
2. Various possible solution for her problem are dependent on the cause
   - In case of change in refractive power it is better to perform retinoscopy and prescribe new glasses having sufficient near add to see very small objects like needle hole or thread margin.
   - Perform a dilated examination to see the lenticular changes and if the cataract is only in grade one or two and patient is achieving N5 with near add then prescribe glasses and if the vision is not improving up to the patient's satisfaction, then perform cataract surgery.
   - Alternately in moderate degree myopes the simplest solution to this problem is just take off the present glasses and thread the needle; because by doing so they are using their natural nearsightedness to see close, hence no accommodation or additional plus power is needed.

> **Note**
>
> This strategy will also be useful when patient try to read very small print, or when it is necessary to read while at the same time patients require distance vision. However the reading material needed to be held closer than the normal reading distance.

Problem 4: A 42 years old asymptomatic emmetrope presented with the complaint of difficulty in focusing the distance objects after reading book for some time. Patient is not wearing glasses for distance or near and has no medical illness. Presently patient feels that it takes a few seconds for his vision to become clear when he looks across the room after reading for some duration. He also feels that words overlap when he read the book continuously for some duration.

1. Explain the etiology of this off and on blurring of vision both in distance and near?
2. How you will manage this case?

Solution

1. This symptom is classical presentation of presbyopia, especially in an emmetrope. The remaining accommodation at 42 years of age is functioning very strongly so that this patient can read for some duration; however due to this extra efforts of accommodation patient's eye takes a few seconds for the accommodation to relax when patient look distance objects. Similarly while reading for some duration the small amount of accommodation gets exhausted and patient feels that words are getting overlapped.

2. To manage this case the options are dependent on the amount and severity of symptoms
   • If these symptoms of blurring off and on are accidental findings by the patient and are not causing any major inconvenience or difficulty; reading glasses can be deferred for some more period of time.
   • However, suppose patient has also noticed some difficulty with small print or would like to eliminate this problem; then reading glasses are recommended.
   • Suppose patient has to perform work on computers and also desire to have crisp intermediate vision then progressive glasses are recommended as the first choice.

Problem 5: A 44 years old emmetrope not wearing any glasses for near presented to the clinic with complaints of difficulty in reading newspaper inside the room especially during early morning or evening time; however, he is able to read the newspaper in balcony in daylight without any glasses. This patient also feels that he faces difficulty in reading the magazine in bed during nighttime; however, the same magazine he can read easily while sitting on table in daylight.

1. Explain the causes of this problem along with the diagnosis.
2. How would you manage this patient?

Solution

1. The most probable cause of these symptoms is weakening of accommodative power of eyes, due to onset of presbyopia at the age of 44 years. These symptoms are occurring because
   • Normally when accommodation power decreases the pinhole effect helps in the ability to read clearly by producing miosis of eyes. Hence this patient was able to read newspaper in daylight. On contrary, normally pupils dilate when surrounding illumination decreases, which cause loss of the pinhole effect; hence this patient was unable to read inside the room.
   • In normal circumstances accommodation is achieved by contraction of the ciliary muscle, which in turn relaxes the zonules and allows the crystalline lens to become more convex. During early morning period the ciliary muscles are mildly slower and until late night the muscle gets fatigued; so this patient has difficulty in reading the newspaper especially during early morning and late nighttime.
   • Usually inside the bed person holds the magazine closer as compared to sitting position during daytime; this decrease in reading distance demands more accommodation power, which this 44 years old patient do not have. Hence this patient faces difficulty in reading the magazine in bed during night time.

2. As this patient is having an early onset presbyopia and has on official work we can manage this patient by prescribing the reading glasses. For an emmetrope at 44 years of age, usually a +1.25 DS power half eye reading glasses will work very satisfactorily. Patient can wear these glasses during reading work by keeping them

Note

In bright sunlight reading is much easier for an emmetropic early onset presbyope because of the pinhole effect. The pinhole effect can be produced either by stimulating the eye with bright light or squinting the eyes.

slightly in front over the nose, so that he can see the distance objects above the glasses.

Problem 6: A 52 years old emmetropic presbyope was using half eye reading glasses since 8 years for reading purposes. He has no history of medical illness or any other ocular problem. This patient walked into the clinic overwhelmed saying that he is capable of reading magazines without his reading glasses on tour, especially when he lay down on seashore.

1. Write an appropriate explanation of improvement in near vision.
2. Is this problem require any additional treatment?

Solution

1. When this elderly emmetropic presbyope is on a tour and lay down on seashore in bright sunlight his eyes get the pinhole effect as discussed in the above problem. Normally on seashore the bright sunlight causes miosis of pupil to produce a significant pinhole effect and this pinhole permits only the central rays (coming from an object) to enter the eye. This effect neutralizes the refractive error and also compensate for the demand of accommodation. Hence this patient is able to read the magazine without wearing his reading glasses.

2. As this pinhole effect is a normal phenomenon and causes no harm to the eyes of patient, no additional treatment is recommended in this case. However, patient can continue to wear his reading glasses in all other situation while reading. Patient must be counseled and explained about the phenomenon of pinhole effect for improvement of his near vision in sunlight.

Problems Related to Refractive and Post-refractive Corrections

REFRACTION

Problem 1: A 65 years old patient having pesudophakia in both eyes came for routine follow-up without any significant complaints. A meticulous cycloplegic refraction was performed on this patient and glasses were prescribed. After a week this patient again came to the clinic with complaint that new glasses prescription given to him are not good and he is facing a lot of difficulties in seeing with new spectacles compare to his old spectacles. This patient has no history of systemic medical illness.

1. What could be the possible cause of non-acceptance of new prescription?
2. How will you manage this case?

Solution

1. To find out the cause of discomfort and non-acceptance of glasses ask the following leading questions to this patient
   - Whether problem of seeing is in one eye or both the eyes?
   - Is their difficulty in seeing at distance, near or both with new glasses?
   - Is there any associated symptoms like ocular strain, tilting of edges of plane object, nausea, sudden blurring?
   - From where these new spectacles were made?

Suppose the patient answers that he is having difficulty in seeing both at distance and near and has no associated symptoms of eye strains then re-evaluate the patient with the old glasses. During re-evaluation examine these points

- Check the power of old glasses.
- Compare the visual acuity with both the old and new spectacles and note down the difference and comfort level (sometimes patient may have better visual acuity and comfortable feel with new glasses).
- Perform a repeat refraction (preferably with cycloplegic drug, e.g. cyclopentolate)

2. Manage the patient according to outcome of examination as follows:
   - Suppose a change in prescription of glasses is must, then advice the patient for new glasses (give complimentary consultation) and also explain him the cause of his difficulty in vision.
   - Suppose the glasses power prescribed were correct but there was an error in making of glasses by optician; handle the situation gently and consult with optician for arrangement of new complimentary spectacles.
   - Suppose the power of new prescription is accurate and also the glasses made are

correct then counsel the patient that sometime a change in power requires adjustment period of one to two weeks, hence do not panic and continue to wear the new prescription.

Problem 2: Two 75 years old patients came together to clinic with complaint of gradual painless diminution of distance visual acuity since few months. A meticulous cycloplegic refraction is done and on subjective refraction best corrected visual acuity with glasses was recorded for both the patients as follows

- Patient A: Distance visual acuity 6/24 and near visual acuity of N12 in each eye.
- Patient B: Distance visual acuity 6/24 and near visual acuity of N6 in each eye.

Considering these abovementioned visual status, explain

1. What is the possible diagnosis of each patient?
2. How will you manage them?

Solution

1. Considering the disparity between distance and near visual acuity
   - Patient A is more likely to have age-related macular degeneration, because in case of age-related macular degeneration, distance and near acuity are comparable. After correction with glasses both the distance and near visual acuity rarely get fully corrected in case of ARMD.
   - Patient B is more likely to have a cataract, because in an early to moderate grade cataract usually a disparity between distance and near acuity is seen where near acuity is always better than distance acuity. After correction with glasses the near acuity is usually corrected in normal range, however, the distance acuity is rarely get fully corrected in case of cataract.
2. Management of these patients include
   - In case of patient A having ARMD the treatment of choice is best correction with glasses and also by low visual aids.

 Note

Suppose a patient present with gradual painless diminution of vision and has both cataract and macular degeneration; then the discrepancy in improvement of distance and near visual acuity can be helpful in deciding which condition is more responsible for the reduced visual acuity.

- As patient B having cataract is not satisfied with distance vision with glasses then cataract extraction with IOL implantation is the treatment of choice.

Problem 3: A young patient having mixed refractive error came for follow-up after a period of two years with complain of slight difficulty in distance vision with existing glasses. Two years back an excellent refraction was performed by you and patient is wearing the same power glasses since then.

1. What type of refraction should be performed to resolve the present problem?
2. Describe the management in this case.

Solution

1. As this patient is having a mixed refractive error and was comfortably wearing the previously prescribed glasses since two years, it means the cylindrical power and axis determined during previous cycloplegic refraction was accurate. This time as the patient is having slight problem in distance vision with existing glasses, means there is no need of changing the cylindrical power or axis in this patient and simple over refraction for correction of spherical power is required to correct the distance vision problem. In over refraction the patient is asked to wear the present glasses and a dry retinoscopy is performed to neutralize the reflexes. New power is recorded and difference in power is considered for prescription.
2. New prescription is dependent on the visual outcome after over refraction.

Suppose over refraction produces an excellent vision in distance, then only a change in the sphere is prescribed along with the existing cylindrical power and axis. Thumb rule of prescription is that do not change the astigmatic error frequently. Difficulty in adjusting to the new prescription will be less in cases where astigmatic power was kept same as compared to the cases where cylinder power (especially cylindrical axis) was changed in new prescription.

> **Note**
>
> Additional advantage of performing an over-refraction is that there is no need to adjust vertex distance (distance between the lens and cornea) in new glasses. Since the new glasses will be fitted in same plane as existing and adjustment of new glasses will be easier for patient. Remember that larger the prescription power, the vertex distance becomes more relevant.

Problem 4: An elderly patient of 85 years age presented to clinic with low distance vision (6/60 in each eye). He is a diagnosed case of age-related macular degeneration (ARMD) and is on medical management. There is no history of medical illness; however, both eye cataract extractions with IOL implantation was done about two years back in right eye and one year back in left eye.

1. Whether routine type of refraction technique will help in improving the visual acuity in this case?
2. Describe an appropriate type of refraction method to improve the visual acuity in this case.

Solution

1. Routine type of dry or wet retinoscopy will not help in this particular case, because the reflexes seen are not very bright and also the patient is not able to appreciate the small changes during subjective refraction. Hence we need to modify the refraction method to improve the visual acuity.
2. Most appropriate refraction technique is to perform the objective refraction under cycloplegia (specifically homatropine) and

selecting large steps of lens power correction in ARMD patients having low vision. Once the objective refraction is done and estimated amount of refractive error is recorded then the subjective refraction power measurement and comparison of spherical and cylindrical powers are done in larger steps like 0.75 to 1 dioptre; not in routine smaller steps of 0.25 D. After changing the power of lenses at every step the patient is asked to compare the visual acuity and then proceed accordingly. Even the axis of cylindrical lens is shifted in steps of 15–20 degrees, not as 2–5 degrees as done in routine refraction method.

> **Note**
>
> There is no role of auto-refractor in these kinds of cases.

Problem 5: An elderly 86 years old patient came to the clinic with complaint of having a lot of confusion about spectacles he needs during daily activities. He has no history of medical illness; however, both eyes cataract extraction with IOL implantation was done about 10 years back. On further investigation four pairs of spectacles were found in a carry bag, which he is wearing for various daily activities.

1. How will you proceed in this case?
2. How will you solve the problem of multiple spectacles?

Solution

1. Primary aim of consultation is to reduce the number of spectacles in this patient which are being used for various activities and simplify the things. Following questions are asked to the patient to understand the real requirement in his daily activities
   - Which pair of spectacle he wishes to wear most of the time?
   - For what kind of activities he requires other pair of glasses?
   - How long he wear other pairs of spectacles?

- Since how long he is using these four pairs of spectacles?

    Answers to these questions will help the practitioner to understand the real requirement of multiple pair of glasses. Based on the answers clinician can decide and accordingly reduce the spectacles which are not really needed by this old man.

2. Management of this problem depends upon the outcome of evaluation of patient and all four pairs of glasses
    - Suppose prescription of all glasses is very old and patient wear most of these spectacles for very short duration then it is better to perform a cycloplegic refraction and prescribe new pair of glasses preferably separate spectacles for distance and near vision. This will reduce the number of glasses to only two pairs from four pairs. Alternately a pair of bifocal glasses having distance and intermediate power and second pair of glasses having only near power can be prescribed.
    - Suppose patient is using these four pairs of glasses regularly and comfortably during various daily activities, then it is advisable to continue all pairs of spectacles as before, because change in pattern may create newer visual problems.

Problem 6: A 65 years old male patient presented to clinic overwhelmed that since a few months he does not require near vision glasses to read newspaper, although he was using half eye reading glasses since 22 years for reading purpose. He has not undergone any medical check up since 6–8 years and also has no symptoms of illness.

1. What are the possible etiologies for improvement in near vision at such an elderly age?
2. How will you manage this case?

Solution

1. Most common phenomenon causing an improvement in reading ability in elderly age group patients is due to acquired myopia. As discussed before the common causes for acquired myopia are
    - Nuclear sclerosis of crystalline lens
    - High blood sugar levels in a diabetic (recent onset) patient.
    - Retinal detachment surgery (recent)
    - Chronic use of medications.

    As this particular patient has no history of recent ocular surgery (specially retinal detachment with scleral buckling), drug intake for longer duration or high blood sugar levels; the probable cause of improvement in near vision is nuclear sclerosis of crystalline lens. Cataract especially of nuclear sclerosis type causes a condition commonly called second sight of nearness because the patient again starts seeing the near objects without reading glasses after wearing the near vision glasses for 20–25 years.

2. To manage this case first evaluate the distance vision with best optical correction and following options are available for this elderly patient
    - Suppose the distance vision improves significantly by optical correction and patient is also satisfied with the amount of vision, then it is better to recommend the progressive glasses for some more year with regular six monthly follow up.
    - Suppose there is not significant improvement in distance vision or patient is not satisfied with the amount of distance vision with glasses, then it is better to recommend the cataract surgery.

Problem 7: An elderly 85 years old patient presented to clinic with visual symptoms due to excessive scratches on present spectacle lenses. On examination the refractive power of present glasses was accurate and a new prescription of same glass power was prescribed.

After a few days patient came with complain of intolerance to new glasses and exaggeration of visual symptoms.

1. How will you evaluate the case?
2. What will be the next step of management?

Solution

1. First we check the power of old glasses on lensometer and also compare the new prescription with the old power of glasses. Once the power of both the old and new prescriptions are checked then
   - Suppose the power of old and new glasses are different, then ask the optician to correct the power of new glasses.
   - Suppose both the power of glasses are the same, then the most likely cause for this problem of intolerance is that the new lenses have a different base curve than that of the old lenses. Change in base curve will affect the accommodation efforts of eye and refractive power of lens, hence will cause intolerance to the patient.
2. Most preferred method to solve this problem is to ask the patient to carry the old lenses to the optician along with new prescription of glasses with specially mentioned note for optician. In this note request the optician to simply duplicate the old prescription including the base curve of lenses.

☐ Note _____

Suppose patient is wearing prisms in old prescription then simply write a note to the optician to duplicate the existing prisms in new lenses.

Problem 8: A 41 years old moderate degree myope recently developed presbyopia presented to clinic with a desire of monovision contact lens fitting. He has no medical illness and contraindications to contact lens fitting.

1. How will you evaluate the case for monovision?
2. What will be your recommendations in this case?

Solution

1. All the basic evaluations for fitting of contact lens are done as discussed in Chapter 10, page 152. In case of monovision contact lens fitting we need to establish which eye of patient is dominant for a successful prescription. Easiest clinical method to determine the dominant eye of patient is as follows
   - Instruct the patient to outstretch both the arms keeping hands one on top of other. Tell the patient to create a small gap between two thumbs of outstretched arms.
   - Then patient is asked to look at a fine object like quotation on wall through this small gap between the thumbs (keeping both the eyes open).
   - Examiner then alternately occludes one eye by an occluder while patient is still looking to the distance object.
   - Patient must be able to see the distance object clearly with one between two eyes. The eye which sees the distance object clearly is termed dominant eye.
2. For a successful monovision contact lens fitting, the recommendations are
   - Determine the dominant eye and prescribe the distance correction contact lens for this dominant eye. A monofocal contact lens of near power is prescribed in fellow eye (non-dominant eye).
   - Alternately bifocal contact lens can be prescribed in both the eyes.

POST-REFRACTIVE CORRECTION

Problem 1: A 70 years old presbyope was comfortably wearing flat top bifocal glasses since 26 years. He developed difficulty in visualizing the TV caption from an intermediate distance with his present glasses. After cycloplegic refraction his glasses were changed from flat top bifocal to progressive type of glasses elsewhere. Now this patient is presented to our clinic with discomfort in vision both at distance and near.

1. How will you evaluate this case?
2. What will be the solution to this problem?

Solution

1. For evaluation of problem
   - First inquire when the patient has been changed from a standard bifocal to

progressive glasses or since how long patient is wearing these new progressive glasses. Usually there is an adjustment period for progressive glasses; some individuals may take approximately 2–3 weeks time period for adjustment of progressive glasses.

- Following problems are asked to decide the cause of patient's difficulty in using progressive glasses:
  - Troublesome inbuilt blur at the sides of progressive glasses
  - Necessity of any abnormal head posture for seeing the distance or near objects

- However, if there is a significant need for the correction of intermediate distance, for example, to see the television; it was reasonable to make the change in glasses from bifocal to progressive.

2. To solve the problem
  - Suppose the patient feels inbuilt blur or require abnormal head posture to see clearly, then check the proper pantoscopic tilt (described in Chapter 7, page 105).
  - Check the power of new progressive lenses by automatic lensometer (to be sure about the fitting of correct prescription).
  - Counsel the patient that usually progressive lenses require some amount of training in viewing the target and also viewing through progressive lenses takes some time for adjustment.
  - Suppose no problem is identified or it is confirmed that patient is unable to tolerate progressive glasses, best option is to change back to standard bifocal flat top glasses.

Note ──────────────────────

Generally when patient is doing perfectly well with standard bifocal and has no complaints, it is better to continue the same type of glasses in new prescriptions.

Problem 2: A 55 years old patient was refracted and prescribed new glasses for both distance and near vision. This patient was previously wearing the D-bifocal glasses and hence made the new prescription in same lens design. After 2–3 days the patient came back with the complaint of having difficulty in reading with the recent prescription received from us; although the distance vision is fine with the new prescription.

1. What are the probable causes for difficult near vision with new prescription?
2. What should be the line of management?

Solution

1. Various situations can cause the reading difficulty in this case.
  - To reach a proper diagnosis some more information is required in this case. Ask the patient whether changing the reading distance (means either keeping the book a little away from eyes or bringing the book a little closer to eye), affects the clarity of reading. Suppose the answer to any one of these situations is yes, means the reading addition given was improper. Always keep in mind that in the making of bifocal lenses, near power is always added with the distance prescription. Suppose the distance prescription is incorrect, then the reading segment prescription will automatically be wrong and patient will have difficulty in reading.
  - Classically position of the upper line for D-bifocal segment is fitted at the level of lower lid margin as described in Chapter 7, page 110. Suppose on inspection the reading segment is found to be fitted too low or too high, then the problem is not in addition power rather the cause is improper fitting of lens in the spectacle frame.
  - Spectacles are verified whether the lower portions of the lenses are fitted with an inwardly angled position (pantoscopic tilt) or not. Proper pantoscopic tilt is

mandatory to read comfortably as described in Chapter 7, page 105.

2. Management of problem
   - Suppose if an improper addition was given in new prescription, then re-examine the patient and give proper addition power.
   - Suppose patient feel more comfortable in reading by pushing the glasses up or lifting the chin up, then reading difficulty is because of improper fitting of glasses in spectacle frame. In these cases the opticians are advised to fit the bifocal segment properly in spectacle frame as described in Chapter 7.
   - Suppose improper pantoscopic tilt was noticed in this case then correction of the pantoscopic tilt will enhance the comfortable reading ability of this patient.

Note

In some individuals spectacle frame slides down from nose while person lowers the head to read a book; so the working position of bifocal near segment is fitted slightly lower than the usual position (i.e. at lower lid margin) in these cases.

Problem 3: A 47 years old emmetrope was presented to clinic with the complaint of recently developed problem in viewing the labels of medicines with his near vision half eye glasses. He was using +1.75 D power half eye reading glasses without any prescription very successfully since one year. He used to purchase the reading glasses from the opticians without any prescription. He has no history of medical illness and also presently has no complaint for distance vision.

1. What are the possible causes for this difficulty in near vision with reading glasses?
2. Outline the solutions to this problem?

Solution

1. Possible causes for difficulty in reading the labels of medicine with present near vision half eye glasses are
   - Whether patient is attempting to see the medicine labels in bright sunlight. If yes,

then the probable reason is that significant miosis in sunlight will cause difficulty in near vision with reading glasses because pinhole effect increases the near vision.
   - Is there any history of purchase of different reading glasses for fine near work, because fine near work requires higher addition power at nearer working distance.

2. Best possible solutions for this problem are
   - Advice the patient to purchase different half eye glasses with stronger power for this kind of fine near work.
   - Suppose patient requires seeing of medicine labels regularly and have multiple half eye reading glasses; then he/she can wear two glasses one above the other for this kind of fine near work.

Problem 4: A 48 years old an office executive who was wearing D-bifocal glasses since many years comfortably is now presented with difficulty in performing the excel work on his computer wearing glasses. The prescription of his bifocal glasses was recently changed about 3 months before and he is having crisp distance and near vision with the D-bifocal glasses.

1. What could be the probable cause for this problem in computer work?
2. Write down the possible solutions for this difficulty in intermediate vision.
3. Describe the tips to remember while prescribing a computer glasses.

Solution

1. Most common cause for difficulty in viewing computer screen clearly is the distance of monitor. The desktop computer monitor is usually situated at a further distance than the normal reading distance. This distance is referred as the intermediate distance of vision; where person is unable to visualize the objects clearly either from the distance portion or near portion of his/her standard bifocal glasses.

2. To correct this problem possible solutions are
   - Prescribe a trifocal lens as discussed in Chapter 6, page 94. Patient is able to view the computer screen clearly and perform excel work comfortably when see through the intermediate segment of trifocal lens. However a small amount of chin lift is required to position the intermediate segment of trifocal lens in visual line of eyes.
   - Alternately progressive lenses can be prescribed, where multiple power will take care of intermediate distance; however a slight chin lift is recommended even for a progressive addition glasses.
   - When patient is not agreeing for either of the above two solutions, then prescribe a separate computer glasses having intermediate correction in top portion and near correction in bottom portion of lenses. For distance vision patient is advised to use a separate spectacle. Patient will see the computer monitor while looking straight ahead, because the intermediate power is fitted in top portion. These computer glasses also eliminate the necessity of chin lift to see the computer screen, hence are useful in patients having neck problems.

3. Remember these points while prescribing the computer glasses
   - Never prescribe single vision glasses having intermediate power, because patient also needs to see near fonts while trying in computer key board.
   - Always prefer progressive glasses as computer glasses, because jumping of images is negligible in progressive glasses.
   - When only computer bifocal glasses are advised, then the near addition look very unusual, because nearly half of near power is required to be fitted in top portion of glasses as intermediate power and only remaining half power will be fitted in near segment.
   - To avoid this unusual looking situation a convenient method to calculate the intermediate power is by use of a near vision test card and slit lamp. Fix the near vision test card in chin rest position of slit lamp; this test card will serve as computer screen. Now gradually change the power of lenses in trial frame until patient comfortably read the smallest line on near test card. This will give the desired intermediate vision with minimum lens power.

> **Note** _____
>
> Suppose patient is suffering from a significant neck problem and feels difficulty in maintaining a chin lift position then both trifocals and progressive glasses are not suitable as computer glasses.

Problem 5: A 62 years old professor is presented with the complaint of difficulty in reading book during taking a class standing against the classroom dice; although professor is wearing the D-bifocal glasses since many years and has clear distance and near vision with glasses. Professor has no history of medical illness or not on any drugs.

1. What could be the possible cause for this problem?
2. How would you manage this problem?

Solution

1. Strongest possibility is that the height of reading dice is such that professor need to read the book at an intermediate distance, which is beyond the reading distance and nearer than distance vision. So professor is unable to read either from distance segment or near segment of his/her present D-bifocal glasses.

2. This problem can be solved by following methods
   - Prescribe the progressive additional glasses or trifocal glasses and replace present D-bifocal glasses.
   - Prescribe a separate pair of glasses (on patient desire) with full distance correction

in the upper portion and add of intermediate correction in the lower portion of D-bifocal glasses; so that professor can see the classroom students from upper portion of spectacles and book with the near segment simultaneously, while taking the class.

> **Note**
>
> Similar management is useful for various professions where person needs distance vision clarity with intermediate correction to read the subject matter kept on the dice.

Problem 6: Patient of age about 45 years working as vegetable vendor presented to clinic with problem in near vision. This patient requires glasses which he can wear continuously during the work. Explain which type of glasses you will prescribe to this patient.

1. Whether a bifocal glass that is fitted with too weak power of addition and why?
2. Whether a bifocal glass that is fitted with too strong power of addition and why?

Solution

1. To this presbyopic patient working as vegetable vendor we will prescribe either the half eye reading glasses or bifocal glasses fitted with weak addition power. Because weaker addition glasses will produce a wider and longer range of reading. This patient does not require reading of book or fine matter, hence weaker addition will work better.

2. Usually bifocal glasses fitted with too strong power are not prescribed because they will create more problems than a too weak fitted bifocal glass. A closer and narrower range of reading produced by too

> **Note**
>
> Suppose half eye glasses are prescribed then patient needs to advise to keep these glasses slightly lower on the nose so that he can see the distance objects from top of glasses.

strong bifocals is less tolerated as compared to longer and wider range of reading produced by weaker bifocal glasses.

Problem 7: A 55 years old golf player presented with the complaint of difficulty in seeing the score card, since few months. However, the player is comfortably wearing flat top D-bifocal glasses since 12 years.

1. What could be the cause for difficulty in viewing the score card?
2. How will you mange this case?

Solution

1. Cause of problem in this case is that usually bifocal addition power is fused in lower segment of glasses and near segment is placed in bottom nasal portion of lens during fitting of spectacles. So normally people read from nasally fitted lower near segment of glasses, because while reading the eyes converge and hence the reading segment lie in front of pupillary center in normal circumstances. In case of golfers they view the score card from temporal side and hence they face difficulty because near segment is fitted nasally.

2. Management of the problem in special cases like golfers near add is required on opposite side of corner of glasses, i.e. temporarily, so that they can read score card while aiming for golf ball straight down. The golfers are fitted with special type of golfer's lenses in one eye and normal fitting in fellow eye as per requirement of golfer (described in Chapter 6, page 93).

> **Note**
>
> Similarly several other professionals like electricians, musicians specially French horn players and watch makers, require near add in top portions of glasses. These bifocal glasses are commonly called occupational bifocals (discussed in Chapter 6 on page no 93).

UNCOMMON REFRACTIVE CONDITIONS

Study these following clinical refractive scenarios which are not so common in routine clinical practice. Plan the strategies to manage these uncommon clinical refractive problems.

Problem 1: A 22-year-old boy came to the clinic for consultation regarding maintenance of his eyes. Presently the boy has no ocular complaints. He had past history of ocular trauma and on examination had no perception of light (PL) in right eye and left eye was emmetropic.

1. What advice you will give to this patient?

Solution

1. It is most important to protect the left eye as this patient is having only one visually useful eye. Following advice can be given to look after the eyes
   - Wear protective goggles while playing contact games like football, cricket or badminton.
   - Wear Plano power anti-reflex coated glasses specifically made from polycarbonate material (non-breakable) for regular work, which give continuous protection from minor ocular injuries.
   - Use preservative free lubricants, because this boy is working on computers for more than 7–8 hours per day.
   - Regular six monthly ocular examinations.

Problem 2: 28 years old patient working on computers for 5–6 hours daily came for an ocular examination to the clinic. Apparently patient is having no visual symptoms, however he occasionally feel foreign body sensation in both the eyes. On detailed examination and after cycloplegic refraction the patient had 6/6 visual acuity in each eye with –1.75 DS power in right eye and plano power in left eye. He also has mild dry eye in both the eyes.

1. How will you prescribe this patient?
2. Will there be any clinical symptoms if we prescribe glasses for this patient?

Solution

1. As we can see that there is significant difference in amount of refractive status of both the eyes in this patient, so it is better to leave the decision on patient whether he wants to wear glasses or not. Prescription of glasses can be done as follows
   - Normally patient is asymptomatic and seeing the distance objects clearly with both the eyes open, because left eye is emmetropic. At the age of 28 years with one eye having moderate degree myopia the patient is comfortable in reading from any distance. Some of patients feel that correcting one eye will not produce any significant improvement in distance vision and hence refuses to use the glasses.
   - On contrary some patient may feel that correction of refractive error in one eye will improve the quality of vision by depth perception and also will not hamper the vision of better eye, so they agree to wear the glasses.

2. When the difference in refractive error between two eyes (anisometropia) of less than 2.5 dioptres is present, it will not produce clinical significant difference in image size (aniseikonia). Hence in this particular case we can prescribe the glasses without producing any new clinical symptoms.

Problem 3: A 50 years old asymptomatic patient walked into the clinic for consultation. On examination when left eye was occluded the distance vision was affected and vice versa when right eye is occluded the near vision gets affected. However, patient is comfortably seeing both the distance and near targets without any glasses binocularly. On performing the refraction patient had –2.25 DS refractive error in right eye and plano power in left eye for distance. Also patient is accepting + 4 DS in right eye and +2 DS power in left eye for near vision.

1. What is the diagnosis of this condition?
2. What kind of consultation you will give to this patient?

Solution

1. This particular patient is asymptomatic because of phenomenon called natural monovision, where patient is comfortably seeing distance objects clearly with one eye (left eye in our example) and vice versa near objects with fellow eye (right eye or myopic eye in our example).
2. Depending on the requirement of patient we can give following advise to this patient having natural monovision
   - Suppose patient require full correction of distance as well as near vision in each eye then we need to advice either bifocal or progressive glasses for this patient, where right eye glasses will have both distance and near powers, whereas left eye glasses will have only near correction power.
   - Suppose patient is happy with present visual status and desire not to wear glasses, then patient will do extremely well even without glasses for some more years.

> **Note**
>
> In natural monovision cases it is always better not to prescribe any glasses.

Problem 4: An elderly 60 years patient presented to clinic with difficulty in seeing the distance and near objects since last few months. Patient is wearing glasses for distance since few years and has no history of medical illness. On examination right eye has a refractive error of –2.5 DS × –1.5 DC × 90° with a near add of +3 DS, whereas left eye has only perception of light.

1. What type of advice you will give to this patient?
2. Does this patient require some special type of prescription for making of glasses?

Solution

1. As discussed above on page 262 protection of eyes specially the right eye having

useful visual acuity is most important in this kind of patients. So we will advice the patient in similar manner as discussed.
2. As the distance refractive power is significant in right eye and left eye has no useful vision, we will prescribe the patient with the prescription having fully corrected power for refractive error on right side column and a balance written in left side column. The optician will understand the meaning of balance and fix an almost matching power of glass in front of left eye also, so that cosmetically both the glasses appear equal and more acceptable. This left eye lens is commonly called balance lens which appear almost equal in thickness and style to its fellow lens. This patient can manage the near vision by simply removing the glasses and keeping the object a little nearer than usual reading distance. Suppose the patient is not comfortable in removing the glasses too often and require near addition, then he can be prescribed bifocal glasses with +3 D addition in both eyes.

Problem 5: An elderly 85 years old patient presented with complaint of reading difficulty with the present bifocal glasses. On examination the distance visual acuity was 6/18 in right eye and 6/12 partial in left eye with present glasses. Patient is wearing an addition of +2.75 DS in both eyes and is having a near vision of N36 with present bifocal glasses. Patient is a diagnosed case of dry age related macular degeneration (ARMD) and is on medical treatment.

1. Describe the management outline in this case.
2. What will be your prescription for this patient?

Solution

1. Normally in emmetrope at this age the maximum near addition given is in the range

of +2.5 to +3.0 DS. As this patient is having ARMD we can consider managing this case on the guidelines of low vision rehabilitation. This patient can be managed by using various low vision optical aids at this stage of disease.

2. Prescription for this elderly ARMD patient include

   • A higher addition of +3.5 to +4.0 DS can be prescribed when patient is getting a significant improvement in near vision and also is mentally prepared to keep the reading objects little nearer than usual reading distance.

   • Suppose a higher addition more than +4.0 DS is required in this case to improve the near visual acuity then we can prescribe separate near vision glasses having high plus power.

Note _____

Suppose near vision further deteriorates, then consider magnification for near objects by using low vision optical aids.

_____

Problem 6: 17 years old young college student presented with complain of difficulty in seeing letters on blackboard, especially when he/she sit on last bench in classroom. There is no history of wearing glasses or any eye examination in past. On examination after cycloplegic refraction the right eye has –5.5 DS refractive error and left eye has –0.5 DS refractive error.

1. Describe this condition in detail.
2. Outline the management strategy for this patient.
3. Write the management of this patient in follow-up visits.

Solution

1. The difference between refractive status of both the eyes is considerably high; hence this condition is called anisometropia. The difference in degree of refractive error is of 5 dioptres, hence when right eye is fully corrected there will be significant amount

of aniseikonia, where patient will see the significantly smaller size images from right eye after full correction of refractive error.

2. To manage this patient initially we need to prescribe trial corrective lenses, means correct the right eye refractive error partially by giving lesser power (say –2.25 DS) lenses than total power (–5.5 DS in our example). Patient is instructed to wear these trial lenses and report after some time about the quality of vision and associated symptoms (if any).

3. In follow-up visit this patient can be managed as follows

   • Suppose patient remains asymptomatic with trial run lenses, we can gradually increase the power of right side lenses (until tolerated by patient) to improve the visual acuity in right eye.

   • Suppose patient shows symptoms of aniseikonia, then we can prescribe contact lens for right eye which will improve the visual acuity and also eliminate the aniseikonia symptoms by abolishing the vertex distance factor.

   • Later on when refractive status of right eye becomes stable and visual acuity has also improved after correction, refractive surgery on right eye is done to correct the anisometropia in this case.

Note _____

Unlike monovision cases always correct the young anisometric patients to prevent amblyopia and other vision related symptoms.

_____

Problem 7: An elderly couple, husband of 65 years age and wife 63 years of age presented to clinic with recent onset difficulty in seeing the distance objects from their present glasses. On examination husband had a large chalazion in right upper eyelid and wife had ptosis of left eye. Both of them had no significant history of systemic medical illness. On performing the refraction a change in spherical power and cylindrical axis was found in respective eyes of both the patients.

1. Explain the cause of change in refractive status on one eye.
2. Describe the course of management in both the cases.

Solution

1. Explanation for change of refractive status in one eye having ocular pathology are

   - In both these cases pressure changes on cornea due to mechanical push of lesion will be seen.
   - In case of husband the large upper eyelid chalazion is mechanically pushing the cornea due to its weight on eyelid and hence a refractive error especially astigmatic type will occur.
   - Similarly in case of wife the left eye ptosis will cause the change in corneal curvature. These changes in cornea can produce astigmatic error (usually irregular astigmatism) due to distortion of cornea.
   - Hence in both the cases these conditions are responsible for recent onset change in refractive status of one eye.

2. Management of problem

   - Surgical removal of chalazion is the treatment of choice, to relieve the mechanical pressure on cornea in case of husband. This will automatically correct the refractive status of right eye; because once the chalazion is removed the cornea will come back to its original shape within a short period of time.
   - Similarly in case of wife correction of ptosis will eliminate the indentation of cornea by left upper eyelid and hence will correct the refractive status of left eye gradually over period of time.

 Note

In these cases correction of refractive error by glasses or other optical means is not helpful.

Index